EVERYDAY
CHINESE MEDICINE

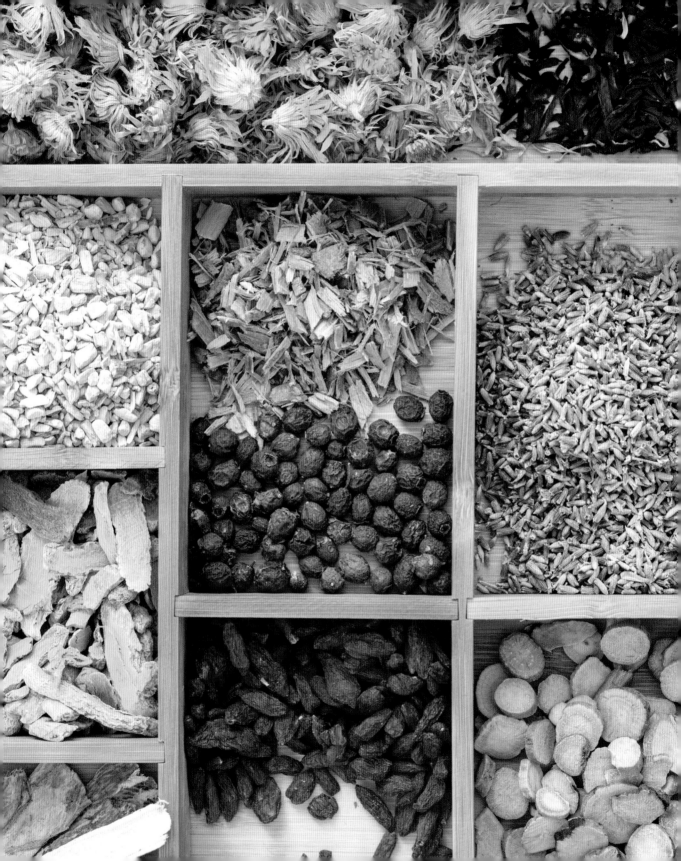

EVERYDAY
CHINESE MEDICINE

Healing Remedies for Immunity,
Vitality & Optimal Health

MINDI K. COUNTS, MA, LAc

PHOTOGRAPHS BY KRISTEN HATGI SINK

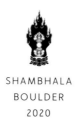

SHAMBHALA
BOULDER
2020

Shambhala Publications, Inc.
4720 Walnut Street
Boulder, Colorado 80301
shambhala.com

Disclaimer: The information presented here is thorough and accurate to the best of our knowledge,
but it is essential that you always practice caution and use your best judgment when consuming
herbs and herbal supplements. Please do not attempt self-treatment of a medical problem without
consulting a qualified health practitioner. Shambhala Publications and the author disclaim any and
all liability in connection to the consumption of herbs and herbal supplements and the use of the
instructions in this book.

9 8 7 6 5 4 3 2 1

First Edition
Printed in China

⊛ This edition is printed on acid-free paper that meets the American National Standards Institute
Z39.48 Standard.
♻ Shambhala Publications makes every effort to print on postconsumer recycled paper.
For more information please visit www.shambhala.com.

Shambhala Publications is distributed worldwide by Penguin Random House, Inc., and its subsidiaries.

Designed by Allison Meierding

Library of Congress Cataloging-in-Publication Data

Names: Counts, Mindi K., author.
Title: Everyday Chinese medicine: healing remedies for immunity, vitality, and optimal health /
    Mindi K. Counts.
Description: First edition. | Boulder: Shambhala, 2020. | Includes bibliographical references and index.
Identifiers: LCCN 2019003465 | ISBN 9781611806502 (paperback: alk. paper)
Subjects: LCSH: Medicine, Chinese—Popular works.
Classification: LCC R601 .C6977 2020 | DDC 610.951—dc23
LC record available at https://lccn.loc.gov/2019003465

CONTENTS

— ◆ —

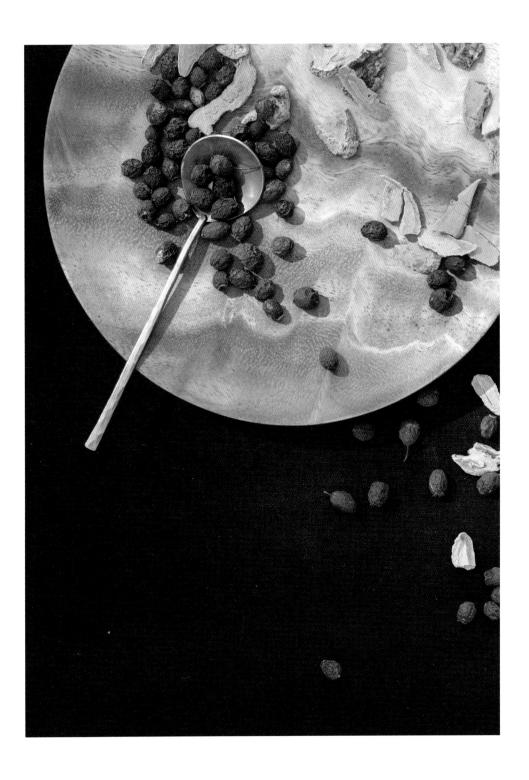

FOREWORD

— ◆ —

I discovered the magic of Chinese medicine more than thirty years ago, and at that time one of the only books available on the topic was the nearly 2,500-year-old *Neijing: The Yellow Emperor's Classic of Internal Medicine*. This is a brilliant text covering all the basic tenants of Chinese medicine which miraculously survived endless wars, dynasties, and more recently, the Chinese Cultural Revolution, during which many priceless ancient traditions were banned.

Today, still alive and strong in its cultural roots and still reaping marvelous results, there is no question that Chinese medicine is a timeless and immensely effective system of medicine. Much of it may seem mysterious and exotic, with its endless references to nature, the spirit, and the seasons, but it captured my attention because it is actually so simple, straightforward, and practical. Its foundation is based on what many in this modern age are missing—awareness of our inherent connection with the natural world. In fact, the ancients believed that if we can observe nature closely enough, we can discover a cure for any disease.

Chinese medicine was originally based on the Five Elements—Fire, Earth, Metal, Water, and Wood—and how they manifest in nature and the cycles of seasons. We, like plants in the winter, begin our life's journey as an embryo in the darkness of our mother's watery womb. We slowly evolve and gather potency as we wait for the warmth of the spring sun. When the time is right, we uncoil and grow a green sprout, shooting toward the warmth of the fiery sun. In the summer we blossom in full color; in late summer, we develop fruit; and in the crisp, metallic autumn, our leaves and fruit drop and rot, returning to the soil. The Chinese knew that the way of nature is no different from the geography and workings of our body, mind, and spirit. At any given moment we may feel deep and flow freely like water, fresh and reborn like a new sprout, hot and explosive like fire, heavy and rich like the mud of the earth, or sharp and cutting like rocks and crystals.

For example, think about how the fire of a fever can burn away toxins and bacteria or how shivering can warm up the body when it's cold. We all know that the bounteous food of the earth nourishes and satisfies us and that the minerals in the soil and water are crucial for the strength and structure of our bones. Water cleanses, cools, and hydrates us, and the growth of plants provides us with food, shade, and oxygen.

In the same way, on an immaterial level, the fire of our loving relationships warms us and contributes to our well-being. Or consider how the satisfaction of a meal with close family and friends raises our immunity against depression. When we mine the gold of our natural gifts and start releasing what no longer serves us (similar to leaves falling in autumn), our chances of rousing our self-worth and confidence escalate. Nowadays, modern science is proving that moments of quiet and solitude (such as with meditation practice) calms our nervous system and reduces stress, while challenging experiences can actually stimulate emotional growth (like how trees and plants grow around obstacles toward the warmth and light of the sun).

The ancient Chinese took these simple facts about physicality and nature and looked deeper. Over centuries they refined their observations and applied them brilliantly to the intricate workings of the human body, mind, and spirit and developed what I describe to my students as a "no-brainer" system of medicine: medicine that covers humankind's myriad ailments, whether physical, mental, or spiritual. Most importantly, this system reveals how to work with and even prevent these ailments. Chinese medicine works not because it is mystical and complex but because it is often simple and obvious.

For example, I once visited a friend in the hospital after she had undergone minor surgery. She was experiencing a sudden gallbladder attack following her procedure, and the doctors were about to wheel her away to remove her gallbladder. I intervened and requested that they wait an hour so I could listen to her pulses and check in with her on an energetic level. They agreed. I then asked her what she had eaten and drunk the night before. She confessed that she'd visited a Japanese restaurant and drunk lots of wine and eaten deep-fried shrimp tempura. Clearly, her poor liver and gallbladder were having trouble processing the alcohol and fat from that delicious meal combined with the strong effects of the pharmaceuticals used to sedate her during her minor surgery. When I took her pulses, she had a simple energy block disturbing the two organs that I suspected was causing the issue in her gallbladder. It took only a few minutes to clear the block, and within an hour the pain and inflammation had disappeared. This was not due to my miraculous healing powers but to simple common sense and a very straightforward method to clear the block. The doctor was clearly mystified and slightly irritated but released her, warning, "You'll be back soon!" But she wasn't. This is just one of hundreds of examples of the power of Chinese medicine to address medical situations with methods to which Western medicine simply does not have access. So imagine the power of combining modern medical science with the ancient, practical wisdom of Chinese medicine!

In this book, Mindi Counts offers us a timely gift from the ancients; a gift full of practical wisdom and knowledge that is tremendously relevant and important to modern-day health and well-being. She has created a comprehensive path to finding the balance and harmony we need to take more responsibility for our health before we fall into patterns of disease.

I have known Mindi since she took my year-long class in Chinese medicine, "The Psychology of the Five Elements," at Naropa University. I think I could rightly say that Mindi is a force of nature—her focus has not just been becoming an accomplished medical practitioner; she has become a kind of worldwide health pioneer. She has started her own foundation, the Inner Ocean Empowerment Project, and has gathered all varieties of health care practitioners to, among other things, bring relief to the slums of India; work with Burmese refugees at border camps; and bring health, education, and aid to remote corners of Nepal. She not only works to provide medical care but aspires to empower the people of those regions to learn skills that will serve the health and well-being of their communities far into the future.

It is clear to me that Mindi's rigorous and adventuresome service work, along with her deep personal dedication to nature, has strengthened her ability to communicate the holistic essence of Chinese medicine and provide access to the wisdom and profundity of this ancient tradition. Her work provides a beautiful bridge between ancient and modern, East and West, and opens a portal of possibility where their diverse ideas and practices can meet, enlighten, and inform each other. What a wonderful world this will be!

MARLOW BROOKS, LAc

Professor at Naropa University

Author of *Singing Our Heart's Song: A Guide to the Five Elements and Plant Spirit Healing*, *Words of the Heart*, and *The Way Through*

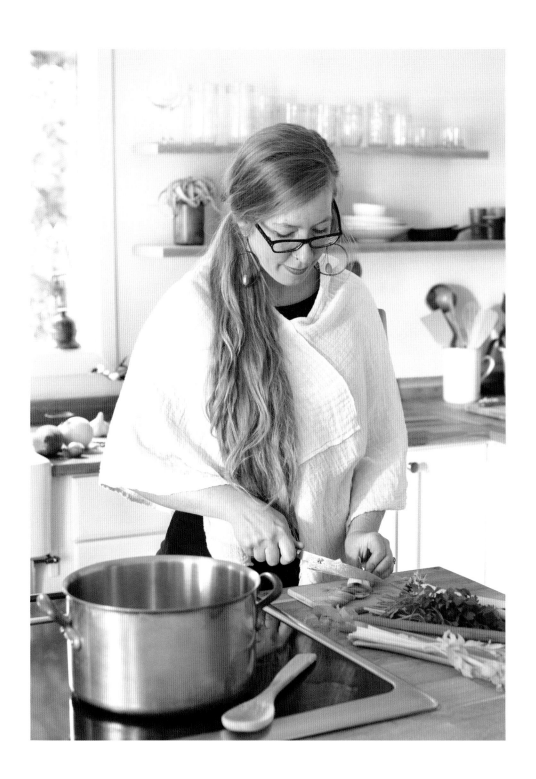

PREFACE

— ◆ —

In September 2008, I was sitting in my car in a parking lot on yet another beautiful day in Colorado. The sun was shining, a slight breeze was blowing, and the mountains that surround this little town I was learning to call home looked ever so inviting. I had the perfect life. I had a sweetie and a couple of rescued dogs. We lived in a cabin in the mountains, just west of Boulder. I was in school studying psychology and working as a caregiver for a family who had a daughter with developmental disabilities. I had an amazing community that I could lean on and also go have fun with. Every weekend was an adventure, as I would explore the mountains, valleys, and rivers of Colorado. And yet, sitting in my car in the parking lot that autumn afternoon, I found myself with tears streaming down my face, unable to truly appreciate any of it.

These were the tears that came from a deep shame of feeling so dissatisfied with myself, despite having all my *t*'s crossed and my *i*'s dotted. These weren't unfamiliar feelings. In fact, grief had been an undercurrent in my life, though it seemed to come on with a bang at least once a year, often during the fall season. If we have to name names, we could call it depression.

In my youth, I had tried antidepressants to change the way I felt, but I found that not only did the pills take away my sadness, they also took with it my joy and inspiration. Much to the dismay of my family and doctor, after several months I had to scratch that idea. By the time I hit my twenties, I had learned to just go with it, to ride the waves of my moods as they came and hope that one day I would find a cure that worked for me. Staying busy was one of the ways I learned to cope with my depression.

When I was twenty-one, I took a college class that shattered every preconception I had developed about my depression thus far. It was called "The Psychology of the Five Elements," and I only took it because of a friend's recommendation, having no idea what the class was about. The next thing I knew, I was sitting on a floor cushion, mesmerized, listening to my teacher, Marlow Brooks, talk about the season of autumn and its relationship to grief and depression. My ears perked up. It turned out to be a class on the philosophy underpinning Chinese medicine.

Marlow explained that "we have internal seasons as well as external ones." She was speaking about autumn as "nature's expression of grief" and how the season can bring about an internal sense of grief also. She said that learning to let go was something nature did in autumn and that we were invited to do the same at this time of year. My teacher explained that some people have a nature that is much like the season of autumn. "In fact," she said, "all people have a nature that could be likened to a season: a Summer type, a Winter type, and so on." I was intrigued and stopped her after class to tell her how much I related to the Autumn type. I wanted to ask how I would know, and what I could do about it.

"You might want to consider seeing a five-element acupuncturist," Marlow replied. A what?! An acupuncturist? I didn't see that coming. At that point I had only heard about Chinese medicine and acupuncture being used to treat pain. I had never had it and didn't know it could help with all the other emotional and seasonal hiccups we were talking about.

Marlow assured me that a five-element acupuncturist could confirm if I were, in fact, more of an Autumn type and could give me a treatment to support the emotional roller coaster on which I found myself each year. So that is exactly what I did.

I saw a five-element acupuncturist every week for eight weeks, and I was shocked to watch myself become the person I used to be and the one I felt I was in my heart. I felt my inspiration, my hope, my delight, and my energy return in such a way that it was almost like magic. I was waking up ready for the day and going to sleep satisfied with myself and my life. It was a complete turnaround from where I'd been just two months prior. The following year, September came without all the debilitating grief and depression. In fact, when my acupuncturist asked how I was doing with September on the horizon, it took me a moment to realize what she was referring to! That was how far I had come in a year.

Through working with my acupuncturist, I learned so much about myself and about nutrition, the seasons, herbal medicine, and practices I could do to support myself even more deeply on the path to healing. I learned about my true nature based on the Five Elements and could see how I had been living a life that, despite looking good from the outside, ultimately wasn't nourishing me. I could see how holding on to the past was disrupting my present life. I learned about my unique balance of introversion and extroversion (yin and yang) and developed a lot of compassion for myself.

I no longer took ownership of my depression as though it was something that defined me. Rather, I saw myself as a dynamic being and recognized that there were places where I could take more responsibility for my health. It was an incredible journey and has ultimately led me here, to writing this book.

Blown away by this change, I eventually became a five-element acupuncturist and herbalist myself. I did this so I could share the incredible healing journey that I experienced with people who also want more from life than what they see. In 2013, I even started taking this system of medicine and its opportunities for healing around the world. I journeyed to places like Thailand, Burma, India, and Nepal, where I gave treatments on reservations and in slums, orphanages, and disaster areas. I held the hands of victims of sex-trafficking, rape, and shootings. I watched this medicine work in all lands, for so many who suffered and were in pain. I watched the light of hope return to sad and empty eyes and a smile break forth once again. I felt how deep the need for healing is in our world. I committed my life to healing and founded my nonprofit Inner Ocean Empowerment Project, an organization that offers the gift of healing to communities in need all around the world. Now I share this gift with you.

Each day in my office, I witness the challenges we face simply by being alive right now. And while Chinese medicine is an invaluable system for healing, this system alone cannot cure all disease in the world. It can however, support our relationship to our health in such a way that suffering and disease become a portal to our awakening rather than a setback. In fact, according to this ancient system of medicine, it is the *strength of the spirit* and not the health of the body that determines the outcome of our lives.

Knowing what I know now about the healing journey, about nutrition, about the incredible gift plants offer us through herbal medicine, and about just how much power there is in physical, mental, and spiritual health, my hope is to empower you with all of these tools and more as you embark on your own healing journey. Lean on me, and trust me when I tell you that you can step into a deeper relationship with yourself and live the life you most want to lead.

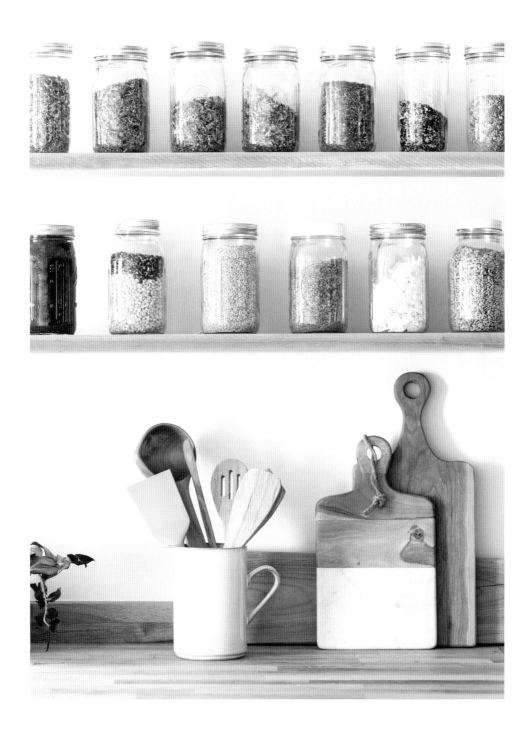

INTRODUCTION

— ◆ —

We are not human beings having a spiritual experience.
We are spiritual beings having a human experience.
—PIERRE TEILHARD DE CHARDIN

Chinese medicine is an ancient, holistic system of medicine that shows us our relationship to and responsibility for the health of our bodies, minds, and spirits. What we eat, what we think, who and what we surround ourselves with, and in general, how we live our lives play a key role in the health and well-being we experience. The Chinese medicine view of health is that we are whole and can find physical, mental, and spiritual balance. The same is true for imbalance. We can experience an illness physically, emotionally, and/or spiritually. In Chinese medicine, patients are never seen as broken and needing to be fixed. Rather, they are always whole and simply experiencing a call to action when unpleasant symptoms arise. Sometimes, finding balance means learning to live well despite such symptoms. Other times, the key to healing is to look at what lies at the heart of our imbalance—what we call the root cause—and work on it at that level.

Chinese medicine and Western medicine differ drastically when it comes to diagnosing and addressing imbalances in our health. There is no doubt that stress and feelings of being overwhelmed contribute to much of our experience of suffering in the twenty-first century. There are also environmental factors, genetic influences, social pressures, and (some rather impossible) standards set by our society that breach our every effort to live well. Chinese medicine considers all of these factors as playing a vital role in our health, as do diet, lifestyle, emotions, climate, and so on. When is the last time your doctor asked you what you were eating or what your childhood was like when you were back in the clinic with your third cold of the season or looking for help with persistent anxiety?

The goal in Western medicine is often to *get rid of* the experience of suffering. With a cold, you are given cold medicine. With persistent anxiety, you are given anti-anxiety medication. The goal in Chinese medicine is vastly different, as we are more focused on coming up with a long-term plan for health care that *prevents* disease and disharmony rather than dodging bullets as they present themselves. This is what makes this system of medicine unique and so life-changing. What if you discovered there were things you could be doing each season, foods you could be eating and practices in which you could be engaging, that would stop that nasty cold from coming back or dissolve years-old depression? The best cure is always prevention, after all.

Another difference between the two systems of medicine is the Eastern use of herbs and natural supplements versus the Western use of synthetic pharmaceutical medicines. While pharmaceuticals are largely made to mimic plant medicines, they have become highly and unnaturally strengthened. However, since they are not natural substances, the side effects of these chemical drugs can sometimes be worse than the symptoms themselves—certainly something to consider before taking them. "Does the benefit outweigh the risk?" is a question often asked in Western medicine. Natural medicines like Chinese herbs have been used for thousands of years and in the last hundred years have been researched extensively. Studies of common Western medical diagnoses have found that many Chinese patent formulas outperform prescription drugs while causing zero side effects.

Western medicine does have some advantages over Chinese medicine—mostly in the case of emergencies and surgery. Sometimes, we need bigger interventions to override life-altering and certainly life-threatening symptoms. Any potentially lethal experiences are best handled by Western medicine because it is designed to get rid of the immediate suffering and put things back in place. Chinese medicine comes in afterward and asks, "Now that the emergency is over, how can we prevent that from ever happening again?" These two systems *together* offer us the best of both worlds: prevention and high-tech responses in case of emergencies.

Chinese medicine takes the approach of supporting you holistically and increasing your self-healing power. Our bodies are quite wise and have all sorts of built-in mechanisms that let us know we are starting to lose balance. For instance, we don't just wake up with stage 4 cancer—there are all sorts of signs and symptoms that show up first, from a loss of energy to lowered immunity. The earlier we can begin to listen to our bodies at the first signs of imbalance, the more likely we can prevent the need for major interventions later.

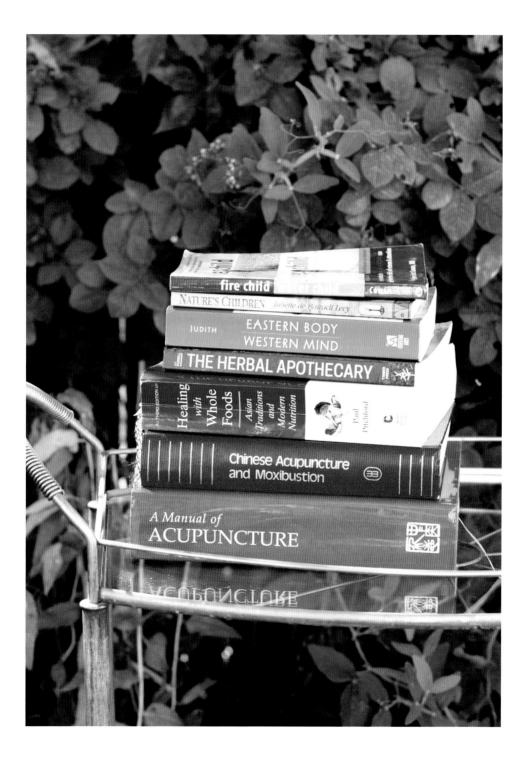

In Chinese medicine, you are invited to increase your curiosity about your symptoms. You can do this by learning to listen to those symptoms and inquire about what they are telling you, rather than simply turning them off. Having an excellent practitioner on board to support you in this journey of making sense of your symptoms will dramatically increase your understanding and your healing. In the West, we tend to have little tolerance for uncomfortable symptoms. When we are young, the second we get a fever (which is actually a good sign that the body is fighting something for us), we are taught to take a fever reducer, thereby immediately inhibiting the body's ability to continue defending itself. If we eat something and get a stomachache, instead of wondering if we are slightly allergic or intolerant to that food, we may take a drug that makes the stomachache go away. This does not mean that we have resolved the root cause of the symptom; rather, we have kept it at bay until the next insult to our system.

The reality is that symptoms are here to tell us that something is out of balance. The more we cover them up, the less we understand what is really going on inside ourselves. Of course, there is a time and a place for cover-ups. If you have a day full of meetings and wake up with a painful, debilitating headache, do what you have to do to get through the day of meetings. But do it knowing that something is still out of balance underneath and needs your attention, even though you have temporarily masked the symptoms.

I am a big believer that learning to listen to your body is an incredibly important skill to develop. If you can learn to open yourself using the experience of symptoms to guide you to the root cause of your imbalance, you will have great success not just in learning the early signs of imbalance but in developing a deeper, richer relationship with yourself. Once you are there, you will naturally become more resilient, and your vitality of body, mind, and spirit will rise tenfold.

DISCLAIMER

I invite and encourage you to work with a practitioner as you delve into this material to support your healing even more deeply. A wonderful practitioner can help you confidently identify your nature according to Chinese medicine, as well as pinpoint any patterns of imbalance you may be experiencing. Most of all, if you are having any health issues, please do consult with your primary health care provider before making any changes to your diet and lifestyle. This book is intended to be used as a tool for you to develop a greater understanding of Chinese medicine and does not replace the incredible benefit of seeing a practitioner of Chinese medicine.

I value health care that is accessible to all, therefore it's important to me to provide a resource that is inclusive. Chinese medicine can be that resource for you. Practitioners have sought many ways to keep this medicine (and its accompanying lifestyle) accessible and affordable. I have done my best to give you many options on how you might incorporate this ancient wisdom into your everyday life. I also encourage you to make use of the wonderful resources listed at the end of this book.

— ◆ —

PART ONE

UNDERSTANDING CHINESE MEDICINE

— ◆ —

PART ONE WILL INTRODUCE YOU to Chinese medicine as a code of best practices for living a balanced life. In modern life, we are seeing an increase in health concerns like toxic stress, addiction, depression, anxiety, autoimmune diseases, and cancer, to name just a few. How do we maintain balance in this kind of world? How do we stay connected to ourselves while giving so much to our families and careers? The system of Chinese medicine came out of a Taoist philosophy that saw a state of health as what naturally arises from a deep connection to the natural cycles and rhythms of the earth. By entrusting ourselves to the wisdom contained in this ancient system of medicine, we can understand some of the greatest challenges of the twenty-first century and learn to navigate them with grace and ease.

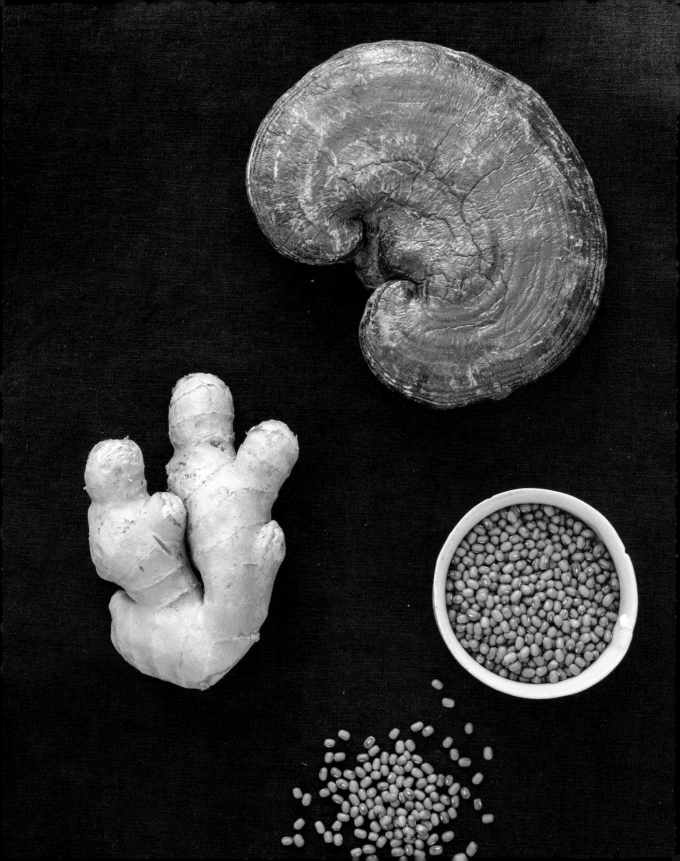

1

CHINESE MEDICINE 101
The Eight Branches

The Eight Branches of Chinese Medicine can be traced back as far as 2600 B.C.E., with each branch pertaining to one aspect of life. They have been found in both of the ancient texts related to Chinese medicine: the *Yellow Emperor's Classic of Internal Medicine (Huangdi Neijing)* and the *Classic of Change (Yi Jing)*. All of the branches together are said to create the foundation for a healthy, happy, balanced life.

As you explore the Eight Branches, you may notice an important theme in Chinese medicine: you are partially responsible for your own health and vitality. This does *not* mean it's all your fault when you experience illness, but rather that you are empowered to support your health in different ways that extend far beyond simply going to the doctor when you are sick. Just as you can participate in your own efforts to become healthy, you can also unknowingly participate in your own imbalances.

Before they know how best to treat you, Chinese medicine practitioners will ask you a number of questions, including what you have been eating, if you have been exercising, and if you have been meditating or cultivating any spiritual practices. All of these elements are considered vital for a healthy and balanced life. The doctors will not simply prescribe a medicine to take your symptoms away. Remember, they are looking for the root cause of your concerns.

Believe it or not, during the sixteenth century, a famous Chinese medicine doctor named Li Shizhen decided to flip the practice of being paid for treating sick patients on its head. He said, "To cure disease is like waiting until one is thirsty before digging a well." Therefore he started a trend of asking patients for a small payment as long as they were healthy. This required that he become an integral part of their lives. When they fell ill, the doctor would treat them *without compensation*. In this groundbreaking system, both patient and practitioner took responsibility for the patient's health. What a different concept from the way it is now! Generally, most of us only show up at the doctor's office when we are ill (and usually have been for some time).

We walk away from the office with medicine that may make us feel better but won't likely get to the root cause of our illness. So we return when the symptoms return.

Doctors of Chinese medicine took partial responsibility for each patient's health care because they not only prescribed herbs and performed acupuncture, but they also advised the patient of the appropriate diet to follow based on his or her constitution and the time of year. They suggested supportive lifestyle changes and nourishing practices to assist patients in finding their unique state of balance. The practitioners also gave each patient the tools needed to participate in his or her own care and prevent future imbalances. The Eight Branches are the foundation of these tools and serve as a blueprint for health and vitality.

1. Meditation

As long ago as the fifth century B.C.E., Taoists practiced meditation as a tool for cultivating inner peace. There is always an aspect of the mind that is quiet, calm, and present; however, it can be masked by thoughts, stories, and emotions that pull us out of the present moment. The mind can be like a toddler, running around from place to place, with an attention span of about one minute. It can easily switch from one emotion to the next. Meditation is not simply the practice of stopping all this chaos and quieting the mind; rather, it is the building of awareness about the mind's habitual nature and the reduction of its distractions. As we build our awareness of the nature of mind, we can learn to watch it the way we watch an airplane fly through the sky, without being tethered to its every whim. We can begin to see ourselves in others and develop immense compassion for all life. The more we practice, the more we reap the benefits of meditation in the short and long term. Some of the many benefits include relaxation, a reduction in stress, better concentration, increased self-awareness, and positive and stable moods. It's important that we gift our minds each day with moments of stillness and intentional time. Meditation could comprise just sitting quietly for a few minutes each day.

SIMPLE MEDITATION INSTRUCTIONS

1. Find a comfortable position to sit or lie down.
2. Soften your gaze or close your eyes completely.
3. Begin breathing naturally, noticing the sensations in your body without forcing anything.
4. Bring your attention to your breath. When you are inhaling, notice how your body expands. When you are exhaling, notice how your body relaxes and grounds. See if you can be present with each inhale and exhale. If your mind wanders, that's OK. Simply bring your awareness back to your breathing without judgment.

Begin by practicing for 5 minutes each day, and then keep extending it so you have longer sessions each time. Notice how this practice influences your day, your emotions, and your life in general.

2. Exercise

Moving our bodies daily is vital to our overall well-being. Physical activity also moves our blood and cleanses our organs. Tai chi and qigong are both ancient forms of exercise used in Chinese medicine for the cultivation of energy. When visiting east Asian countries, you will see groups of people coming together to practice these movements every day. Even if you don't know these two ancient practices, walking, running, swimming, dancing, hiking, playing sports, and even stretching are all wonderful forms of exercise. Movement helps us to move the energy in the body and also to create new energy for the body to use. Each day should include some form of movement to keep the body supple and the blood flowing. The more we find ourselves in jobs that require us to sit and think rather than use the physical body, the more we need to make a special effort to incorporate movement into each day. Otherwise our bodies can stagnate and develop aches and pains.

3. Nutrition

Food is like medicine. It can nourish us to our very bones, bring us back from illness, and give us a tremendous amount of energy for living. Imagine taking the wrong kind of medicine at the wrong dosage three times each day. What would you expect to happen eventually, if not right away? You would expect to get sick. Not knowing which foods to eat at what time of year and for what kinds of imbalances, not to mention eating food from unknown sources—where it was grown, how the animals were treated, if/what chemicals or preservatives were used—puts us in this same territory. Many of us are getting sick. Returning to natural, unprocessed, whole foods that match your constitution, align with the season, and support you through any imbalances you may be experiencing is the most direct way to find balance. Through this lens, each meal provides an opportunity to heal from the inside out and to prevent illness rather than be vulnerable to it.

4. Cosmology

Cosmology refers to the foundation of any spiritual tradition that reveals the core beliefs of how we human beings came to exist and what helps us to thrive. In Taoist cosmology, human beings are not seen as separate from the natural world but rather as a manifestation and integral part of it. Therefore, to cultivate a state of balance, we must look to the natural world around us and mimic the rhythms and cycles we see. For instance, if it's wintertime, we should try to align with what we see happening around us: it's a darker time of year, animals are hibernating, trees are drawing in their sap, and there is a pause in growth. To mimic that, we might save some of our own energy, hibernate a little, sleep a bit more, and otherwise conserve energy so we can enter springtime renewed. We can learn to use this deep connection to the natural world to benefit our health and strengthen our bodies, minds, and spirits.

5. Feng Shui

Just as we can benefit from finding balance inside ourselves by meditating, exercising, and eating a diet that is aligned with nature, we can benefit from creating a similar balance outside ourselves. This is called feng shui, and it encompasses the practice of enhancing health through the environmental balancing of the home, office, garden, and other sacred spaces. Feng shui reminds us that even though we may separate ourselves physically from the landscape, we are not, in fact, separate. We are a part of the ecology we find ourselves in, and the more connection we can build with it, the more balanced we will become. Learning permaculture, growing some of your own food, getting to know your neighbors, shopping locally, and generally caring for the earth are all ways we can develop strong feng shui. We can even use it to cultivate specific energetic invitations, such as for abundance, career enhancement, fertility, and health. For example, if you wanted to call more abundance into your life, you could place a piece of wood (nature's symbol of abundance) in the area in your home that corresponds to abundance (the southeast corner). Feng shui reveals that making this change opens the energy of your life to abundance.

6. Bodywork

Touch is vital to our overall health. The physical practice of being touched in a therapeutic way allows us to relax deeply and experience the release of tension on all levels. Bodywork gifts us with a number of amazing endorphins (feel-good hormones) most especially, oxytocin. Oxytocin is sometimes referred to as the "love hormone," as the body releases it when we experience physical affection such as hugging, holding hands, or lovemaking. We also get oxytocin when in physical contact with an animal such as petting a dog or cat. By supporting the movement of energy in the body, we can move the energy of the mind and spirit too. You would be surprised to find how much your thoughts and feelings can change after a bodywork session! Some of my favorite types of bodywork are acupressure, massage, *tui na*, shiatsu, Rolfing, craniosacral therapy, and reflexology.

7. Herbal Medicine

Chinese herbal medicine has been around for thousands of years as a vital tool for maintaining health throughout the life cycles and seasons. Eating medicinal plants from the earth allows us to be in direct relationship with the earth. In addition to a diet that is in sync with our nature, herbal medicine can target specific health imbalances and enhance the healing benefits of meals. Thanks to the early practitioners of Chinese medicine, the precise energetic nature of many plants, animals, and minerals was tested and recorded. These practitioners also discovered that each medicine has a particular affinity for a specific organ or system. As you can imagine, a vast legacy of information was left behind and is now available for our reference.

This branch of Chinese medicine is gaining popularity in the West as we not only recognize the limitations of synthetic pharmaceutical drugs but also witness their repercussions. From teas to tinctures, herbal medicine both enhances our health by supporting us in resolving imbalances and prevents future ones.

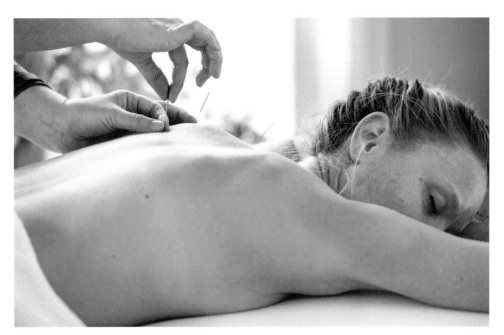

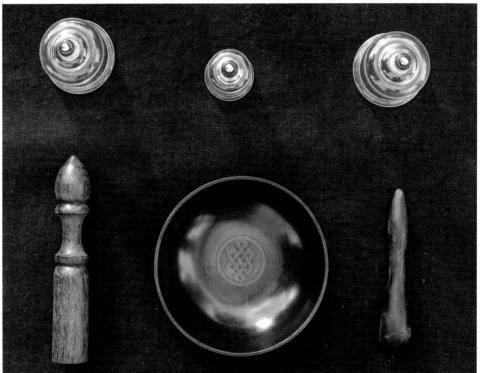

8. Acupuncture

The final branch of Chinese medicine is also the newest of the eight (though still more than two thousand years old)—the practice of acupuncture. Acupuncture is the art of inserting very fine, sterile needles just under the skin in strategic places to nourish, calm, or otherwise direct the movement of energy. This ancient art form has been found not only to reduce pain but to influence myriad systems in the body, mind, and spirit. From anxiety to leaky gut syndrome to depression to inflammation, acupuncture treats us on many levels. While this practice can certainly address everyday imbalances, I have found it to be most beneficial when used as a tool for prevention. Acupuncture can also be done without needles (called acupressure) by stimulating the same points on the same meridians but using your fingers and massaging the points instead. To become a licensed acupuncturist requires many years of study and at least a master's degree in America. It's important to find a skilled acupuncturist and one you connect with easily. (For more information on how to find an acupuncturist, see the "Resources for Delving Deeper" section at the end of this book.)

INTEGRATIVE HERBAL MEDICINE

It is important to note that I do not use only Chinese herbs in my practice. Because I am from the West, I am naturally inclined to learn about and use the herbs I see growing all around me. Not only that, but I was introduced to Western herbal medicine first and studied it extensively before learning about Chinese herbs. There is no denying that Western herbal medicine is in its infancy compared to Chinese herbal medicine. In fact, some of the formulas I mention in this book have been patented and documented to have been used for thousands of years. Research about Western herbs is just now coming to the forefront, showing their efficacy, potency, and affinity for certain conditions, some of which are above and beyond the current measures of Chinese herbs. As such, I will include Western herbs that also support everyday imbalances and serve to complement the Chinese herbs described. There is a complete list of herb and food energetics in Appendixes B and C.

CHINESE MEDICINE THERAPIES

Chinese medicine includes supportive therapies to acupuncture and bodywork such as moxibustion, *gua sha*, *tui na*, acupressure, and cupping. These adjunctive remedies enhance our healing capacity when used alongside the Eight Branches.

While many practices call for you to work with a practitioner, there are some that you can learn and begin doing every day to support your healing. Here I will introduce you to those that are safe to perform at home, will enhance your nervous and immune systems, and will bring you closer to your unique state of balance. Many of these tools are most useful when applied at the earliest sign of an imbalance.

Moxibustion

In addition to performing acupuncture, a Chinese medicine practitioner almost always burns moxa in a therapy called moxibustion. This is an ancient practice known to increase energy in the body and warm it up. The plant burned is *Artemesia vulgaris*, otherwise known as mugwort. Practitioners burn it on strategic areas of the body, including acupuncture points and along meridians where chi is stuck and/or depleted,

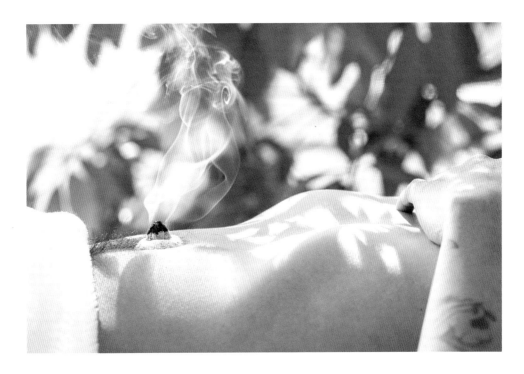

giving rise to pain, coldness, edema, fatigue, and other imbalances. Moxa comes in many forms, including raw leaves, salves, topical tinctures, and pressed into pencil- to cigar-size sticks. For home use of moxa, I recommend using a tiger warmer (more on this in the next section). Thousands of years ago, moxa was placed under a patient's pillow to bring about dreams, visions, and insight, as well as to eliminate nightmares.

Jade Facial Roller

This is a hand-held facial massage tool that is used to increase circulation in the face and neck, increase absorption of skin care products and reduce fine lines, wrinkles, under-eye swelling, and dark circles. It works by supporting lymphatic drainage away from the face. The roller is typically made with two smooth jade stones, one at each end. Depending on the size of the area you are working on, you can use either the small or large end. To use, simply massage your favorite skin cream or oil onto your face and neck and, using the roller, make small sweeping motions from the center of your face, out toward your hairline or down toward your neck. Do this for about five minutes each morning. If you tend to have puffiness under your eyes or red, irritated skin, you can put the roller into the freezer overnight and use it cold the next morning.

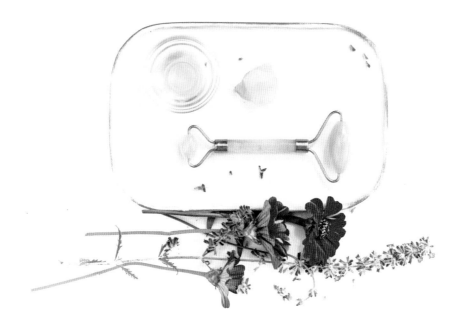

Tiger Warmer

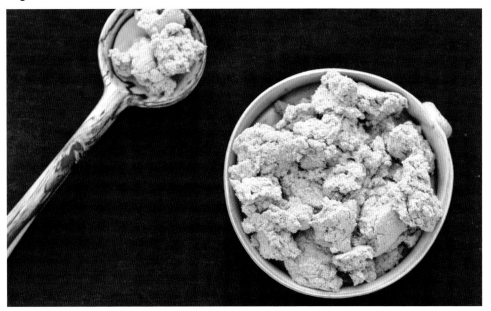

Due to the risk of burning yourself during moxibustion, it is safest to work with a practitioner. However, there are some safe and effective ways to practice moxibustion without that risk. My favorite method requires a tiger warmer. This small metal tube suspends a burning moxa stick just far enough away from the skin that you can treat acupressure points, meridians, sinuses, muscles, and organs that need support without burning yourself. Tiger warmers are used to heal everything from pain to diarrhea to sinus congestion.

TOPICAL OILS

When it comes to using a jade roller or tiger warmer or practicing gua sha (loosely translated as "to scrape until you see redness"), acupressure, or cupping, I recommend using topical oils to support your skin while performing the therapy. It's important to use oils that mimic those your skin has naturally. I find that jojoba is the most similar in this regard, and it is easy to use in these therapies. After jojoba, my favorite oils to use are almond, sesame, and coconut.

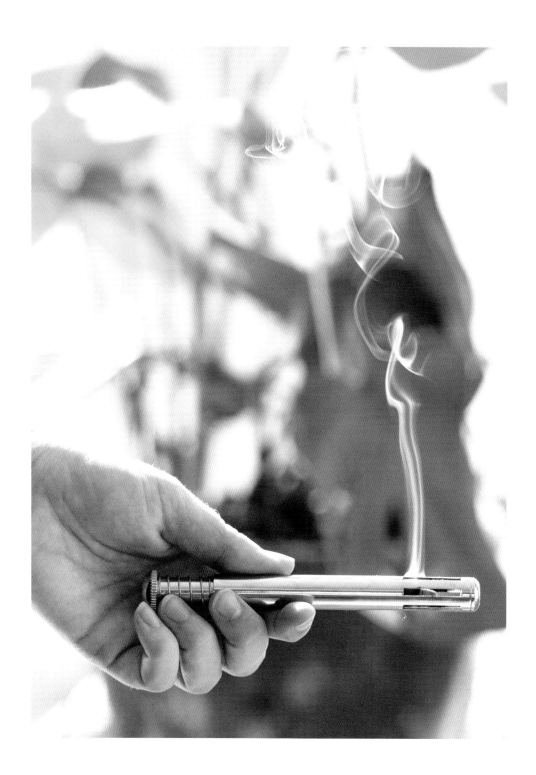

You will need a tiger warmer, a lighter or match, and pressed moxa sticks that fit the warmer you have. Tiger warmers come in small and large sizes, depending on what you are treating; I prefer large as it is the most versatile. Suspend the moxa stick inside the metal tube of the warmer, ensuring that the fit is tight and the moxa stick won't slide out, and light the end. Insert the suspended and burning moxa stick and tube inside the larger metal tube, keeping the lit end of the moxa stick visible through the holes at the end of the tiger warmer. This ensures that the stick will stay lit because it has access to oxygen. Frequently test the heat at the end of the warmer on the back of your hand to make sure it feels warm to hot but not burning. Press the tiger warmer directly on the acupressure point, meridian, or area you wish to treat, moving along the meridians in a sweeping, circular, or tapping motion. Do this until the area you are treating becomes pink and feels hot, indicating an increase in circulation. Then slip the moxa stick out of the larger metal tube and place the lit end in water. Save the stick to use again. Repeat 1 to 3 times each day until symptoms resolve. Expect to see results in 24 to 72 hours for acute symptoms and 4 to 6 weeks for chronic symptoms.

Gua Sha

This practice of strategically "scraping" body surfaces is performed to relieve pain, reduce inflammation, increase circulation, and boost the immune system. Traditionally this is done with a small, flat jade stone with rounded edges, which can be used on the body, muscles, acupressure points, and/or meridians to release heat, toxins, and so on. You usually scrape in the direction of the meridians only until you see small red dots (called petechia). These red dots indicate that blood has been brought to the surface of the skin, where it is able to release the heat and toxins. Chinese medicine calls this "raising the *sha*," which is said to eliminate stagnation and inflammation in the blood and protect the immune system for days or even weeks after the treatment. You can easily learn to do this at home for certain conditions, such as when you are feeling vulnerable to a cold, have tight or sore muscles, or are feeling inflamed in a particular part of your body. For chronic conditions such as cancer or autoimmune disease, or if there are lumps, cysts, or fibroids, I recommend working with a practitioner before performing gua sha.

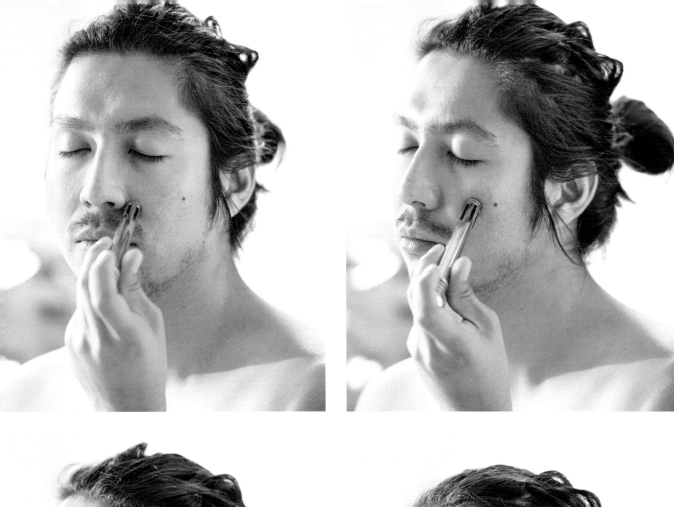
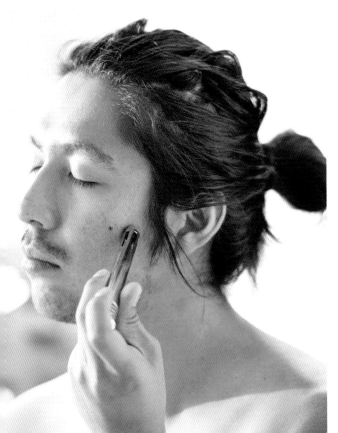
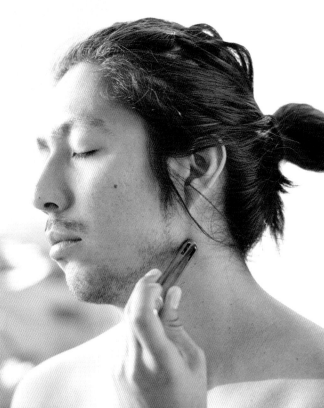

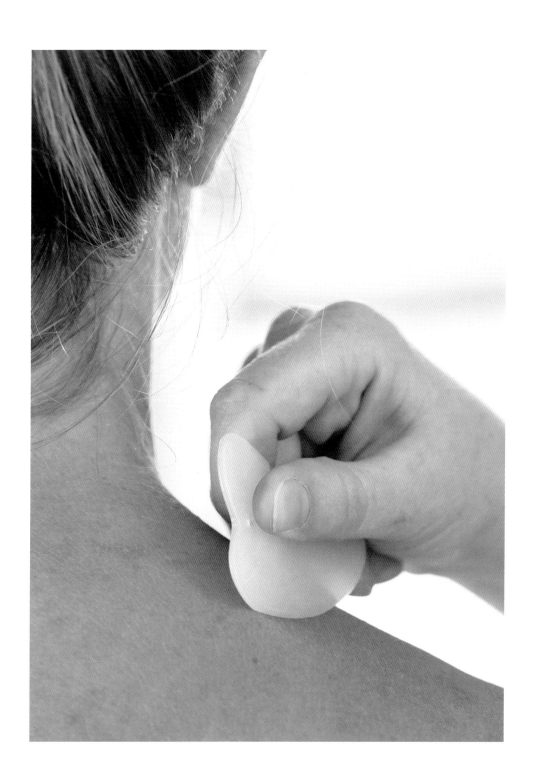

To do gua sha at home, you will need a jade stone with rounded edges, or you can use an Asian soup spoon. I also recommend using an oil like jojoba to protect your skin and support the smooth flow of chi and release of sha.

To start, locate the point, meridian, or area of pain or inflammation you will be working on, and put enough oil on the area so that it feels somewhat slippery. Grip the stone or spoon in your hand and place it on the skin at a 45-degree angle with about three pounds of pressure (the amount it takes to use a can opener). Briskly begin to "scrape" the area repeatedly until you see small red dots forming. Stop once you see this reaction, and do not repeat until they are completely gone. The photos below show a gua sha treatment for the common cold, allergies, and asthma; due to the location of the treatment, another person was needed to perform the gua sha.

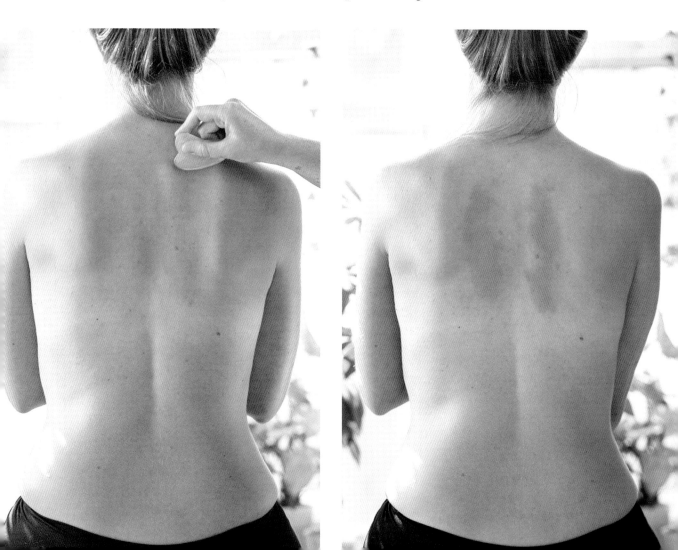

Acupressure

Acupressure points are places in the meridians where a patient's energy can collect and cause a disruption in the harmonious flow of chi. This can cause any number of symptoms, from emotional imbalances to physical imbalances like pain and inflammation. Learning to stimulate or sedate the acupressure points supports the return to an appropriate flow of energy and therefore a reduction in symptoms. As such, acupressure point prescriptions are given later in this book to provide you with personal tools to treat common imbalances. Note: acupressure points are the same places in the meridians that acupuncturists use as acupuncture points; however, you can use them to treat yourself with your hands rather than needles. If you were to see an acupuncturist as well, he or she would likely use these same points.

If you are working with an acupuncturist, ask your acupuncturist which points they would recommend you work on at home. If you are not, then the first thing to do with acupressure is to discover which points would be most appropriate to stimulate. For a comprehensive approach to this, keep reading to discover your constitution and any patterns of imbalance you might be experiencing. For quick reference, turn to Appendix A for a list of my favorite acupressure points and their descriptions. To utilize the appendix, simply choose 3 to 5 points to stimulate during each session. They can be the same each time or you can rotate, depending on what you are working on.

The best way to find and treat an acupressure point is to locate it, using the charts in Appendix A. Feel around the place suggested by the dot on the chart. Using your fingertips, notice where you feel a slight ache or tender place in the vicinity of the dot. This is usually where the acupressure point is. Once you have located it, you can stimulate the point using about three pounds of pressure (the amount it takes to use a can opener), massaging vigorously in a clockwise direction for approximately 60 seconds. You can stimulate the same point on each side of the body at the same time, but I recommend stimulating different points separately. Repeat this treatment anywhere from once per day to once per week until you notice results (typically 24 to 72 hours for acute conditions and 4 to 6 weeks for chronic conditions). Do not perform more than one treatment in a day (3 to 5 points total).

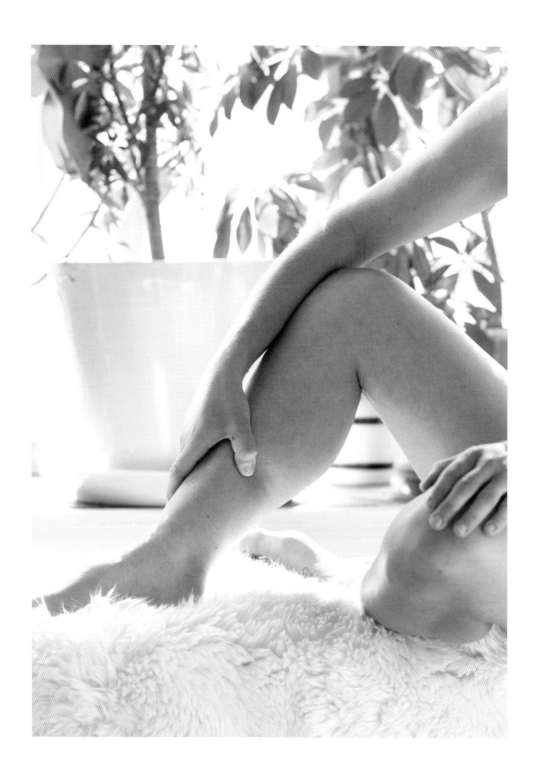

Tui Na

The practice of working with chi energy in the meridians is done only with your hands, sometimes using lotion or oil. Tui na is similar to giving a massage, but instead of focusing on muscle groups, you focus on the meridians that run through the muscles. For instance, if you are having bowel issues like constipation or diarrhea, you can use tui na to massage the Large Intestine meridian from end to end. You can massage, tap, brush, and/or squeeze the meridians to achieve the desired effect. If the large intestine is overactive, as in the case of loose stools, you can massage the Large Intestine meridian in the opposite direction of chi flow to slow the chi in the meridian. If it is underactive, as is typical in cases of constipation, you can massage the meridian in the direction of chi flow to help move the energy to induce a bowel movement.

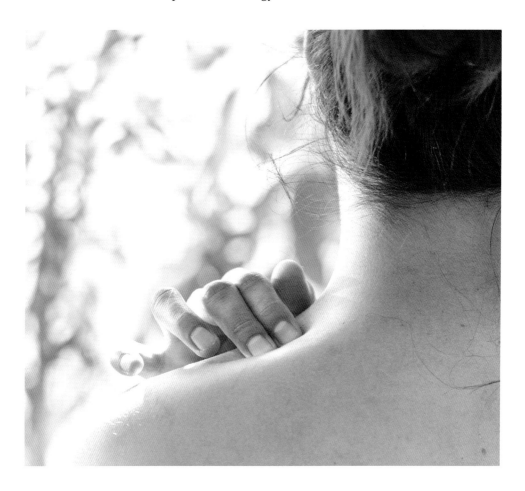

Cupping

Cupping is an adjunctive therapy used only by acupuncturists and bodyworkers. This is the ancient practice of stimulating circulation and pulling toxins from a particular area on a patient's body by creating suction with a vessel and placing it strategically on areas of pain, inflammation, stagnation, and so forth. While I don't recommend you do this on yourself at home, it is worth having a practitioner do it for you. Cupping relieves pain, calms the nervous system, and helps even the oldest and most stubborn injuries to heal. Sometimes you are left with small circles of bruising after the cups have been removed, and the lightness or darkness of these bruises indicates the level to which the stagnation and/or injury occurred. This means that the darker the bruise, the deeper the injury or stagnation, and the greater the healing opportunity. The bruises heal over the course of a few days or a week and leave you with more free-flowing energy. Of note, cupping can also stimulate detoxification by pulling toxins from deep in the tissues and releasing them into the bloodstream for elimination. Be sure to drink plenty of water after cupping therapy.

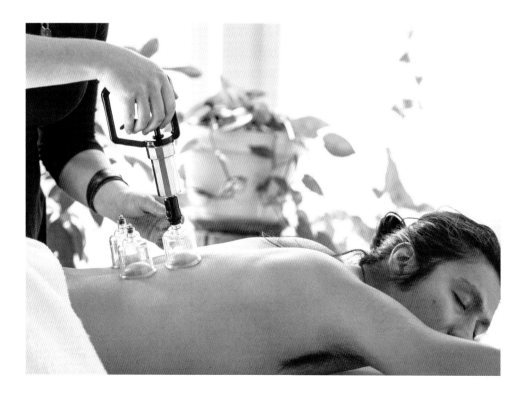

CHI—LIFE FORCE ENERGY

All living beings, including plants and animals, have a life force that is energetic and resilient. We each have our own life force that is unique to us and yet very similar, even across species. A toddler's life force is different than a dog's life force, but both are animated with personality, preferences, and aversions, and both have the will to stay alive and avoid suffering. This life force energy is called *chi* in Chinese medicine, and an understanding of it shows how this system of medicine can impact so many different kinds of people and illnesses.

Imagine you were born with a bucket of energy in your hand. This bucket reflects the energy your parents shared with you at conception and during your development. If they had a lot of energy, ate and drank well, shared moments of loving connection, and generally took care of themselves, then they likely had a lot to give you. The opposite is also true. They had less to give if they were exhausted, didn't eat a great diet, and were stressed or overworked; if your conception came at the end of a long, hard period in their lives; or if you were last in the line of many children. The energy you were born with is called *jing qi*, and Chinese medicine practitioners assess this energy because it sets the foundation for the energy you will have in your life.

Whatever amount of energy you were born with, however, is not the only determining factor for the energy you will have access to throughout your life. We derive energy from a multitude of resources and experiences in our world, including the food we eat; the water we drink; the air we breathe; the loving relationships we have; the habits we form (such as rest, meditation, and movement); and even the contact we have with plants and animals. Because of this, we can, in effect, add to a bucket that may have started out a little low.

Throughout our lives, we will draw from the energy bucket, and how we live our lives determines how much energy we draw. The goal is to replenish it faster than we take away from it. If you live a high-intensity, stressed-out life that is incongruent with the energy you have available, you may first find yourself addicted to things that will bring you temporary feelings of energy (like caffeine), but you will end up exhausted and depleted. Rather if you live your life well, preserving your energy when possible and replenishing it frequently, you will have enough energy for the life you want to live.

Meridians

The chi bucket is a metaphor for the human body as chi lives everywhere inside us. Chi lives inside each cell, organ, and tissue, and it runs like a multitude of rivers from the head to the toes and back. These reservoirs of energy were mapped and studied extensively by practitioners almost three thousand years ago, and today we refer to them as *meridians*. There are two meridians that act like oceans and twelve that act like rivers, drawing chi from and returning it to the oceans.

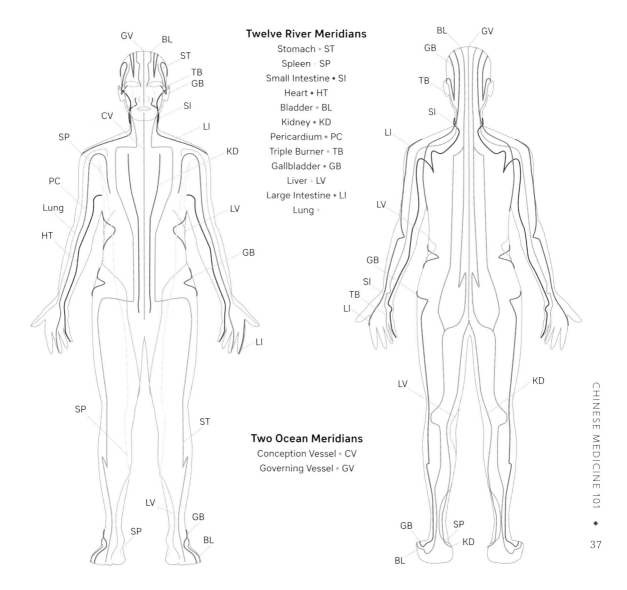

Twelve River Meridians

Stomach • ST
Spleen • SP
Small Intestine • SI
Heart • HT
Bladder • BL
Kidney • KD
Pericardium • PC
Triple Burner • TB
Gallbladder • GB
Liver • LV
Large Intestine • LI
Lung •

Two Ocean Meridians

Conception Vessel • CV
Governing Vessel • GV

Each meridian reflects a relationship to an organ and/or system in the body. This means that when an organ or a system is functioning well, it will produce plenty of chi to flow in its corresponding meridian. And when the meridian is flush with chi, it will keep the organ or system nourished and functioning well. Not only that, but if an organ or a system is struggling, another organ or system will often step in to compensate for the imbalance. These kinds of things happen in the body all the time and reveal the interconnected relationship between all the organs and systems.

When chi is flowing freely through the meridians, we feel fantastic, energetic, and at home in ourselves in such a way that we feel we can be and express who we truly are. We have limited physical discomfort, and when life throws us curveballs, we bounce back quickly. However, when chi gets stuck, we feel emotionally vulnerable, physically uncomfortable, and sensitive to life's ever-changing tides. Everything we do to care for ourselves (or not) impacts our chi and therefore our meridians. Acupuncture is the practice that works directly with balancing the chi in the meridians. When we receive this therapy, we can often feel our own chi and its movement along our meridians. It's quite spectacular!

Yin and Yang

The two foundational qualities of chi are yin and yang. Most of us have heard of the concept of yin and yang, which draws from ancient Chinese texts (more than eight thousand years old) and can be used to describe the nature of all things in life. The Chinese character for *yin* literally translates as the "dark side of the mountain," whereas the character for *yang* translates as the "light side of the mountain." The best metaphor for yin and yang is introversion and extroversion, as these are familiar concepts in the West. Introversion is a quieter and more contracted energy, whereas extroversion is a louder and more expanded energy. Here are a few examples of the qualities associated with yin and yang:

Yin	Yang
Moon	Sun
Feminine	Masculine
Passive	Active

Yin	Yang
Intuitive	Logical
Creative	Intellectual
Dark	Light
Cold	Hot
Moist skin	Dry skin
Submission	Dominance
Contracting	Expanding
Downward	Upward
Night	Day
Soft	Hard
Stillness	Movement
Water	Fire
Valleys	Mountains
Feeling, emotion	Thought
Right-brained	Left-brained
Left-hand dominance	Right-hand dominance
Receiving	Giving
Nurturing	Protecting
Flexible	Rigid
Introverted	Extroverted
Dampness	Dryness
Cooler body and personality	Warmer body and personality
Aloof, dreamy	Hyperactive, focused
Timid	Aggressive
Fearful, insecure	Impatient, irritable
Pale complexion	Ruddy complexion
Soft voice	Loud voice

As you can see, yin and yang describe the everyday energetic qualities of the world we live in and our experiences. Energy lives on a continuum and is constantly shifting the way day turns to night and back into day again. Nighttime brings about a yin experience, then as the sun comes up, the yang experience of daytime grows. When the sun sets, we move from yang back to yin, and the cycle continues.

Yin-Yang Cycle

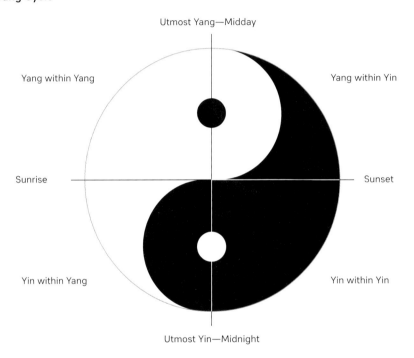

The seasons follow their own rhythm of yin and yang, winter being the most yin of all the seasons, and summer being the most yang. Everything in between is a mixture of the two. Spring, for instance, is the movement from a mostly yin experience (winter) to a mostly yang experience (summer). Even the places we live have a yin or yang energetic quality to them. Places that are sunny and warm all the time are much more yang in nature, whereas places that are rainy and cold all the time are much more yin. Of course, there is every variation in between.

You can see how each moment of life can be characterized by whether yin, yang, or a mixture of these energies is at play. It's important to note that nothing in life is ever completely yin or completely yang, as neither state is ever static—they are fluid energetic states. Why is it important to know the yin-yang state of things? Because each of us has a yin nature and a yang nature that are always in flux. For instance, although you may feel drawn to a yin environment, that does not mean you are a completely yin-natured person. You undoubtedly have some yang qualities within you, even though you might lean toward yin, at least at this moment in your life. Each of us has our own unique quantities and expressions of yin and yang energies within, and that is part of what makes us different. The more familiar we are with our unique energetic qualities, the more appropriate our life decisions will be for enhancing our health.

Twenty-first-century Westerners live in a predominantly, energetically yang society. This means we have endless opportunities, activity buzzes around us constantly, and productivity is highly rewarded. Although some people who are quite yang in their energy do well in this environment, those with a more yin nature can find this level of activity challenging. In fact, many clients come to me because they are exhausted, overstimulated, and often even addicted to substances that help them cope with this level of busyness. It's clear to me that they are trying to conform to a life that is not congruent with their nature. Sadly, these clients often feel like something is wrong with them and not the other way around.

The most common concerns I treat in my office are anxiety and depression, and these diagnoses are two sides of the same coin: anxiety being the yang expression of stress and depression being the yin expression. Many of the symptoms associated with these imbalances come from this feeling of incongruence between their authentic nature and the lives they find themselves living. This split between what many of us need energetically and the activities we participate in makes it easy to understand why addiction is so rampant. In particular, addiction to stimulation and stimulating substances such as coffee, sugar, and alcohol, and activities such as TV, video games, and even exercise like extreme sports. These habits undoubtedly increase our energy (albeit temporarily) and may even make us feel much more extroverted than we really are. However, when we forsake our energetic needs, we will always pay a price.

If you know that you have a mostly yin nature, it's important to do things every day that will support your yin-yang balance. If you have not extended yourself enough (for example, working too long in a yin environment, being too sedentary), you may need to invoke more yang practices to find balance. The same need for balance is true if you feel you have a mostly yang nature. When you notice you have overextended, be sure to recoup your energy by adding in nourishing yin activities.

YIN ACTIVITIES: Sleeping and napping, eating slowly, cooking meals slowly, baking, spending one-on-one time with friends or family, reading books, taking baths, going on slow walks in nature, meditating, doing yin yoga, getting a massage, doing light gardening, playing cards or other low-key games, spending quiet time with loved ones or alone, playing instruments, drawing/painting

YANG ACTIVITIES: Socializing with a group, exercising (such as aerobics and weight lifting), participating in competitive and/or team sports, performing hard labor, running, playing, dancing, singing, having a potluck, planning a vacation

MENSES AND THE MOON

Women are gifted with the opportunity to cycle through yin and yang monthly (and psst: men have similar cycles too!). Menstrual cycles follow cycles similar to that of the moon, and if we are in tune with the natural world, we will either be ovulating or menstruating on the full and new moons, respectively. During menstruation is the most yin time of the cycle, as it is dominated by the yin hormone estrogen. Then as the cycle moves toward ovulation, the yang hormone progesterone begins to dominate, giving us access to increasingly more yang energy.

I see many women in my practice who feel overwhelmed and anxious during specific times in their cycle. After mapping out their energetic patterns along with the days of their cycle, we can see that their feelings of being overwhelmed often come at a phase during which they are ruled by mostly yin energy. Yet their lives are still moving full speed ahead. I believe this is where most premenstrual syndrome (PMS) symptoms—irritability, sadness, anxiety, depression, anger, fatigue—come from.

Knowing what is happening in our bodies energetically empowers us to do what we can to care for ourselves and tend to those deeper needs. If you are menstruating, try honoring your cycle phases by transitioning into a more yin time during those first two weeks (slowing things down, taking breaks when possible, limiting yang activities, and so on), then gradually increasing your yang activities for the second half of your cycle (returning to the full scope of work, scheduling social outings, and otherwise engaging in the world in a more extroverted way). Learning to live in accordance with our natural energy is the first step toward health.

2

THE FIVE ELEMENTS AND
YOUR CONSTITUTION

In addition to the qualities of yin and yang, the ancient Chinese recognized that energy could be classified further into the Five Elements. This philosophy dates back almost eight thousand years. Interestingly, you can find similar descriptions of energy in other cultures, as in Indian, Native American, Tibetan, and Mayan traditional medicine. These elements provide a language with which to describe the unique and dynamic energy of everything in our world.

FIRE ELEMENT	This literally refers to the element of fire, the sun, and that which creates heat.
EARTH ELEMENT	Earth refers to the soil that holds nutrients, plants, and trees in the ground.
METAL ELEMENT	Rocks, minerals, and compost are all considered part of the Metal element.
WATER ELEMENT	This refers to the water of our planet—oceans, rivers, lakes, precipitation, and so on.
WOOD ELEMENT	This refers not only to the wood found in trees but also to the sturdy, fibrous structure of all plant life.

All life on earth is dependent on the Five Elements. For instance, a seed attempting to grow must have access to Water to germinate; Wood so it grows a strong structure and roots for its coming leaves, flowers, and fruit; Fire so when it sprouts it will grow toward the sun; Earth so the soil can hold the roots and structure; and Metal so it is continuously nourished by the minerals in the compost.

The early Taoist philosophers observed that these elements described not only physical entities all around them but also something energetic. Upon deeper observation, they discovered that the elements are not fixed states of energy but rather are constantly changing and are more akin to phases than to fixed conditions. These phases can be seen in all life on earth. Using our plant metaphor, a plant would have a period of incubation (Water), growth (Wood), maturation (Fire), harvest (Earth), and death (Metal). This knowledge led to the discovery that nature's way of moving through the elements matched the cycles and rhythms of the seasons. As a consequence, each element became associated with a season.

Additionally, it was observed that the seasons provided a similar experience for plants, animals, and humans alike. Granted, it's important to note that these observations were recorded during a time when people lived close to the land and were dependent on the rhythms and cycles of the seasons. If they had tried to grow rice in winter or harvest fruit in spring, they would have risked their health and the survival of their community. This is what the ancients observed:

WINTER is a time for incubation.

SPRING is a time for birth and growth.

SUMMER is a time for maturation and celebration.

LATE SUMMER is a time for harvesting.

FALL is a time for letting go and returning to the earth.

Even though in the West most of us live indoors now, the seasons still impact us. Not only are we affected on the outside by bundling up in winter and wearing sunscreen in summer, but we are also affected on the inside. Seasons impact our emotions, organs, and systems too. Taoist philosophers found an example of this when they observed that the lungs, large intestine, and skin experienced health challenges during autumn that weren't noticeable during the other seasons. One of the biggest differences was that it is often drier and cooler in autumn. The philosophers also noticed that in the natural world, autumn is a season of letting go, declining energy, and shedding what is no longer alive in us, the same way trees do. When this happens, the emotion that naturally arises in response to letting go is grief. Therefore, the lungs, large intestine, and skin became the organs and tissues associated with Autumn and the Metal element, and grief became the related emotion.

Since each organ is related to a particular season, we can target our support for certain emotional imbalances, organs, or systems to maximize our healing at certain times of the year. For instance, the emotion of anger and the liver and gallbladder are associated with the Wood element and the Spring season. When spring arrives, the body's energy begins to move in a different way. Usually we are more active and more extroverted than we are in winter. As such, the liver and gallbladder begin to work harder to move the energy in our bodies to match the increased demand for energy. If we have any stuck energy, toxin buildup, or repressed emotions, this will be very noticeable during a season when we need more energy. This feeling of "stuckness," whether physical or energetic, is what can lead to anger. Since the liver and gallbladder's primary job is to move energy in the body, Spring would be the best time to support these organs and any emotional imbalances associated with the Wood element.

According to Chinese medicine, understanding what is happening in nature and knowing what to expect from each season provides an essential guide for how to stay healthy and get the most out of each day. According to this ancient system, if you look outside and see that it's winter, you should also be experiencing Winter on the inside. If instead you find yourself with more Summer-type energy, you are likely to experience incongruence and, eventually, imbalance. Learning to live in accordance with the seasons is the second step toward health.

It is not just the seasons we need to consider when trying to improve our health and vitality. Practitioners of Chinese medicine observed many years ago that each organ also has a daily high point of energy as well as a low point. These points have been documented as a roughly two-hour window in each twenty-four-hour period. This information serves us well when it comes to supporting specific organs. If we know that heart time is between 11 A.M. and 1 P.M., would it be nice to know what we can do during that window to maximize support for our heart?

Meridian Clock

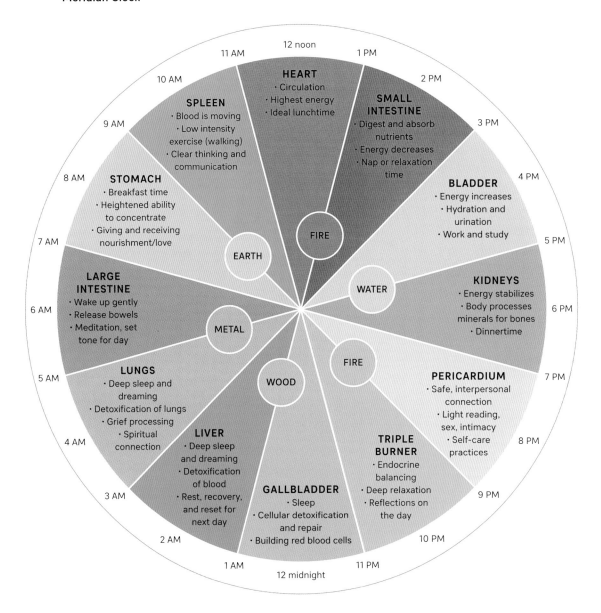

Five Element Associations

	Water	Wood	Fire	Earth	Metal
SEASON	Winter	Spring	Summer	Late Summer	Autumn
EMOTION	Fear	Anger	Joy	Worry	Grief
YIN ORGAN	Kidneys	Liver	Heart, pericardium	Spleen	Lungs
YANG ORGAN	Bladder	Gallbladder	Small intestine, triple burner	Stomach	Large intestine
BODY PART	Bones	Tendons, ligaments	Blood, sexual fluids	Muscles, fat	Skin
SENSE/ORGAN	Hearing/Ears	Sight/Eyes	Speech/Tongue	Taste/Mouth	Smell/Nose
FLAVOR	Salty	Sour	Bitter	Sweet	Pungent

YOUR CONSTITUTION

We are made up of all five of the elements, and we cycle in and out of different elemental phases throughout our lives. That being said, according to Chinese medicine, each of us embodies a unique combination of the elements within us, which is called our *constitution*. The constitution is the energetic imprint we are born with. As we ebb and flow through life, our qualities of energy can also ebb and flow. However, the underlying current of our constitutional energy will, for the most part, always be the same.

It's important to note that *we need all of the elements* present in our world to find balance in our bodies, minds, and spirits, as well as in our families and communities. Each person and his or her unique constitution bring something unique to the table that provides balance *for* and seeks balance *from* other constitutions.

The constitution can be viewed as our medicine offering to the world. Let's look at plants for a moment, as they are very similar in this regard. There isn't a single plant on earth that doesn't carry within it the ability to heal *something*. For example, the bark from the cinchona tree heals malaria, turkey tail mushrooms (*Coriolus versicolor*) can shrink tumors, and even those little yellow dandelions that shoot up in every nook and cranny of your lawn can cool down a fever and help detoxify the blood. Every single plant has medicine, and humans are no different.

There is no other medicine, nor will there ever again be medicine, like what you have to offer our world. You are truly unique and a vital gift to the planet. You don't come here with a unique energetic imprint just so you can hide away in your home all your life. You are born with a divine purpose that can be traced back to and manifests out of your constitution. (Sadly, length restrictions will not allow us to explore the process of uncovering your purpose in depth. You will have to stay tuned for my next book!)

There is great wisdom in learning about your constitution and patterns of imbalance *before* uncovering your purpose. A famous psychologist named Abraham Maslow created what we know as the "hierarchy of needs" in the early 1940s. His hierarchy depicts, in order of importance, the shared global human needs.

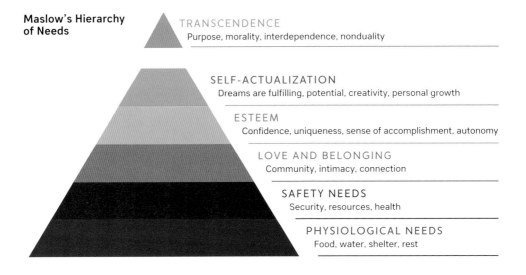

Maslow's Hierarchy of Needs

TRANSCENDENCE
Purpose, morality, interdependence, nonduality

SELF-ACTUALIZATION
Dreams are fulfilling, potential, creativity, personal growth

ESTEEM
Confidence, uniqueness, sense of accomplishment, autonomy

LOVE AND BELONGING
Community, intimacy, connection

SAFETY NEEDS
Security, resources, health

PHYSIOLOGICAL NEEDS
Food, water, shelter, rest

Our most basic needs for survival live at the bottom of the hierarchy, and as we work our way up, we find the more complex needs. When we are sick or in pain, our very survival is challenged, and we often cannot possibly think of anything more complex than getting through the day. Fulfilling survival needs relates to the balancing of the Water element. As we heal, we can then work our way toward establishing feelings of safety in our minds, our bodies, and our lives. Working on our safety includes putting systems in place to prevent us from returning to survival mode by building personal, financial, and health resources. This stage relates to the Wood element.

As we enter the Fire stage, we can work toward fulfilling the need for love and belonging through family, friends, and intimate relationships. This provides us with a sense of being connected to the larger landscape of our lives. Feeling as though we belong is a need that is largely unmet in our culture and one that is absolutely vital. Beyond that, we can enter the stage of the Earth element, which is a key stage for individuation and taking ownership of who we are. At this stage we may feel inclined to take career risks that highlight our strengths and accomplishments. We may make bigger decisions about what we want to get out of life versus finding ourselves always at the other end, making do with others' decisions about our lives. Our personal power grows in this stage.

Maslow's final stage in the hierarchy relates to the Metal element and describes a state in which we want to become the best possible version of ourselves. He referred to this stage as that of self-actualization, and it represents the development of a personal connection with the divine, God, Goddess, you name it.

A few years before Maslow died, he realized he had made a mistake. He hadn't completed the hierarchy, as one level was still missing. So in 1970, he added another need at the very top; he called this the need for transcendence. He was defining *transcendence* as the need all humans have at some point in their lives to live a life of purpose (and he acknowledged that purpose usually included service). He explained that this need does not typically come to the surface until we have met (even if only partially) most of our other needs lower in the hierarchy. This final stage of transcendence can also be likened to homing in on the unique balance of all the elements within us so that in some sense we can simply be present and no longer strive.

I'm sure after looking at this hierarchy of needs, you can see why it would be strange for me to give you information to guide you toward your purpose and offering to this world if you are waking with debilitating anxiety every day. You must work your way through your needs in an order that makes sense, that fills your cup along the way, and that gives you the tools to make your way to your own version of evolution. The book you hold in your hands contains these tools. If after some time spent with this material, you begin to feel the pings of "What is my purpose?" and "What am I doing with my life?" then you will probably be interested in the next book I'll be writing, which will cover this very material: your constitution, your purpose, and how to manifest it into an offering for our world.

Knowing your constitution serves you in a number of ways, including:

1. Knowing how to support your body, mind, and spirit by supporting the elements that are most prominent in your constitution
2. Knowing how to prevent health imbalances by supporting the most challenged organs in your constitution
3. Having insight into your unique energetic imprint that will guide you toward your purpose and offering to the world
4. Developing compassion for yourself and others as you learn about critical elemental differences that make each of us important and unique

As a practitioner, I always want to know which elements are in each client's constitution because that will set the foundation for the treatment plan as well as his or her health and life goals. One of the surefire ways to know the elements present in your constitution is to consult someone who has studied the Five Elements extensively, most notably a Five Element acupuncturist. This professional will listen to you, look at you, and even smell you to accurately diagnose your constitution. In the interest of discovery and supporting you in learning more about yourself, I have provided a quiz at the end of this section that will give you some insight into your constitution. However, I cannot guarantee that it will be 100 percent accurate. For this, you will need to see a qualified practitioner.

Once you know your constitution (whether through seeing a practitioner or through your own studies), a part of your healing strategy should always include the foods, herbs, and practices that best support that primary element and season. For example, if you discover you are primarily a Wood constitution, I recommend that you include nourishing your liver and gallbladder in regimens throughout your whole life and especially in spring. While it is enticing to flip straight to the chapter on your constitutional element, I invite you to follow along through all the chapters to better understand how to use this information in your day-to-day life. As a rule, practitioners always seek to find balance in the individual and his or her true nature first, followed by attuning the person to the corresponding season. Working in this order ensures that we don't undermine the nature of a patient. I recommend you follow a similar path as you work your way through this book.

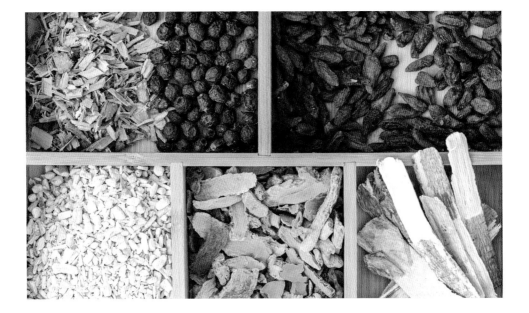

Quiz

For each question, select one answer out of the five options. Remember that since we are assessing your constitution and not just a sudden uprising of symptoms, you need to read these statements as though you are looking at a *lifetime of patterns*. For instance, one of the questions reads, "When it comes to a large social gathering . . . _____." The options include "No thanks," "Bring it on," and so forth. When you answer, choose the response that reflects something that you have noticed for most of your life as opposed to something you have felt on occasion. For example, we have all had times when we feel antisocial and want to reject an invitation, but is that your usual reaction to large social gatherings? Or would that be rare for you? You will want to give it the highest score if it is your primary reaction.

After you have taken the quiz, tally up the numbers in each column. You will end up with five columns of numbers. Take the highest number and note the element that it is associated with. This element will be considered your *primary element* and therefore, your constitution. If you have a tie between two elements, then consider it a wonderful opportunity to learn about both of the elements that show up strongly in your constitution. Regardless of having a tie, it's important to learn about all of the elements, since you are made up of all of them, and they each play a pivotal role in your life.

Five Element Quiz

	1	2	3	4	5
My dominant emotion is:	Fear	Anger	Joy	Worry	Grief
I identify as:	An extreme introvert	Mostly extroverted	An extreme extrovert	Half introvert/half extrovert	Mostly introverted
I prefer company to be:	Minimal and quiet	Focused on a task	One on one	An intimate gathering of lots of close-knit family and friends	A gathering of people that have room to do things on their own and together
When it comes to a large social gathering:	No, thanks.	What's our goal?	Bring it on!	Wait, who will be there?	I can take it or leave it
I am mostly afraid of:	Death	Not meeting my life's goals	Not being loved	Not belonging	Not being connected
My Achilles' heel is:	Dogmatism	Feelings of being stuck/held back	Impulsiveness	Worry and self-doubt	The need to be right
I know I'm stressed out when I:	Get extremely tired and can't get enough sleep	Feel angry and exhibit addictive behavior, even with work addiction	Feel anxiety, have heart palpitations, and experience insomnia	Do not digest food properly (Every meal is an obstacle.)	Get frequent colds and sinus infections, asthma
What's most important to me and my work:	Truth	Justice	Connection	Sharing	Fairness
I'm really good at:	Using my imagination, creating art	Problem solving	Communicating	Anticipating others' needs, establishing routines	Seeing the big picture
I'm not so good at:	Being frivolous	Not fixating on a goal/plan	Being serious	Setting/reading boundaries, handling change	Making mistakes

	1	2	3	4	5
My family and friends come to me for:	Serious talks, words of wisdom	Decision making, planning	Love, play, adventures	Nurturing, compassion, listening ear	Inspiration, spiritual guidance
I consider myself:	Articulate and deep (I just want to know.)	Highly creative and intuitive (I just want to create.)	A people person with no shortage of passions (I love life.)	A natural caretaker (I just want to help.)	Self-disciplined and organized (I just want to serve the greater good.)
On a Friday night, I prefer:	To stay home with a book	To work late and get ahead for next week	To go out and socialize	To have people over for a community dinner	To attend a ceremony or ritual to commemorate someone or something
I wish all beings:	Would just listen to their own truth	Would just do something for the world	Could be happy	Could have their needs met	Could feel connected, not alone
My leadership style is:	Within the comforts of my home or office	Front line, alone if necessary	I prefer to have one good friend by my side	Collaborative, or equal leadership in a group	Quiet and with integrity, but I'll get big and loud if I need to
I am at my best when:	I'm given full creative license and space	I'm in charge	I get to follow my bliss	I get to be of service to others	My life mimics my core values
I love my:	Alone time	Work	Spontaneity	Routines	Guiding principles
My natural pacing for life is:	Slowest—it's more important to focus on quality	Fast—let's get it done so we can move on	Quick—how much can we fit into one lifetime?	Average—I'm no faster or slower than those around me	Slow—it's more important that we not miss anything
I have an aversion to:	Chaos	Pushy people	Attention stealers	Clinginess or neediness	Authority and misuse of power

	1	2	3	4	5
Physically I feel:	I am not as adept as others, and I don't care.	I'm really strong and have lots of stamina.	Great! I can do anything!	I have to work hard to keep fit.	I'm okay. I can get stronger if I put my mind to it.
My body type is:	Average. Weight goes to my belly but doesn't touch my legs.	Athletic, sinewy. My weight is evenly distributed.	Sexy/ good-looking. I like to dress to show my body.	Fluctuating. I have challenges with my weight, which typically settles in my belly, hips, and thighs.	Tall and lean with a long neck. I can gain weight mostly in my hips.
Totals					
KEY	1 = Water	2 = Wood	3 = Fire	4 = Earth	5 = Metal

PATTERNS OF IMBALANCE

Once you have discovered your elemental constitution, you will have an idea of how best to use this book to support yourself throughout the many phases of your life. But that's not all you will need to find balance in your world. In addition to your constitution, you also need to know which patterns of imbalance you are experiencing. While patterns *may* reflect some aspect of your constitution, often they reveal something completely different about you, like your Achilles' heel. Patterns are best understood as a collection of symptoms that often end up with a Western medical diagnosis such as pain, depression, anxiety, or high blood pressure. However, if you look at these patterns through the lens of chi and the Five Elements, you can begin to understand them in a different light. Instead of "pain," you can see where chi is stuck and learn how to get it moving. Instead of "chronic fatigue syndrome," you can see where chi is depleted and learn how to replenish it.

Learning about the most common patterns of imbalance will guide you to a direct understanding of how your chi is impacted by your diet, lifestyle, environment, genetics, and so on. Guiding principles that address the pattern of imbalance presenting in your life include recommendations for specific dietary, lifestyle, and environmental changes. While there is a total of sixty-two patterns of imbalance in Chinese medicine, there are only about twenty that I see frequently. If you find that you have multiple patterns of imbalance, or you can't differentiate your pattern of imbalance based on the information that follows, then I recommend working with a qualified practitioner before proceeding with treatment principles.

Understanding the Language of Chinese Medicine

The language used to describe patterns of imbalance can help us to understand how elements, organs, and systems can lose their natural balance. The common terms Chinese medicine practitioners use to describe the state of chi in a person, an organ, or a system are *yin*, *yang*, *deficiency*, *dampness*, and *stagnation*.

GENERAL CHI DEFICIENCY: When our chi is abundant, we feel abundance in body, mind, and spirit. We awake looking forward to the day; we feel aligned physically, mentally, and spiritually; and we have enough energy to do the things that are important to us. It's just like a river that is full and wide and flowing downstream. When we experience a loss of chi, the river goes down and the banks are exposed. We feel this deficiency on all levels and may develop symptoms that include fatigue, shortness of breath, spontaneous sweating, a swollen tongue with teeth marks on the sides, and a weak pulse. General chi deficiency does not happen overnight but is a condition that develops over a long period of time. Any organ can experience chi deficiency.

In addition to general chi deficiency, there are more specific types: yin chi deficiency, yang chi deficiency, and blood deficiency.

YIN CHI DEFICIENCY: Also a chronic pattern, yin chi deficiency usually presents after long-term exposure to high-output activities, stressors, and lifestyles, without the appropriate yin to keep us balanced. This is where we may find ourselves feeling "tired but wired." When yin is deficient, yang gets to take over. Thus, yin deficiency often produces yang symptoms such as dry skin and hair, night sweats, excessive thirst, dry mouth or throat, poor memory, weakness (especially in the lower back and knees), restlessness, sleep disturbances, irritability, anxiety, and muscle aches.

YANG CHI DEFICIENCY: As with all chi deficiency patterns, yang chi deficiency takes a long time to develop. Often, though not always, it is preceded by yin deficiency. Burning the candle at both ends is most often what leads us to developing these patterns. Instead of the tired-but-wired feeling we get with yin deficiency, yang deficiency leaves us feeling just plain tired. When yang is deficient, yin gets to take over. This leads to symptoms such as low energy and stamina, low libido, afternoon crashes in energy, cold hands and feet, a desire for warmth, feelings of all-over weakness, fears, phobias, and panic attacks.

BLOOD DEFICIENCY: Water that flows through a healthy river is teeming with life and abundant in minerals. Can you imagine water that is empty of life and minerals? That would be akin to the pattern we call blood deficiency in Chinese medicine. Not only can blood deficiency reflect a low level of blood (as in cases of anemia), but it can also reflect a deficiency in nutrients typically found in the blood. When we have plenty of nutrient-rich blood flowing through our veins, every organ is nourished, and the mind and spirit flourish also. We feel at home in ourselves and look vibrant, from rosy cheeks to shiny hair, moist skin, and healthy nails. When the blood is deficient, anxiety is one of the first symptoms we notice. Additionally we may experience heart palpitations; brittle and dry hair, nails, and skin; sleep disturbed by active dreams or nightmares or a lack of REM sleep; exhaustion; a pale complexion; and sadness.

DAMPNESS AND PHLEGM: While *dampness* may be unfamiliar in Western medical terminology, Chinese medicine refers to it as the root of many imbalances, such as high cholesterol, metabolic disorders, chronic fatigue syndrome, fibromyalgia, allergies, and even cancer. Dampness refers to a level of internal humidity that develops when the spleen does not function well. Dampness then accumulates in the digestive system and lungs. It can cause mucus, phlegm, a wet cough, diarrhea, and generally low energy. If left unaddressed for a long time, dampness can become what is referred to as *phlegm* in Chinese medicine. Phlegm is the progression of dampness into congealed fluid that can further disrupt the function of other organs and systems.

STAGNATION: Stagnation occurs in a river that is low or has areas of debris where the flow is blocked. Patterns that fall under this category are indicative of chi or blood that is no longer flowing as well as it could be and is therefore stagnating in either the meridians or the organs. Most often this results in pain, emotional instability, feeling stuck, frustration, and/or depression. For women who have menstrual cycles, this can show up as the classic symptoms of PMS. The organ most susceptible to stagnation is the liver, which is responsible for the smooth flow of all chi in the body.

Tongue Diagnosis

Much information can be gleaned from looking at your tongue: from the quality of your blood to the strength of your liver to the challenges of your digestive system. It is one of the key tools in understanding all of these patterns. Tongue diagnosis is often the differentiating factor between two similar patterns.

Practitioners diagnose your patterns of imbalance by not only hearing what symptoms brought you in, but also by looking at your body, skin, hair, and nails, listening to the sound of your voice, listening to your pulses, palpating your organs and meridians, and looking at your tongue. Since you aren't able to listen to your own pulses (it would take many years of practice before you could), the best way to self-diagnose patterns of imbalance is to make a list of the symptoms you are experiencing, categorize them based on the most common patterns presented in the following pages, and having a look at your tongue to match it to the pattern. The tongue diagnosis diagram is reflective of the most common patterns practitioners see. All of the information you gain from your symptoms and your tongue will *mostly* fit a single pattern but sometimes more than one.

The best way to begin diagnosing your tongue is to start having a regular look at it in the mirror. It's best to do this in the morning before you have eaten and brushed your teeth or tongue. Notice your tongue's general appearance, its shape and colors, and any coating it may have. Notice if there are cracks in the surface and, if so, where they are located. If you look at the underside of your tongue, there are two blood vessels, which should be full, blueish, and about an inch in length. Once you have gotten an idea of the general state of your tongue, check it once every week or two as you begin to apply changes to your diet and lifestyle and most certainly if/when you begin working with a Chinese medicine practitioner (changes to your tongue don't happen rapidly).

Tongue diagnosis often includes descriptions such as light red, pink, pale, red, purplish, wet, dry, swollen, thin, teeth marks, red tip, white coating, yellow coating, cracked, or peeling. Each of these descriptions gives you information that guides you toward a pattern of imbalance diagnosis. A chart of the most common tongue patterns is provided for your reference.

Tongue Diagnosis: Which Tongue Are You?

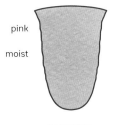

pink

moist

NORMAL

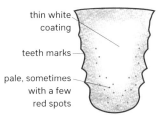

thin white coating

teeth marks

pale, sometimes with a few red spots

CHI DEFICIENCY
Fatigue, poor appetite, spontaneous sweating, shortness of breath, overthinking, worrying

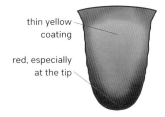

thin yellow coating

red, especially at the tip

HEAT
Feel hot, sweat easily, thirsty, constipated, irritability, red skin irritation/rashes

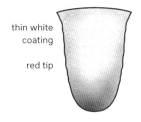

thin white coating

red tip

CHI STAGNATION
Stressed, tendency to be depressed and upset, unstable emotional state, PMS, lots of sighing

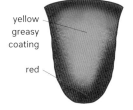

yellow greasy coating

red

DAMP HEAT
Skin problems (red and weepy), urinary infections, clammy skin, irritability, joint aches

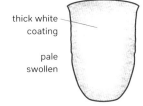

thick white coating

pale swollen

YANG DEFICIENCY
Feel cold easily, pale complexion, back pain, tendency to panic, emotionally low, impotence, infertility, deep exhaustion

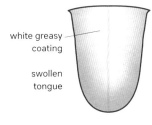

white greasy coating

swollen tongue

DAMPNESS
Bloated, fullness in chest and abdomen, feel heavy and lethargic, difficulty waking

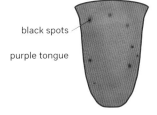

black spots

purple tongue

BLOOD STAGNATION/STASIS
Cold limbs, varicose veins, painful legs, headaches, chest pain, liver spots, lack of skin luster, gynecological pain

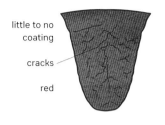

little to no coating

cracks

red

YIN DEFICIENCY
Hot flashes, sweating at night, insomnia, irritability, ringing in the ears, "tired but wired"

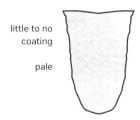

little to no coating

pale

BLOOD DEFICIENCY
Dizziness, fatigue, heart palpitations, poor concentration and memory, insomnia, PMS

The tongue is considered to be a map of the body's major organs, from its base relating to the kidneys to its tip relating to the lungs and heart. Therefore, in addition to the descriptions of your tongue, a practitioner is also interested to see if there are changes to the tongue's appearance in specific places. Notice that when the tongue map provided is flipped upside down, it follows the way the organs are situated in your body.

Tongue Map

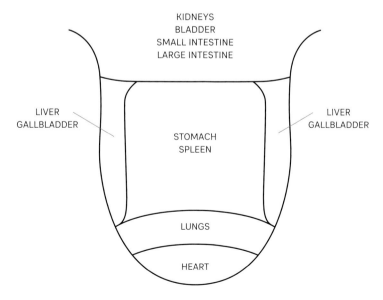

KIDNEYS
BLADDER
SMALL INTESTINE
LARGE INTESTINE

LIVER
GALLBLADDER

LIVER
GALLBLADDER

STOMACH
SPLEEN

LUNGS

HEART

Together, symptoms, tongue diagnosis, and a pulse picture (obtained from a practitioner) will guide you to the pattern of imbalance you are likely experiencing. The most common patterns of imbalance I see in my practice are listed in the tables by element.

Water Element Patterns		
ORGANS	Kidney (Yin Organ)	
PATTERNS	Yang Deficiency	Yin Deficiency
SYMPTOMS	Chills and aversion to cold; cold limbs; feelings of fear; bright pale complexion; asthma; apathy; lethargy; cold and sore lumbar region; cold and weak knees; loose stools, especially early morning ("cock's crow diarrhea"); copious, clear urine; frequent urination; incontinence; edema; memory issues; ear and/or hearing challenges; spermatorrhea	Tired but wired, five palm heat (hands, feet, and face all hot), malar flush or red cheeks, night sweats, afternoon fever, constipation, dark urine, thirst, soreness in knees and lumbar region, low-pitched tinnitus, poor memory, dizziness, feelings of fear, sexual dysfunction (premature ejaculation and/or nocturnal emission), tendency toward addiction, chronic urinary tract infections (UTIs), ear and/or hearing challenges
TONGUE	Pale, flabby, with thin white coating	Red with little or no coating, likely cracked
HOW WE GOT HERE	Burned the candle at both ends. Began depleting kidney chi (milder experience of symptoms) and then kept going until cold signs began to appear. Kidney chi deficiency led to kidney yang deficiency.	Burned the candle at both ends. Overwork, overstimulation, stress, and even too much sex can lead to kidney yin deficiency. Often too much yang activity and not enough yin activity. Without the rest and restoration to balance yang, the body begins to burn up fluids and signs of heat increase.
WESTERN MEDICAL DIAGNOSES	Low sex drive, infertility, adrenal fatigue, chronic fatigue syndrome, hypothyroidism, polycystic ovary symptom (PCOS), menopausal symptoms, obsessive-compulsive disorder (OCD), tendency toward addiction, autoimmune conditions	PMS, low libido, attention-deficit disorder (ADD) or attention-deficit/hyperactivity (ADHD), autoimmune conditions, adrenal fatigue, chronic fatigue syndrome, insomnia, hyperthyroidism, menopausal symptoms, fibroids, infertility
NUTRITIONAL PRINCIPLES	Bitter Pungent Warming Tonifying Slightly astringent *Avoid salty and cooling*	Salty Neutral Slightly cooling Calming Moistening *Avoid warming and astringent*

Wood Element Patterns		
ORGANS	Liver (Yin Organ)	
PATTERNS	Liver Chi Stagnation	Liver Fire Blazing
SYMPTOMS	Emotionally backed up; irritability; constant sighing; moodiness; tendency toward addiction; constipation, diarrhea, or switching between the two; irritable bowel syndrome (IBS); allergies; pain; headaches/migraines (especially on the sides of the head and around the eyes); distention and pain in the chest and hypochondriacal region	Irritability; red face and eyes; angry outbursts; high-pitched tinnitus; dizziness; temporal headaches/migraines (especially on the sides of the head and around the eyes); thirst; bitter taste in the mouth; constipation; dream-disturbed sleep; dark, yellow urine
TONGUE	Can be normal	Red body, redder sides, with a dry yellow coating
HOW WE GOT HERE	Liver chi stagnation is due to holding on to the past, not forgiving, not expressing real feelings, and not moving on. These emotional symptoms begin to affect the physical body as the two cannot be separated. With liver chi stagnation, patients often complain and/or are negative much of the time because whatever happened to them in the past has been left unaddressed and now colors their world. Instead of expressing how angry/scared/sad they are about something, they complain (and sigh) a little each day to slowly release the pressure they have built up inside. Stress will exacerbate this pattern.	As a consequence of unresolved liver chi stagnation, significant heat signs and the pattern of liver fire blazing can develop. This pattern is unmistakable in its presentation of heat as it is a *truly* excessive pattern, and the heat signs are everywhere. There tends to be a lot of irritability and impulsiveness with this pattern.
WESTERN MEDICAL DIAGNOSES	PMS, post-traumatic stress disorder (PTSD), depression, IBS, allergies, fibromyalgia, chronic fatigue syndrome, insomnia, low libido, infertility, PCOS, endometriosis, eating disorders, bipolar disorder	Irritability, bipolar disorder, acute trauma, PTSD, cold sores/herpes, constipation, insomnia
NUTRITIONAL PRINCIPLES	Sour Neutral Pungent Sweet *Avoid warming*	Cooling Bitter Moistening Calming *Avoid warming and astringent*

→

Wood Element Patterns (continued)	
ORGANS	**Liver (Yin Organ)**
PATTERNS	**Liver Blood Deficiency**
SYMPTOMS	Blurry vision, floaters in the eyes, pale complexion, dizziness, pale lips, tight tendons, weak muscles, muscle spasms and cramps, brittle nails
TONGUE	Pale, especially on the sides
HOW WE GOT HERE	Deficiency of protein in the diet and/or poor overall diet, sluggish or weak digestive system, blood loss due to hemorrhage, and long-standing kidney chi deficiency can all cause blood deficiency in the liver.
WESTERN MEDICAL DIAGNOSES	PMS, amenorrhea, anemia, dysmenorrhea
NUTRITIONAL PRINCIPLES	Blood-building Warming Tonifying Salty

Fire Element Patterns

ORGANS	Heart (Yin Organ)		
PATTERNS	**Heart Chi Deficiency**	**Heart Blood Deficiency**	**Heart Yin Deficiency**
SYMPTOMS	Heart palpitations, fatigue, shortness of breath, spontaneous sweating, pale complexion, feelings of cold, a desire for warmth	Heart palpitations (more pronounced in the evening); poor memory; dream-disturbed sleep; feelings of being easily startled; dull, pale complexion; pale lips; dizziness	Heart palpitations, mental restlessness, feelings of being easily startled, poor memory, fever, hot flashes (more pronounced in the evening), night sweats, and five palm heat, dry mouth and throat
TONGUE	Normal to slightly pale	Pale and slightly dry	Red with no coating, possible red tip or red spots
HOW WE GOT HERE	Often occurs after a period of chronic sadness or excessive negative emotions. Since the heart is the home of shen (spirit), emotions can significantly disrupt the heart's function. If left unaddressed, this can turn into heart yang deficiency (more extreme coldness, more sweating, cold limbs).	Too much mental activity, overthinking, and worry combined with an insufficient diet turns the pattern of spleen chi deficiency to heart blood deficiency. Chronic worry and anxiety disturbs shen, which depresses the heart's function and leads to a deficiency in the blood that moves through it. Severe hemorrhaging (such as in childbirth) can also cause heart blood deficiency.	Chronic anxiety, worry, and a busy lifestyle can damage the yin, dry up the body's fluids, and eventually cause yin deficiency.
WESTERN MEDICAL DIAGNOSES	Anxiety, blood pressure issues (mostly high, but sometimes low), tendency toward addiction, depression	Anxiety; depression, PTSD; blood pressure issues (mostly high but sometimes low); insomnia	Anxiety, high blood pressure, tendency toward addiction, insomnia
NUTRITIONAL PRINCIPLES	Warming Pungent Calming *Avoid cooling and salty*	Blood-building Calming Sweet	Bitter Neutral Moistening Calming *Avoid salty and warming*

◆

Fire Element Patterns (continued)		
ORGANS	**Heart (Yin Organ)**	
PATTERNS	**Heart Fire Blazing**	**Heart Phlegm Fire**
SYMPTOMS	Heart palpitations, mouth and tongue ulcers, mental restlessness, agitation, impulsiveness, dream-disturbed sleep, bitter taste in the mouth, thirst, fever	Severe mental health imbalance, heart palpitations, restlessness, thirst, feelings of oppression in the chest, dream-disturbed sleep, agitation, confusion, red face
TONGUE	Red with a very red tip, possibly swollen with red spots, possible yellow coating and midline crack	Red with redder tip, swollen tip, thick yellow coating, often with a deep heart crack
HOW WE GOT HERE	Trauma, chronic anxiety, constant worry, being in a state of fight-or-flight for a long time, and chronic depression can all lead to heart fire. The emotional aspect to this pattern leads to chi stagnation, and chronic stagnation leads to fire. Liver fire can often turn into or include heart fire signs. Therefore, any of the causes of liver fire (anger, resentment, or frustration) can also cause heart fire.	Trauma, especially emotional trauma (excessive and chronic worry, fear, shame, or guilt) along with a diet with excessive amounts of phlegm-inducing foods (dairy, sugar, greasy foods, alcohol) and/or overeating in general are usually responsible.
WESTERN MEDICAL DIAGNOSES	Anxiety, bipolar disorder, tendency toward addiction, high blood pressure, insomnia, cold sores	Anxiety, bipolar disorder, high blood pressure, insomnia
NUTRITIONAL PRINCIPLES	Cooling Bitter Calming Moistening *Avoid salty, sour, and warming*	Cooling Bitter Astringent Calming *Avoid moistening*

$\rightarrow$

Fire Element Patterns (continued)		
ORGANS	Heart (Yin Organ)	
PATTERNS	Blood Deficiency	Blood Stagnation/Stasis
SYMPTOMS	Dizziness, anemia, restless leg syndrome, problems with focus and concentration, musculoskeletal pain	Body aches (general or local), fixed pain, chest pain. **For women's health imbalances:** fixed pain in the lower abdomen relieved by warmth; dark, clotted menstrual discharge; aversion to cold; late or absent period; back pain; diarrhea; vomiting; nausea; loss of appetite
TONGUE	Pale, otherwise normal (The blood vessels on the underside of the tongue may appear empty or be difficult to see.)	Purplish, dark or purple spots, possible swelling or distension of the blood vessels on the underside of the tongue
HOW WE GOT HERE	Since blood is formed out of food, an insufficient diet and chronic stress can often lead to blood deficiency. Most at risk are vegetarians or vegans, those on a restrictive or low-fat diet, and nursing mothers. Spleen chi deficiency can lead to blood deficiency via worry, overthinking, and anxiety. Liver chi stagnation can also lead to blood deficiency, especially when emotions go unexpressed.	Blood stagnation is a thickening or clotting of the blood in the body. A general achy feeling can arise from the area of stagnation, often from chronic inflammation of the body, usually from poor diet, stress, or an unhealthy lifestyle (like excessive alcohol or drugs). If left unaddressed, this can become blood stasis, which has fixed, stabbing pain.
WESTERN MEDICAL DIAGNOSES	Insomnia, depression, anxiety, skin conditions (especially dryness), headaches/migraines, chronic fatigue syndrome, infertility, chronic pain, arthritis, women's health imbalances (such as fibroids, PMS, midcycle spotting, amenorrhea, PCOS, and cycles longer than 35 days)	Pain, arthritis, fibromyalgia, endometriosis, PCOS, fibroids, acute trauma, mania, cancer, congestive heart failure
NUTRITIONAL PRINCIPLES	Blood-building Tonifying Salty Sweet *Avoid sour and pungent*	Cooling Sour Bitter *Avoid warming and astringent*

◆

Earth Element Patterns		
ORGANS	Spleen (Yin Organ)	
PATTERNS	Spleen Chi Deficiency	Spleen Yang Deficiency
SYMPTOMS	Little or no appetite, abdominal distention after eating, weakness and heaviness in limbs, sallow complexion, loose stools, nausea, stuffiness in chest and epigastrium	Lack of appetite, abdominal distention after eating, bright white or sallow complexion, weakness in the four limbs, loose stools (often with undigested food), aversion to and feelings of cold, edema
TONGUE	Normal or pale with swollen sides; teeth marks; and a thin, white, sticky, greasy coating	Pale, swollen and wet with significant teeth marks, sometimes with a white coating
HOW WE GOT HERE	Excessive cold and raw foods, irregular and excessive eating, or eating lots of carbs and not a lot of protein combined with excessive mental activity and worry, overwork, and eating on-the-go (or while stressed) all deplete spleen chi. This is common in students and very active businesspeople. If left untreated, this deficiency can create dampness that leads to lumps, cysts, nodules, and in some cases, cancer.	When spleen chi deficiency is unaddressed, spleen yang energy is compromised, leading to an excess of yin symptoms (hence the edema, coldness, and so on).
WESTERN MEDICAL DIAGNOSES	Anxiety, ADD/ADHD, IBS, leaky gut syndrome, gas and bloating, diarrhea, asthma, fatigue, chronic fatigue syndrome, fibroids, infertility, PCOS, OCD, yeast/Candida infections, cancer	Anxiety, eating disorders, leaky gut syndrome, diarrhea, yeast/Candida infections, fatigue
NUTRITIONAL PRINCIPLES	Sweet Neutral Warming Slightly astringent *Avoid moistening and cooling*	Warming Bitter Pungent Slightly astringent *Avoid cooling and salty*

→

Earth Element Patterns (continued)		
ORGANS	Stomach (Yang Organ)	
PATTERNS	**Stomach Yin Deficiency**	**Rebellious Stomach Chi**
SYMPTOMS	Stomachaches; little or no appetite; fullness after eating; slight fever or feelings of warmth, especially in the evening; dry mouth	Nausea, belching, hiccupping, lack of appetite, stomachaches, spontaneous sweating
TONGUE	Red, peeling in the center	Possibly normal (This condition is often an acute experience or the progression of another pattern and may not affect the tongue.)
HOW WE GOT HERE	Eating at irregular times, especially late at night before bed, or eating too quickly or while worrying can deplete stomach chi, over time burning up the stomach fluids and creating a yin deficiency.	Often this pattern develops due to overwork, stress, pregnancy, eating foods that are difficult to digest, a digestive system lacking in good bacteria (not enough probiotics), or as a response to stomach yin deficiency that has turned into stomach fire. A diet with foods that irritate you (but are not necessarily allergic to) also creates heat that burns up fluids. If left unaddressed, this deficiency can turn into stomach fire and blood stagnation in the stomach.
WESTERN MEDICAL DIAGNOSES	Anxiety, constipation, heartburn, stomach ulcers	Nausea/vomiting, heartburn, anxiety
NUTRITIONAL PRINCIPLES	Slightly cooling Moistening Neutral Sweet *Avoid sour and warming*	Sweet Neutral Salty Calming *Avoid pungent and sour*

Metal Element Patterns		
ORGANS	Lung (Yin Organ)	
PATTERNS	Lung Qi Deficiency	Lung Yin Deficiency
SYMPTOMS	Grief; shortness of breath upon exertion; weak cough; thin, watery sputum; weak voice; lack of desire for speaking; spontaneous sweating; aversion to cold; bright white complexion; smoking addiction	Dry cough or cough with sticky sputum, dry mouth and throat, grief, hoarse voice, low-grade fever or heat sensation in the evening, malar flush, night sweats, five palm heat
TONGUE	Pale or normal	Red, peeling with cracks in the lung area (late stage)
HOW WE GOT HERE	Unresolved grief, especially carried down through the family, can lead to lung chi deficiency. Children who grew up in a smoking household often wind up with this pattern. Chronic use of antibiotics, especially at a young age, depletes the lung chi and wei qi.	If left unaddressed, lung chi deficiency and stomach yin deficiency can develop into lung yin deficiency. Additionally, due to the relationship between the lungs and kidneys in Chinese medicine, chronic overwork and adrenal fatigue (kidney yin deficiency) can lead to this pattern.
WESTERN MEDICAL DIAGNOSES	Allergies, asthma, skin conditions, chronic or recurrent colds and flu	Allergies, asthma, skin conditions, chronic or recurrent colds and flu, chronic fatigue syndrome, insomnia, tendency toward addiction (especially to smoking)
NUTRITIONAL PRINCIPLES	Pungent Tonifying Moistening Warming *Avoid cooling*	Slightly cooling Moistening Sweet Neutral *Avoid warming and astringent*

$\rightarrow$

Metal Element Patterns (continued)		
ORGANS	Large Intestine (Yang Organ)	
PATTERNS	Damp Heat in the Large Intestine	Heat and Dryness in the Large Intestine
SYMPTOMS	Stomachaches; intestinal cramps; urgent diarrhea; mucus and/or blood in the stool; foul-smelling stools; burning anal sensation (especially after a bowel movement); scanty and dark urine; long-standing grief; fever; spontaneous sweating; thirst (not necessarily a desire to drink); heavy sensation in the body and limbs	Long-standing grief, constipation, dry stools, emotional "backup," slight fever, scanty and dark urine
TONGUE	Red body, sticky yellow coating	Thick yellow coating (possibly dark)
HOW WE GOT HERE	Consuming too many hot and greasy foods or foods with bacteria the body doesn't know how to handle can lead to this pattern. Unprocessed grief, relentless worry, and anxiety can also lead to damp heat in the large intestine. When there is an emotional component (almost always), there may be liver chi stagnation as well.	Unprocessed grief and other emotions can lead to this pattern. Children and adults who had difficult childhoods often wind up with constipation due to heat and/or dryness in the bowels. Constant stress burns up the fluids in the body, and the inability to express feelings constricts the bowels. This can also happen from overconsumption of hot and astringent foods.
WESTERN MEDICAL DIAGNOSES	Diarrhea, IBS	Constipation
NUTRITIONAL PRINCIPLES	Sour Astringent Cooling *Avoid moistening and sweet*	Moistening Slightly cooling Pungent Sweet Salty *Avoid astringent and warming*

As you can see, there are many overlapping patterns. For instance, allergies are listed under multiple patterns. This is why Chinese medicine is so unique: no two people are ever treated exactly the same, even if they have the same Western medical diagnosis. Someone with allergy symptoms could likely be diagnosed with either lung chi deficiency or liver chi stagnation as the pattern behind the symptoms, and the treatment strategies will be entirely different. Even two people who both present with lung chi deficiency will be treated differently. One person may have asthma, whereas the other may have a cough and eczema. These two people will be treated and given dietary feedback and practices that are radically different from one another.

SEASONAL RECIPES, HERBS, AND PRACTICES

NOW THAT YOU ARE FAMILIAR WITH YOUR CONSTITUTION and potential patterns of imbalance you may be experiencing, Part Two will introduce you to how to use this information to support your return to health for the rest of your life. From nutrient-dense recipes to herbal medicine to nourishing practices, you will gain access to all of the healing secrets I impart to all my clients. As you read through Part Two, keep your constitution in mind, as that and the current season will be the areas of your focus. For instance, if you have a Fire constitution but are currently in winter rather than summer (the season associated with the Fire element), you will not want to drop all of the recommendations for Winter to support your constitution. In fact, I would recommend primarily focusing on the season in which you find yourself and adding the foods, herbs, and practices that best support your constitution on a limited basis. Do this until it's summer (or the time of year when your primary element has the most energy), and then you can really go for it without depleting yourself or getting out of sync with the seasons.

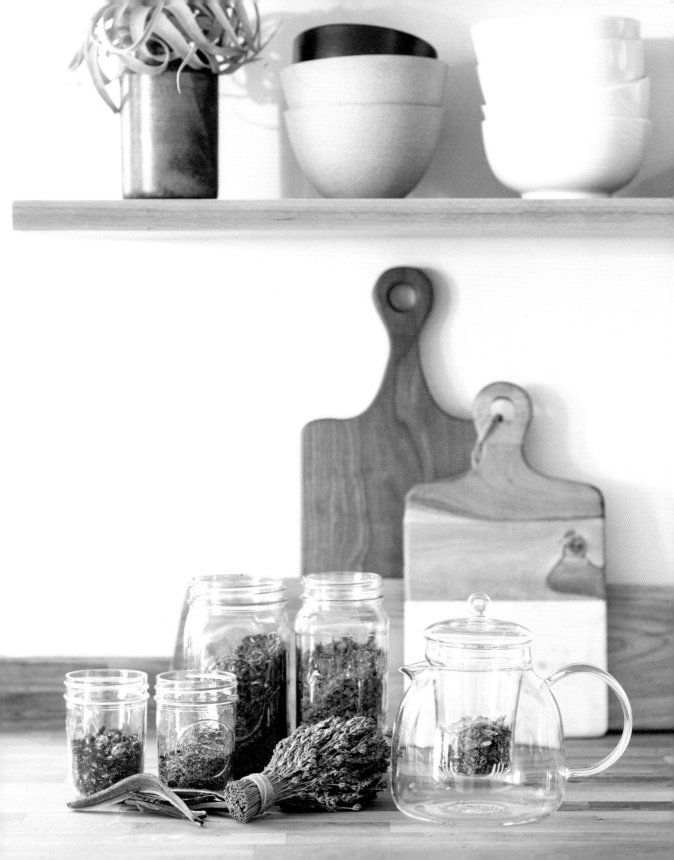

PANTRY GUIDELINES

Each season brings with it a new and magical array of foods to add to our diet for optimal nutrition. We want to eat foods that the earth provides each season in as close to their natural state as possible. This practice ensures that we get the most out of our diet. Foods that travel far to get to us and then sit on the shelves at a supermarket will lose their nutritional value in a short time (which is why many foods are stabilized with preservatives, and we don't want that).

In fact, before beginning working on your pantry, I recommend giving it a little cleanup and clear out. Check expiration dates on everything and throw out whatever has been sitting around for more than a few months. There is vitality in food, and age certainly depletes that vitality. So have that mind-set when you are going through your pantry and fridge *before* you bring in more of the food suggested in the following chapters. Ask yourself, "Does this food still have life force in it?" If it was processed to death, the answer is no. If it has been living on your shelf or in your fridge for more than three months, the answer is no (aside from grains). Eating healthfully means eating "fresh-fully"!

I will recommend guidelines for getting the most out of each season through your diet. Recipes unique to the season are key to waking up the different energies in the body at their most important times of year. How do you know what to eat during each season? Although this book will give you that information, a quick way to figure it out is to go to your local farmers market. Everything you see there are the things that are growing and ripening around you right now. This means their nutrient content is as dense as it will ever be; they didn't travel far to get to you, and they have not been preserved. In addition, eating according to what's in season lowers your carbon footprint and allows you to support local farmers and businesses—a win–win proposition.

The guidelines in the following chapters may ask for flexibility with this rule. Sometimes when you need to rebalance your system, you may have to forego a couple of fresh local foods that are ripe at the moment in order to reset and return to eating completely with the seasons at a later time.

We will discuss the organs that are most closely associated with each time of year and how best to care for them. If you have noticed some imbalances in your health and want to correct them through nutrition, there will be more specific suggestions on how to do this in each chapter focused on the organ and system that needs support.

Buying your produce and animal products from a local market can sometimes be outside your budget. There are a couple of ways around this. First, you can go to the farmers market just to see what is ripe and available at the moment. Then take that information with you to your supermarket and replicate it in your purchases there. Second, many farms need labor and are willing to give food in exchange for it, especially during the most prominent harvest weeks (late summer and early fall). I have spent many days volunteering at local farms in exchange for fresh produce and animal products. It also gives you the opportunity to build community as well as get your hands in the soil. Also, in most urban and suburban areas you can find a local discount grocery store where many local organic products wind up as they near their expiration date.

CRAVINGS

Understanding nutrition means learning about the foods we crave. Often (though not always) the foods you crave indicate an underlying deficiency in your diet. For instance, if a client tells me he is craving potato chips, I will undoubtedly assume he has either a fat and/or salt deficiency in his diet. If a woman tells me all she can think about is chocolate before the start of her cycle, I will wonder if she has a Water element imbalance such as a magnesium deficiency (the highest mineral content in a chocolate bar). Sugar cravings are often indicative of a dopamine deficiency, which is mostly dependent on the Earth element finding harmony.

Sugar and alcohol addiction are so alike biochemically that I often treat them similarly. One way to address sugar/alcohol cravings is to incorporate cinnamon into your diet as it tricks the brain into thinking it has just received sugar. Good Earth tea is one of my favorite herbal teas to prescribe for sugar cravings. Consume one to three cups each day with one or two tea bags in each cup of hot water, especially at times when you are tempted to go for sugar and/or alcohol. There's more on addiction on page 254.

KITCHEN STAPLES

Kitchen staples are items you will use every single day to prepare nutritious meals based on the principles of Chinese medicine. The following staple items reflect not only Chinese medicine but also our current challenges with regard to food and water sourcing, nutrient density, the use of organic versus inorganic foods, and so on. It is absolutely vital to know where your food and water come from and how they have been treated. With the prevalent use of pesticides and genetically modified foods, you need to be your own food advocate and fill your pantry with the highest quality ingredients you can find and afford.

Water

Water is vital. It is something we should be drinking all day long. It helps to keep us "in flow" and prevent the daily exposure to toxins from becoming concentrated inside the body. Water not only supports the bladder and kidneys, but it helps every single cell in the body to function at its best and detoxes the rest.

Depending on where you live, your tap water may not be the best option for you. In the West, we add a lot of chemicals to our tap water to "clean it up," we also take out the vital nutrients we need when we filter water to the extreme. If you live near oil and gas industry facilities or certainly any fracking sites, your water may be even more compromised.[1]

I cannot emphasize this enough: It's vital to have good water quality since it is so vital to your health. Do a little research to see if there are any companies tapping local springs and testing the spring regularly (and not treating it with unnecessary chemicals). Or for a solution that is more affordable, consider connecting a ten-stage filter to your tap and re-mineralizing your water with mineral drops. Throughout this book I will recommend water to nourish specific organs, unwind patterns of imbalance, and use in recipes. As much as possible, include your best option for water in each of these instances.

HOW MUCH WATER SHOULD YOU DRINK?

In general, you should be drinking half your body weight in ounces per day. For example, if you weigh 150 pounds, divide that in half and you have 75 pounds. Change this to ounces. Your minimum daily water intake should be 75 ounces (a little more than nine cups) per day.

COFFEE ADDICITION

Coffee, while many of us like it, should be used in moderation by someone who is healthy and not at all in cases of Wood imbalances. The reason it becomes addictive is because it seems to lighten mood. Partly that is because coffee is wildly bitter on the Chinese medicine flavor spectrum, and this turns up the Fire element in the body, making us feel happier and more energized. But sadly, once the effects wear off, we are left with even worse symptoms, most notably tiredness, irritation, and frustration. Try switching out coffee for roasted dandelion root, burdock root, chicory root, rose, or jasmine tea.

Oil

Oils comprise an exceedingly important staple item in your diet. Just like water, every cell in the body depends on fat to be able to function properly. The brain basically sits in a bath of fat! Fats get a bad rap because they have been tampered with so heavily and associated with deterioration of heart health. But good oils actually provide the heart with excellent lubrication and are naturally anti-inflammatory. Fun fact: Bottles of oil used to be delivered to homes long before milk delivery began. It was a staple item in every household and was used every day. These bottled oils were plant-based—mostly olive, flax, and sesame.

Today, we have turned this extremely life-giving and healthy product into quite a toxic food. Many oils from the supermarket have been tainted with heat, treated with chemicals, refined, bleached, deodorized, and laden with preservatives so they stay clear and last for years. But guess what? Oil was not meant to last for years.

Because oil is a natural product, it is fragile and does go rancid, especially quickly when it is exposed to heat and sunlight. That's why you should buy oils fresh and use them liberally and right away. When purchasing, look for oil in a dark glass bottle with some or all of the following words on the label: cold-pressed, organic, unrefined, and extra virgin. When cooking with the recipes in this book (and even when cooking in general), I recommend using oils of this quality.

My Favorite Oils	My Least Favorite Oils
Olive	Soybean
Avocado	Canola
Butter	Vegetable blend
Ghee	Corn
Tallow/lard	Hydrogenated/refined
Cocoa butter	Palm
Macadamia nut	Sunflower
Coconut	Safflower
Almond	Peanut
Walnut	Rice bran
Flax	Margarine
Sesame	Shortening

Sweetener

For the most part, I don't use sweeteners in my kitchen. Fruits are naturally sweet, and they have generally become enough for my taste. It's amazing what a banana can do to a dough or a date to a nut milk or sauce! There are times, however, when sweetener can become medicinal, like when you catch a cold and want something to lubricate your throat, or if you just spent the day outside in the hot sun and are feeling fatigued. Something sweet will give you a boost of energy and moisture. When selecting sweeteners, look for those that come straight from the earth and have very little processing such as a raw local honey, molasses, or maple syrup.

Meats and Animal Products

Let me stress again how important it is to always know where your animal products come from. In the Western world, industrial animal farming has led to not only inhumane practices but also to exposure to toxic chemicals like antibiotics and synthetic hormones. Additionally, animals that are mistreated will build up cortisol, a stress hormone, and store it in their tissues.[2] Then you consume the milk and milk products, as well as the meat of those animals and are undoubtedly exposed to their stress hormones. If you eat meat and animal products, it is important to get local, organic, pastured, grass-fed, and humanely slaughtered animals from farmers you trust. Some of my favorite nutrient-dense proteins are grass-fed beef, buffalo, lamb, and turkey, as well as wild, sustainably caught salmon.

THE CHOLESTEROL MYTH

Animal products, especially red meat and butter, get a bad rap for being high in saturated fat and thereby causing high cholesterol. High cholesterol is often blamed as the root source of heart disease and heart attacks in the West. I can't tell you how many of my clients are on statins (the number-one drug prescribed to treat high cholesterol) and told to go on a low-fat diet to lower their risk of heart problems. Cholesterol is not all bad. In fact, having low cholesterol can be dangerous: Nearly every cell in your body is dependent on cholesterol to function.

Having high cholesterol also does not equate to having eaten too many animal products.[3] Rather, this diagnosis more closely reflects the function of the liver than that of the heart. The liver's job is both to produce about three-quarters of the body's cholesterol and to eliminate excess cholesterol. Therefore, when patients come to me with high cholesterol, it tells me first and foremost that their liver could use detoxification. I often recommend a liver-supporting diet (see page 147); exercise; a diet with fewer saturated fats; and liver-cleansing herbs and supplements such as bupleurum, milk thistle, garlic, and vitamin B_3 (niacinamide).

Vegetables and Fruits

I always recommend organic produce, grown as locally as possible in order to limit toxins like pesticides and the currently unknown safety risks of genetically engineered foods,[4] as well as to avoid a heavy carbon footprint. When you are eating local and organic, wash your produce gently versus scrubbing it extremely clean. The produce carries what are called soil-based organisms (SBOs) that are nature's probiotics. Probiotics nourish the body's overall health by providing good bacteria that support the optimal functioning of our digestive and immune systems. If you could just eat a spoonful of truly alive dirt each day, you would get the same health-promoting effect, but something tells me you won't follow that advice!

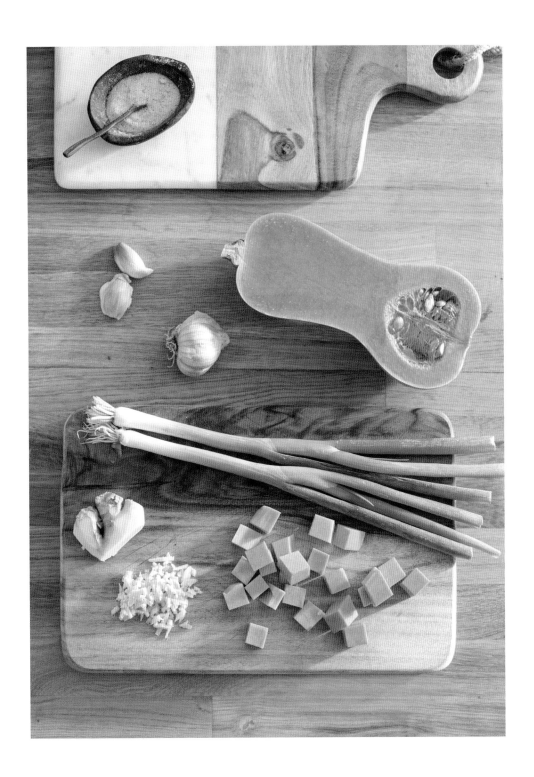

Grains

Why are *grains* getting a bad rap? All the most popular diets these days are eliminating grains, although grains are a part of traditional diets all around the world and have been for years. Many people find that if they eat grains, they feel sluggish, as though the food just sits in the stomach. Some report brain fog, gas and bloating, headaches, mood changes, and other unpleasant symptoms after eating grains.

In modern society, most people are struggling with spleen chi deficiency. And since the spleen (together with the stomach) is responsible for breaking down food with the appropriate enzymes, breaking down the more complex structure of grains has become harder and harder. If you are someone who struggles with eating grains, try cutting them out temporarily while you support the function of your spleen and stomach. When you reintroduce them into your diet, be sure to cook them properly and perhaps take additional digestive enzymes at first to help your body get used to breaking them down again. If you have an increase in unpleasant symptoms after eating grains, it's possible you have developed a food allergy or intolerance to them. (More on food allergies/intolerances on page 282.)

Another aspect to consider in relation to grains is your ancestry. If you know where you came from, you can make some guesses as to which foods you will likely have an easier time digesting. For example, if you have Mexican ancestry, you are more likely to digest corn well; if you have Asian ancestry, you are more likely to digest rice well.

If you do enjoy grains and find that you derive energy from them, know and trust their sourcing, and can digest them well, here are a few of my favorite grains that are also the most nutritious (the gut's probiotics love them): whole rye, quinoa, oats, barley, millet, brown rice, buckwheat, and spelt.

Legumes

Legumes provide certain B vitamins as well as many minerals to your diet. They are rich in fiber and tend to have a lower glycemic index than grains. Similar to grains, however, some people have no trouble digesting them, and others get a lot of gas, bloating, and discomfort from eating them. If you can make sure that your legumes are organic, are soaked and cooked properly, and are not causing you any trouble, then enjoy them. However, if you have taken all the steps to ensure proper preparation and they still cause you digestive distress, then you may have an allergy/intolerance

Soaking and Sprouting		
Seeds/Nuts/Grains/Legumes	How Long to Soak	How Long to Sprout
Seeds		
Pumpkin seeds	8 hours	1–2 days (24–48 hours)
Sesame seeds	8 hours	1–2 days (24–48 hours)
Sunflower seeds	8 hours	2–3 days (48–72 hours)
Nuts		
Almonds	2–12 hours	2–3 days (48–72 hours)
Brazil nuts	3 hours	Do not sprout
Cashews	2–3 hours	Do not sprout
Hazelnuts	8 hours	Do not sprout
Macadamias	2 hours	Do not sprout
Pistachios	8 hours	Do not sprout
Walnuts	4 hours	Do not sprout
Grains		
Amaranth	8 hours	1–3 days (24–72 hours)
Buckwheat	30 minutes–6 hours	2–3 days (48–72 hours)
Millet	8 hours	2–3 days (48–72 hours)
Oat groats	6 hours	2–3 days (48–72 hours)
Quinoa	4 hours	1–3 days (24–72 hours)
Beans and Legumes		
Adzuki beans	8 hours	2–3 days (48–72 hours)
Black beans	8–12 hours	3 days (72 hours)
Chickpeas	8–12 hours	2–3 days (48 –72 hours)
Kidney beans	8–12 hours	5–7 days (120–168 hours)
Lentils	8 hours	2–3 days (48–72 hours)
Mung beans	24 hours	2– 5 days (48–120 hours)
Navy beans	9–12 hours	2–3 days (48–72 hours)
Peas	9–12 hours	2–3 days (48–72 hours)

or a deficiency in the enzymes needed to break them down. (Check out the Soaking and Sprouting guide.) Some of my favorite legumes are chickpeas, black beans, kidney beans, lentils, mung beans, adzuki beans, and fava beans.

Nuts and Seeds

These foods can be an excellent source of fats and proteins, as well as many vital minerals. Human beings have been eating nuts and seeds for hundreds of thousands of years. Not only are they dense in nutrients, but they also provide a little roughage in the digestive system to help eliminate toxins. In general, make sure to eat them raw and soaked as much as possible before assessing if you can tolerate them or not. Because seeds and nuts are rich in fat, only purchase them from places where they have been refrigerated and keep them refrigerated at home as well. Some of my favorite and most nutrient-dense nuts and seeds are walnuts, sesame seeds, sunflower seeds, almonds, and pumpkin seeds.

ON BEING A VEGETARIAN

We live in tricky times when it comes to eating other animals and their products. To start, animals are not treated well in industrial farming settings. Then there is the environment, which is negatively affected by the meat industry. That being said, human beings have evolved largely as meat eaters.

The body takes animal protein, fat, and cartilage and immediately puts it to use (perhaps especially when we are recovering from mental or physical illness). The body also builds neurotransmitters that are vital to mental health and uses proteins and fats to heal wounds and fight sickness. The general rule of thumb is that if you are living a vegetarian/vegan lifestyle and having health problems, it is worth looking into your diet. Have your iron as well as your cholesterol checked (low cholesterol is more dangerous than high cholesterol).

If you want to stick with your lifestyle no matter what, then it's important to supplement your diet to meet the nutrient needs of your body. Consider eating a blood-building diet (see page 96), taking B$_{12}$, and a multimineral supplement.

CLEANSING

Many of us are well aware of the increase in toxic load these days, even if we ourselves haven't experienced some of the unpleasant symptoms of increased exposure. This awareness seems to have led to an increased desire to cleanse. The body does have built-in mechanisms for constant cleansing; the lungs, kidneys, large intestine, lymphatic system, skin, liver, and gallbladder are primary cleansers. Are they doing enough for your body given the global increase in toxins? The answer to this question is different for everyone. Ultimately, it depends on your individual experience of stress, diet, age, degree of health (or stage of disease), hormones, toxin exposure levels, pH balance, and circadian rhythm. Supporting your body's natural detoxification system is, after all, the best way to reduce your overall toxic burden. Here is how you can do that every day:

- Reduce your overall exposure to toxins by eating organic, whole foods.
- Drink half your body weight in ounces each day.
- Drink warm lemon water first thing in the morning.
- Exercise daily.
- Sweat often, especially through exercise, use of saunas and steam rooms, and hot baths.
- Take milk thistle seed extract (250 to 500 milligrams) each evening, thirty minutes before bed.
- Take magnesium citrate (150 to 800 milligrams, depending on bowel tolerance) each evening, thirty minutes before bed.
- Take a Nourishing Bath (recipe on page 107) each night, if only for 30 minutes.
- Perform a Detox Bath and Skin Brushing (see pages 85 and 242) one night each week.
- Choose one nourishing practice for the current season to do each day.
- Reduce your exposure to stress.
- Build up your personal resources (breathing techniques, meditation, visits to a therapist, making art or music, time in nature, community time, and so on) to manage unavoidable stress.

I am often asked, "How do I know when I need to do a cleanse?" The answer is two-fold. Sometimes I think we just *know*. We feel stuck or gummed up. Or we know we have been eating foods and drinking beverages that aren't good for us. Other times we start having subtle symptoms like a skin breakout, a sensitive stomach, or headaches. Women may notice changes in their cycles. Perhaps the cycle becomes more painful, or there are clots in the blood. When you start to see these kinds of things happening, consider doing a cleanse.

When we are cleansing, we have the opportunity to cleanse on all three levels—body, mind, and spirit. Often we are more familiar with the physical practices of cleansing from food. But mind and spirit cleansing can be integrated into this practice by taking a bit of extra time and space for ourselves and/or adding spiritual practices to our days. In addition to cleansing with food, think about what it would be like to cleanse from technology, to cleanse your environment, to cleanse your sleep, to cleanse your schedule, and to cleanse your social life. If you try this, you can make the most of your cleanses and be intentional and thorough when you consider carving out the time and space for them.

Another question I am asked is, "When is a good time to cleanse?" The truth is any time of year is a good time; however, each time of year has its own strengths and challenges. If you cleanse in the winter and eat the cold, raw foods of summer, you will undoubtedly find yourself feeling cold and depleted at the end of the season. However, it might seem easier to cleanse in the winter because schedules are often less demanding at this time. Perhaps instead, consider cleansing with bone broth and warm, cooked veggies. It is important to evaluate the time of year and the symptoms you are experiencing, because they will determine which organs need the most support and which foods are freshest and best to support them in the cleansing process. (For answers to cleansing questions and more, see Appendix E.)

This bath is excellent to incorporate into your weekly routine to stay ahead of any toxin build-up and to eliminate excess stress hormones from your system. For a more targeted cleanse, this bath can be taken 3 to 5 days in a row.

4 to 8 cups Epsom salt

1 cup baking soda

¼ cup Detox Tea (page 155): mix together only the dry ingredients (omitting cayenne) and tie into a cheesecloth bag

4 capsules digestive enzymes (break open and sprinkle into water)

10 drops total of one or two of the following essential oils: geranium, lemon, rosemary, ginger, or lavender

Add all the ingredients into hot bathwater as the tub is filling up. After soaking for 30 to 45 minutes, dry off and skin brush (see page 242) before finishing with a lukewarm shower. Plan to rest or go to bed soon afterward.

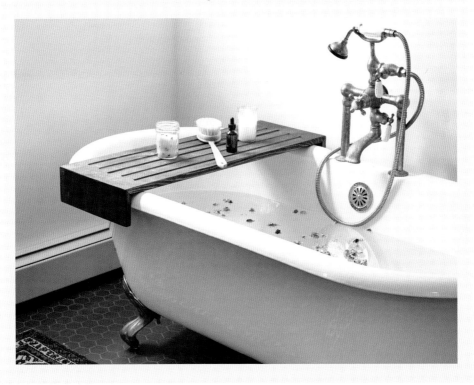

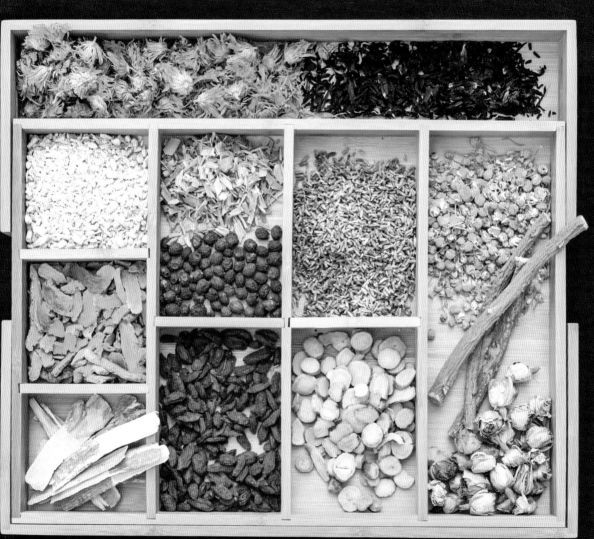

CHINESE HERBAL MEDICINE AND NUTRITIONAL PRINCIPLES

Herbs have always been an integral part of medicine around the world, and Chinese herbal medicine is one of the most ancient systems. (I always smile when I hear people call Chinese medicine "New Age.") The first documents on Chinese herbal medicine were written around 2800 B.C.E. by Shen Nong. Many of the formulas he wrote about are still used today, and his language on herbal energetic properties is now widely recognized. In addition to plants, Chinese medicine also includes the use of minerals, bones, and other natural substances.

One of the most important contributions Chinese medicine has made to both herbal medicine and nutrition has been the attribution of energetics (the five flavors, temperatures, and actions) to foods and herbs. This has given us a tremendous amount of understanding of how foods and herbs can be used medicinally and directly impact certain organs and systems. For instance, if you are experiencing symptoms that are both hot (inflamed) and dry, it's best to not only avoid hot and dry foods and herbs but also to incorporate more cooling and moistening herbs. We will use these descriptions of flavors and temperatures in the following pages as I introduce you to the world of Chinese herbal medicine. As with all Taoist principles, foods and herbs are never 100 percent one flavor, temperature, or action. Rather, they exist on a continuum and can be found in multiple categories. For instance, vinegar is both bitter and sour, and citrus peel is both bitter and sweet.

THE FIVE FLAVORS

The five flavor categories of herbs represent the way herbs taste when you put them in your mouth. When herbs taste a certain way, you know they will have a specific impact on the body and its energy. For instance, when something tastes spicy you can assume your body temperature will go up slightly, you will feel a rise in energy, and you may also produce mucus in response. The five flavors are important because we can use them to induce or reduce the anticipated responses.

The flavors pungent and sweet are considered to be more yang in nature (increasing energy), whereas bitter, salty, and sour tend to be more yin in nature (reducing energy). Foods and herbs that do not fit these five categories are usually labeled "bland."

THE HERB WITH ALL FIVE FLAVORS

One magical Chinese herb is known as the "five flavor herb" and is used to balance a significant number of ailments due to its versatile properties: schisandra. Schisandra berries make a wonderful digestive aid and can bring balance to the body, mind, and spirit during times of stress (see more about schisandra on page 239).

Bitter

Related to the Fire element and said to enter the heart and small intestine, bitter is perhaps one of the least favorite flavors in the West. Bitter presents as slightly sharp with a mostly cooling temperature and drying action (although some ancient texts refer to bitter as bringing warmth to the heart but coolness to the liver). Therefore, it is excellent when excessively moist or damp conditions such as yeast/Candida infections, mucus, swelling anywhere in the body, tumors, cysts, and edema are present.

The body's response is often to begin producing digestive fluids in response to bitter flavor. This is why Digestive Bitters, an ancient herbal remedy that has been used for thousands of years around the globe, is so helpful when drunk before meals. It stimulates digestion and can also induce peristalsis to treat sluggish digestion and/or constipation (recipe on page 181). Often, the bitter flavor is found in the protective coating of certain foods like citrus fruits and the outermost layer of cabbage. The following are some of the bitter foods you will find.

HERBS AND SPICES: Burdock root, chamomile, chicory, coptis, dandelion root, echinacea, elderflower, hops, marigold, nasturtium, pau d'arco, rose, schisandra, valerian, white pepper, yarrow

VEGETABLES: Alfalfa sprouts, artichoke, asparagus, carrot tops, celery and celeriac, dandelion greens, endive, escarole, lettuce, mustard greens, radish greens, rhubarb, scallions, turnip, watercress

FRUITS: Cacao, capers, citrus (lemon, grapefruit, orange), bitter melon, papaya

GRAINS AND LEGUMES: Amaranth, buckwheat, oats, quinoa, rye

PROTEINS: Liver, organ meats

OILS: Olive oil

CONDIMENTS AND MORE: Coffee, slightly charred foods (as from the grill), vinegar

Sweet

Related to the Earth element and said to enter the spleen and stomach organs, sweet is perhaps one of the favorite flavors in the West. Sweet presents as a soft, pleasant flavor that relaxes us, increases our endorphins (anti-stress and pain-relieving hormones), and builds our energy. As a more yang flavor, sweet foods and herbs strengthen us and treat any kind of deficiency; generally speaking, they bring warmth to our bodies. Speaking of sweet, we are referring here to *nature's* sweet taste and not the refined sugar taste we are all too familiar with.

Slightly sweet foods are easy to digest (with sugar actually starting a breakdown process). Complex carbohydrates, which serve as the center point for many traditional diets, are considered sweet flavored, as are dairy products from cows, goats, and other animals. Not only are sweet foods recommended during late summer, they can also be used during autumn and spring, as they moisten the lungs and calm an overactive mind, restless heart, and agitated liver.

HERBS AND SPICES: Ashwagandha, astragalus, licorice, schisandra, spearmint

VEGETABLES: Beets, cabbage, carrots, chard, cucumbers, eggplant, mushrooms (button and shiitake), peas, potato, string beans, squash, sweet potato, tomatoes (technically a fruit though often treated as vegetables in the kitchen), yams, zucchini

FRUITS: Apples, apricots, bananas, cherries, coconut, dates, figs, grapes, mango, melons, mulberries, papaya, peaches, pears, plums, strawberries

GRAINS AND LEGUMES: Barley, corn, millet, oats, rice, sweet rice

NUTS AND SEEDS: Almonds, chestnuts, coconut, pine nuts, sesame seeds, sunflower seeds, walnuts

PROTEINS: Beef, chicken, duck, eggs, goose, lamb, pork, tofu

OILS: Almond, flaxseed, olive, sesame

CONDIMENTS: Molasses, rice syrup

Pungent

Related to the Metal element and said to enter the lungs and large intestine, pungent represents those flavors that create heat when they hit the tongue. Due to this, pungent foods and herbs are also called acrid or spicy and are said to be very warming, to awaken the senses (ever eaten something too spicy and felt like your head was going to explode off your body?), and to disperse stagnation in the body by moving energy. They can also be considered diaphoretic as they can induce sweating, which is one of the many reasons they are known to have powerful immunity-boosting qualities.

Pungent foods naturally stimulate digestion and metabolism, clear congested sinuses, improve circulation, and relieve gas. They can help the body break down oily foods better by emulsifying the fat in them. This flavor is also known to stimulate a sluggish liver and increase blood circulation. Pungent foods and herbs should be used with caution in cases of severe deficiency and certainly in cases of heat and inflammation.

HERBS AND SPICES: Angelica, anise, basil, black pepper, caraway, cardamom, cayenne, chamomile, chilies, chives, chrysanthemum, cinnamon, cloves, coriander, cumin, dill, elderflowers, fennel seeds, garlic, ginger, horseradish, lavender, magnolia, marjoram, mugwort, mustard seed (whole and powdered), nutmeg, parsley, peppermint, rosemary, sage, schisandra, spearmint, tangerine peel, thyme, tulsi, turmeric

VEGETABLES: Cabbage, celery, fennel bulb, green onions, kohlrabi, leeks, mustard greens, onions, radishes (all, including daikon and radish leaves), scallions, sweet peppers, taro, turnips, watercress

FRUITS: Kumquats

CONDIMENTS AND MORE: Kimchi, wine (all kinds)

Salty

Related to the Water element, salt enters the kidneys and bladder. Salty is a familiar flavor in all world cuisines. It combines slightly bitter and slightly sour to create a savory taste. Salty herbs and foods do not taste like the table salt that comes from mines. Rather, the salty flavor in nature is much milder and indicative of a high mineral content in the foods and herbs in which it is found. Salty has the effect of moving fluids in the body via the kidneys and is said to bring heat from the exterior of the body deep into the interior. This function takes away some of the impact of cooler temperatures in autumn and winter and can therefore be used more during these seasons.

Common table salt is not as nutrient-dense as natural sea salt and is often overused. Too much salt and the body retains water, the kidneys and bladder tighten, and you are left thirsty but unable to expel water efficiently. The proper amount, however, keeps you hydrated, supports detoxification, and softens hard lumps and stiffness. Salt also provides a centering quality in the body, mind, and spirit, as well as strengthens mental clarity and concentration.

HERBS AND SPICES: Chickweed, nettles, oatstraw, schisandra, violets

VEGETABLES: Seaweeds (bladderwrack, dulse, kelp, kombu)

GRAINS AND LEGUMES: Barley, millet

PROTEINS: Clams, crab, cuttlefish, duck, oysters, pork, sea cucumbers, shrimp

FRUIT: Umeboshi

CONDIMENTS AND MORE: Capers (in brine), Celtic sea salt, gomasio, kimchi, miso, pickles, sauerkraut, soy sauce, tamari

Sour

Related to the Wood element, sour enters the liver and gallbladder, and it is not a popular flavor in the West except as a rare condiment (or prank). When we taste sour flavor, the body reacts immediately by closing pores and drying up all the fluids in the mouth (hence, the involuntary puckering). In fact, sour flavors are meant to make us retract as an evolutionary survival tactic so that we and other animals don't eat all the fruits and vegetables from plants before they have a chance to ripen.

Sour is often both cooling and astringent, relieving any heat in the body, moving stagnation, drying dampness, and stimulating digestion by promoting bile flow and the secretion of digestive enzymes. Eating foods or drinking tea with sour herbs can counteract the effects of a rich, greasy meal by acting as a solvent. Sour flavors usually come with high levels of antioxidants, such as those found in citrus fruits and berries. Antioxidants support the immune system, especially in times of transition like spring and autumn.

HERBS AND SPICES: Black tea, blackberry leaves, citrus peel, elderberry, green tea, hawthorn, lemon balm, milk thistle, red peony, rose, rose hips, royal jelly, schisandra

VEGETABLES: Leeks, tomatoes

FRUITS: Blackberries, crab apples, cranberries, grapefruit, grapes, green apples, huckleberries, lemons, limes, mangoes, oranges, papaya, pears, pineapples, plums, pomegranate, pomelo, strawberries, tangerines, umeboshi

GRAINS AND LEGUMES: Adzuki beans

DAIRY: Cheese, kefir, plain yogurt

CONDIMENTS AND MORE: All fermented dishes, olives, pickles, sauerkraut, sourdough bread, vinegar

FOOD AND HERB TEMPERATURES

The three temperature categories of foods and herbs refer not only to the way they taste, but more to the warming or cooling effect they have on the body. Heating herbs increase the body's temperature, and cooling herbs lower it. You can use these temperature profiles to restore balance when you have become too cold or too warm. The temperatures of foods and herbs are described as warming, neutral, and cooling. Neutral foods and herbs can be used anytime.

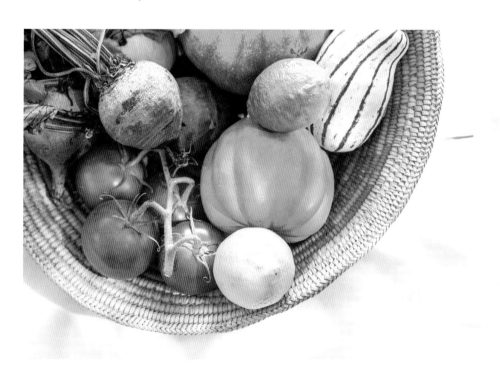

Warming Foods and Herbs

HERBS AND SPICES: Allspice, basil, black pepper, caraway, cardamom, cayenne, chilies, chives, cinnamon, cloves, coriander, cumin, fennel seeds, garlic, ginger (fresh is warm, dried is hot), horseradish, mustard seed, nutmeg, oregano, rosemary, saffron, star anise, tarragon

VEGETABLES: Fennel bulb, leeks, mustard greens, onions, peppers (whole green or red), pumpkin, radishes, scallions, shallots, spring onions, squash

FRUITS: Apricots, cherries, coconut meat, dates, peaches, raspberries

GRAINS AND LEGUMES: Black rice, sticky rice

NUTS AND SEEDS: Chestnuts, pine nuts, pistachios, walnuts

PROTEIN: Beef, chicken, eels, lamb, mussels, trout, venison

DAIRY: Butter, goat's milk

CONDIMENTS AND MORE: Brown sugar, coffee, wasabi

Neutral Foods and Herbs

HERBS AND SPICES: Licorice

VEGETABLES: Artichoke, beetroot, cabbage, carrots, cauliflower, peas, potatoes, shiitake mushrooms, string beans, sweet potato, turnips, yams

FRUITS: Apricots, crab apples, figs, pineapples, pomegranate

GRAINS AND LEGUMES: Adzuki beans, black beans, chickpeas, corn, fava beans, kidney beans, lentils, peanuts, red beans, rice, rye, soybeans

NUTS AND SEEDS: Almonds, flaxseed, hazelnuts, pistachios, pumpkin seeds, sesame seeds, sunflower seeds

PROTEINS: Carp, duck, eggs, goose, herring, liver (beef), oysters, pork, quail, salmon, sardines, scallops, shark, tuna, whitefish

OIL: Olive oil

DAIRY: Cheese, cow's milk

CONDIMENTS AND MORE: Coconut milk, olives

Cooling Foods and Herbs

HERBS AND SPICES: Cilantro, dill, green tea, hops, marjoram, parsley, peppermint, thyme, vanilla

VEGETABLES: Alfalfa sprouts, asparagus, bamboo shoots, bitter gourd, celery, chestnuts, cucumbers, daikon radishes, eggplant, green leafy vegetables (kale, spinach, Swiss chard), lotus root, mushrooms, seaweeds (bladderwrack, dulse, kelp, kombu), spinach, tomatoes, water lettuce

FRUITS: Apples, bananas, grapefruit, grapes, lemons, mango, melons (especially winter melon), oranges, papaya, pears, plums, pomelo, star fruit, strawberries, tamarind, tangerines, watermelons

GRAINS AND LEGUMES: Barley, buckwheat, millet, mung beans (especially sprouts), soybeans, wheat, wild rice

PROTEINS: Clams, crab, cuttlefish, egg whites, sea cucumber, shrimp, snails, tofu

OIL: Sesame oil

DAIRY: Yogurt

CONDIMENTS AND MORE: Capers, honey

FIVE FOOD AND HERB ACTIONS / PROPERTIES

The five properties of foods and herbs refer to the actions they have on the body in regard to energy levels and body fluids. Properties of foods and herbs can be used to support producing more fluids, drying up too many fluids, lubricating dry tissues, increasing or decreasing energy, and building healthy blood. We refer to these actions as moistening, astringent, tonifying, calming, and blood-building.

Moistening

These foods and herbs have a moistening effect on the body and can therefore be used to lubricate tissues and organs when they have become too dry. Herbs with this property are also called demulcent. Incorporating moistening foods increases the protective coating in the upper respiratory system, as well as the "third lung" (skin), making us less susceptible to dryness.

HERBS AND SPICES: Aloe vera, comfrey, licorice, marshmallow root, oatstraw, plantain, slippery elm, Solomon's seal, violets

VEGETABLES: Avocado, celery, cucumbers, seaweeds (bladderwrack, dulse, kelp, kombu), squash, sweet potato

FRUITS: Apples, pears

PROTEINS: Herring, oysters, salmon, trout, tuna

DAIRY: All kinds

CONDIMENTS: Oils

Astringent

These foods and herbs have a drying effect on the body as they draw out fluids, close pores, and shrink tissues. This supports the creation of a healthy barrier on the tissues and in the lungs when there is none or in cases of excessive fluid production. Some astringent foods and herbs also act as diuretics by increasing urination.

HERBS AND SPICES: Basil, bay leaf, black tea, blackberry leaves, caraway, cinnamon, coriander, dill, fennel seeds, green tea, marjoram, nutmeg, oregano, parsley, poppy seeds, rosemary, saffron, turmeric, vanilla

VEGETABLES: Avocado, broccoli, cauliflower, lettuce, peas, potatoes, sprouts

FRUITS: Apples, bananas (green), cranberries, lemons, pomegranate

GRAINS AND LEGUMES: Quinoa, rye, wheat

PROTEIN: Chicken

Tonifying

These foods and herbs are highly nutritive and can therefore serve to increase energy and promote general well-being. By tonifying and strengthening the body's organs and systems, they can be taken more frequently to combat exposure to daily stress and prevent depletion.

HERBS AND SPICES: Burdock root, cinnamon, codonopsis, dandelion root, hawthorn, licorice, marjoram, nettles, parsley, radix ginseng, royal jelly

VEGETABLES: Alfalfa sprouts, artichoke, asparagus, peas, potatoes, squash, sweet potato, yams, zucchini

FRUITS: Apples, apricots, avocado, bananas, cherries, dates, figs, grapes, lemons, limes, longan, mangoes, mulberries, pears, persimmons, pineapples, pomegranate, watermelons

GRAINS AND LEGUMES: Barley, millet, mung beans, oats, rice, sweet rice

PROTEINS: Beef, clams (freshwater), crabs, cuttlefish, duck, duck eggs, eggs, fish (most), goose, octopus, oysters, pork, rabbit, sardines, tofu

DAIRY: Cheese, cow's milk

CONDIMENTS: Honey, molasses

Calming

These foods and herbs help to ground energy, providing a spectrum of effects from mild relaxation to full-on sedation. They are best used in cases of high stress, anxiety, and insomnia as they can lower cortisol and adrenaline levels. They are also called nervines.

HERBS AND SPICES: Catnip, chamomile, chrysanthemum, lavender, lemon balm, poria, schisandra, valerian

VEGETABLES: Cucumbers, spinach, zucchini

FRUITS: Goji berries, longan, melons

GRAINS AND LEGUMES: Mung beans

SEEDS: Black sesame seeds, chia seeds

DAIRY: Small amounts of cow's or goat's milk

Blood-Building

These foods and herbs support the building of red blood cells and increase the nutrient density of the blood. Animal-based foods that are rich in hemoglobin (like red meat) are not the only supports for building blood. Plants that are rich in chlorophyll ("plant hemoglobin") also support blood building.

HERBS AND SPICES: Alfalfa leaf tea, angelica, bupleurum, burdock root, dandelion root and leaves, ginseng (notoginseng), nettles, parsley, yellow dock

VEGETABLES: Beets, carrots, dark leafy greens, pumpkin, seaweeds (bladderwrack, dulse, kelp, kombu), sweet potatoes

FRUITS: Apricots, berries, cherries, dates, grapes

GRAINS AND LEGUMES: Black beans, brown rice, kidney beans, oats, quinoa, red lentils

NUTS: Pistachios

PROTEINS: Beef, buffalo, eggs, elk, liver (beef)

CONDIMENTS AND MORE: Molasses, nutritional yeast

CHINESE HERBAL PREPARATIONS

When it comes to making medicine, herbalists use the following parts of plants and trees: leaves, flowers, stems, seeds, roots, fruit, rhizome (laterally growing root), and bark. The part that is used determines which preparation method is used to extract the medicine from the plant. In general, the lighter the plant material, the less intensive the extraction method. The heavier and more dense the plant material, the more intensive the extraction method.

Leaves and flowers: Light
Fruit, stems, and seeds: Medium
Rhizome, roots, and bark: Heavy

Parts Two and Three use terms like *infusion* and *decoction* to describe the best way to consume particular herbs. These terms reflect how the medicines were extracted from the herb and prepared for use. For oral preparations, there are many ways to extract the nutrients from plants as well as best ways to consume them. Some plants release their healing powers in a moment's time during extraction, and others need hours and hours of macerating and steeping to give up the goods. So I will recommend the extraction method best suited to the herb and the specific constituents we are trying to draw out. As you will see, you can implement some of these methods yourself, whereas you will likely need to seek out a trained herbalist and/or apothecary for others. Note that the following is not a complete list of herbal preparations, but rather the ones I use most frequently in my home and office.

Light extraction method: Hot infusion
Medium extraction method: Hot infusion or decoction
Heavy extraction method: Decoction

GRANULES: A MODERN-DAY METHOD FOR CHINESE HERBAL MEDICINE

The most popular modern way to prepare and consume Chinese herbs is in granular form. Here the herbs are first made into a decoction, then the water is evaporated, leaving behind an herbal powder. The powder is then used to make a hot tea, without a tea bag. Granulated herbs need to be prepared in an herbal pharmacy by someone skilled in this method. The reason granules are so attractive in our modern world is because you can prepare and consume them quickly, without intensive cooking methods. However, to get the maximum benefit of the herb, you do have to drink the sludge of herbs found in the bottom of your cup!

Measuring Herbs

Herbs are best measured by weight rather than volume as that allows for more specificity in dosage. For instance, the volume of leaves is quite large compared to the volume of roots. I recommend using a scale and weighing in grams. A table with specific dosage parameters in grams is featured in Appendix B. In general, herbs can be prepared like this:

Herbs measured by weight: 0.5 to 5 grams herb per 8-ounce cup of water

Daily dosage = 3 to 4 cups, depending on the herb and the condition being supported (see Appendix B for specific recommendations)

Decoction: Herbs and water are brought to a boil and then simmered for 30 minutes. This is the gold standard for consuming herbs in Chinese medicine.

Hot infusion: Herbs are steeped (like a cup of hot tea) for 15 to 20 minutes (sometimes longer depending on the herb).

Note that it is rare for an herbalist to prescribe only one herb to a client. Typically decoctions are prepared with about a week's worth of herbs, and the patient is instructed to consume between 2 and 4 cups of the decoction each day. There are generally between six and sixteen herbs in one custom formula and between 3 and 12 grams of each herb. The average formula is about 100 to 120 grams total, for a week's worth of herbal medicine support. Each herb in the formula will interact with the others and round out the benefits. For instance, let's look at cinnamon. This is a wonderful sweet, pungent, and warming herb, but it can also be drying, which may not be best for someone who is already experiencing dryness. Therefore, we can pair cinnamon with a moistening herb such as licorice to round out the formula's actions and energetics.

Additionally, there are no true protocols when it comes to Chinese herbal medicine. Herbal formulas are prescribed to individuals and are therefore created for each unique person, his or her constitution, and the health challenges that are present.

That being said, some patent formulas are tried and true when it comes to certain patterns of imbalance, and I will mention them as appropriate. However, depending on the person taking the formula, even a patent formula might need to be modified to match the constitution and unique needs of the person taking it. On a related note, while ancient Chinese medicine holds a reputation of using potentially rare or endangered animals in their medicinal formulas, this practice is now very rare. Modern research has shown most practitioners that there are equal alternatives we can use without using animals to make medicine. (For more resources on Chinese herbal medicine and places to purchase herbs, see the "Resources for Delving Deeper" section at the end of this book.)

NUTRITIONAL SUPPLEMENTS

Nutritional supplements consist of natural products that contain vitamins, minerals, and amino acids. It's important to know why I may recommend nutritional supplements for certain times of year and certain health imbalances. As I mentioned before, I am an integrative health care practitioner and find it most helpful to use modern research while also practicing an ancient and holistic system of medicine. The recommendation for nutritional supplements begins with understanding the common issues with our soil.

Plants draw nutrients and water up from the soil through their root systems, and when we eat the plants, we receive a vast array of nutrients from them. Over the last hundred years, our soil has been depleted by unsustainable farming practices, clear-cutting (leaving behind no natural compost), and climate changes (global warming). Because of these critical issues, our depleted soil has led to plants that are also depleted of the nutrients they once had in abundance.[1]

In addition to soil depletion, we are now at a record-high degree of exposure to environmental and food toxins. Without adequate vitamins and minerals in our diet, many of us are finding it difficult to detox from these poisons at the same rate as we take them in. Because of this exposure to toxins coupled with soil depletion, I often recommend nutritional supplements (especially if you are experiencing health imbalances) to supplement the loss of minerals and vitamins in food. If you are able to get lab work done, you can now be tested for specific nutritional deficiencies and supplement your diet in a way targeted to your unique challenges. It's important to choose good-quality nutritional supplements that are free from chemicals, fillers, and dyes. (For more information on good-quality nutritional supplements and labs, see the "Resources for Delving Deeper" section at the end of this book).

DOSING FOR HERBAL MEDICINE AND NUTRITIONAL SUPPLEMENTS

Because each of us is truly unique, dosing for herbs, formulas, and nutritional supplements is also unique. Proper dosage depends on many factors, such as your constitution, presenting symptoms, patterns of imbalance, digestive system strength, allergies and intolerances, and the potency of the preparation. As such, there is no one magical dosage to treat a presenting imbalance! I will give you the recommended dietary allowance (RDA) of the herbs and nutritional supplements I introduce. Note that in natural medicine we tend to recommend what is called a *therapeutic* dosage for conditions that require them. This is often a higher dosage than the RDA that has been shown to have tremendous health benefits. However, therapeutic dosages should only be prescribed by a qualified practitioner.

SEASONAL PRACTICES

Each time of year requires not only that we eat properly and take the appropriate herbs, but also that we move our bodies and use practices that will allow our bodies to come into greater alignment with our needs and with what is happening in nature during that season. Our lives have become so focused on thoughts and mental performance that our bodies are often last in line for attention. Therefore, in each seasonal section I will provide ways to include your body in the practices. In my life, I like to choose at least one movement practice, one hands-on practice, and one spiritual practice to do each day throughout the year. I find that this keeps me centered, healthy, and in touch with my greater purpose. It also gives me energy and helps me to reset when I've been knocked off balance. I invite you to do the same as you travel through each season with me in the following pages.

CALL TO ACTION

If you are anything like me, you want to be in the know. We live in difficult times where we cannot blindly trust what we are told about what is healthy or not, about medications we have been prescribed, or even claims made by people in power. In a big way, each of us is being called to be our own advocate in the twenty-first century and to question the things we may have, at some point, taken for the truth.

I still remember being a child and assuming that everything sold in a supermarket *had* to be healthy in order to be sold there. I also vividly remember the first time I learned about how horrifically animals were (and still are) being treated in the food industry; I was shocked, and it filled me with such shame for all the years that I ate meat and other animal products without knowing. This information is not obvious; you have to go digging for it, which means you have to want to be in the know, and you have to have the necessary resources (like time, energy, money, education, the Internet, a computer, and the intellectual and emotional capacity) to get there.

Our individual health is not something that can be assessed as separate from the health of our planet. We are completely interconnected with and interdependent on the earth. When we hear the mind-blowing news that a collection of plastics the size of the state of Texas was found in the ocean, or the tragic news of yet another school shooting or natural disaster, it's perfectly normal to feel sad, scared, angry, confused, helpless, or any number of other feelings. In fact, our mutual acknowledgment of this collective experience of suffering will only bring us deeper into our own hearts and closer to each other. It is this shared honesty that heals the many divisions. *It is okay to grieve for the state of our world.*

If beyond that grief you feel the call to get involved, then I urge you to reach out to the causes that speak to you the most. There is certainly no shortage of causes and places in need. If you can't give monetary support, consider giving time and volunteering. If you can't give time, consider becoming educated on the cause so you can share with others what you have learned and how *they* can get involved. And if you can't become educated on the subject, prayers, intentions, and well wishes go a long way and are always needed. Service is, after all, not an action we perform but a state of mind. If you have a service state of mind, then everything you do becomes a gift to our world.

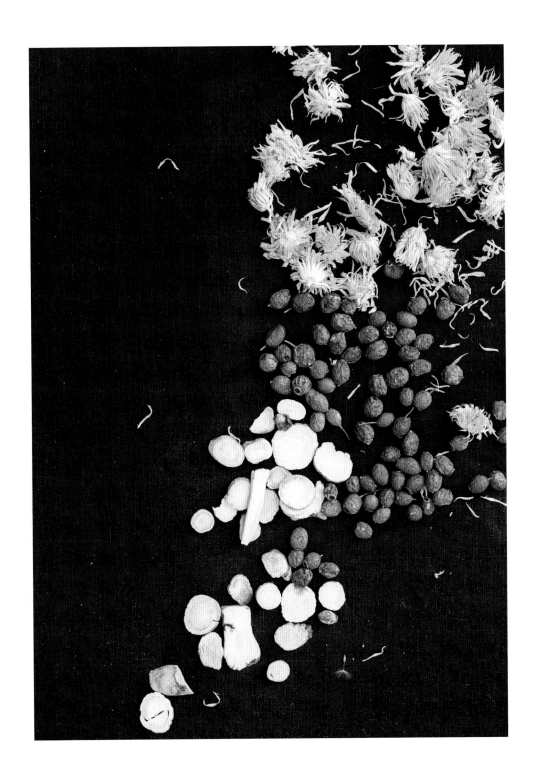

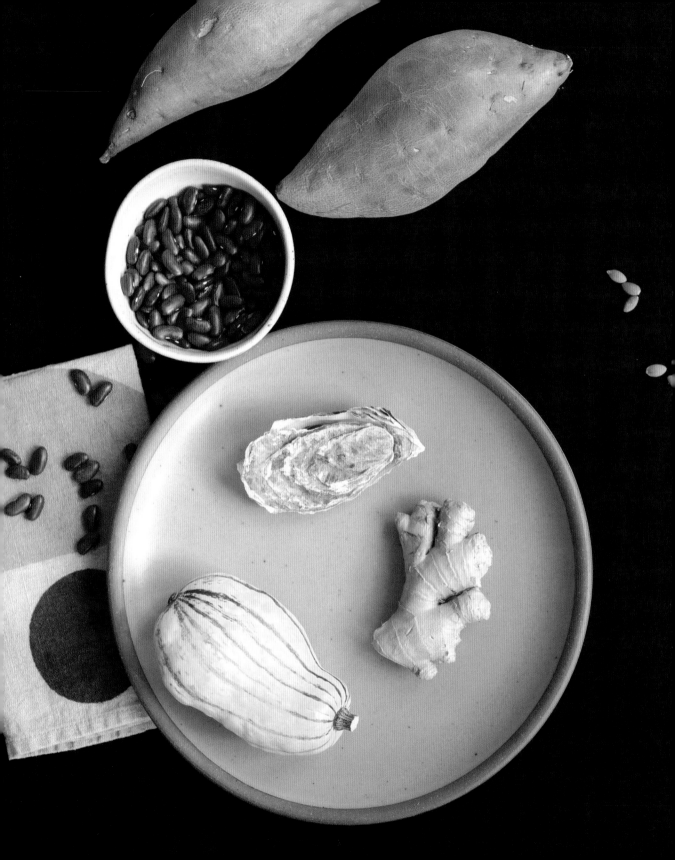

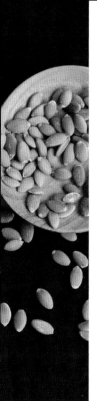
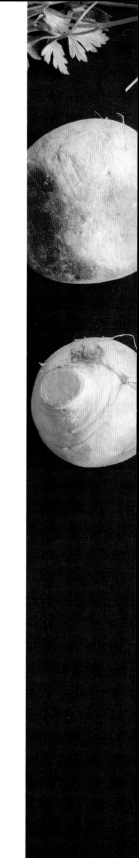

WINTER AND THE WATER ELEMENT

WINTER SOLSTICE (DECEMBER 21) THROUGH SPRING EQUINOX (MARCH 20)

Don't think the garden loses its ecstasy in winter.
It's quiet but the roots are down there riotous.

—RUMI

— ◆ —

Winter is a time of year that, after letting go in autumn, we have shed all that is no longer serving us and have gotten back down to our essence. We can look around and see the people and practices we know and love. It is a time of year for reflecting on what is most important to us, a time for *slowing down* and spending quiet, intentional time with ourselves.

As the most yin of all the seasons and elements, Winter is a time for relinquishing aspects of our relationship to the outside world and instead turning our energy and attention inward. If we are lucky enough to live in a place where the arrival of winter is evident (cooler weather, snow, and so on), it is a wonderful calling home to ourselves and an invitation to begin conserving our energy; something we can mimic what is happening with the plants and animals at this time. Trees draw in their sap. Animals slow down their movements and even their heart rates when they enter hibernation. Winter is a time for incubation when most of our energy can be spent internally and only on the most vital of processes—that of restoring ourselves in preparation for spring.

DEEP LISTENING

In many places around the world where winter means snow is coming, the season brings a quiet so deafening and so utterly still that you can hear a single leaf fall from a tree branch. If you slow down and stay quiet enough, you can hear this and all the other subtle stirrings of your body, mind, and spirit this time of year.

Winter is darker than most seasons because there is less sunshine and often more precipitation. Both of these things contribute to an increase in water and therefore the energy of the Water element. For many, this time of solitude and slowing down can feel either like a welcome breath of fresh air or like a deeply uncomfortable invitation. As our activities and stimulation are minimized, we are left with the stillness (or chaos) inside ourselves. When fear comes up in response to winter, it can highlight a part of our being that needs tending, most especially our Water element.

THE WATER ELEMENT

Winter is the season when the element of water holds the most prominent energy. Here we are talking simply about water as you know it: the kind you drink, the kind you swim in, and the kind you see falling from the sky when it rains. Streams, lakes, rivers, oceans, aquifers—it's everywhere. Water is so vital to life that while we can go for many weeks without food, we will die in only a few days to a week (max!) without water. Just like the earth, we are also largely made up of water. Sixty percent of the human body (70 percent of the earth's total surface) is pure water. Suffice it to say that we are largely watery beings.

Water is a transformative substance, and when it runs over any other element, it changes it. For example, water changes fire rapidly by putting it out. Although it takes longer to change other elements like metal (rocks, sand, and so on), water changes them nonetheless (think of the Grand Canyon). In the soil of the earth, water can be so readily available that it becomes muddy or so minimal that the soil is dry like the sand in a desert.

Water is always seeking the lowest point of gravity. In any given vessel, it will drop to the bottom without hesitation. Yet a tiny movement from below can change the current and flow of water for miles, creating ripples throughout or even a tidal wave. The same can be said of people too! In the same way that water seeks gravity, people who have a lot of Water in their constitution are truth-seekers. They are not built for using up energy frivolously but rather for getting to the bottom of things. They often have a strong desire for periods of solitude and silence and can return with one epiphany that, just like water, can change the current of their family, their community, and their society. This is the power of the Water element.

NOURISHING BATH RECIPE

This bath is wonderful to incorporate into your daily or weekly routine, especially if you are feeling cold, fatigued, or overwhelmed. The Epsom salt will increase the flow of your blood and lymphatic fluid while the baking soda reduces inflammation and restores your body to neutral pH. The essential oils will nourish your spirit and transform your state of mind.

2 cups Epsom salts

1 cup baking soda

10 drops total of one or two of the following essential oils: lavender, frankincense, vanilla, cinnamon, rose otto, or ravensara

2 tablespoons raw local honey

2 tablespoons sweet almond oil

Add all the ingredients into hot bathwater as the tub is filling up. After soaking for 30 to 45 minutes, dry off and skin brush (see page 242) before finishing with a lukewarm shower. Plan to rest or go to bed soon afterward.

WATER CONSTITUTION

ARCHETYPE: THE PHILOSOPHER

People with significant Water in their constitution often go by the motto "Slow and steady wins the race." They move about the world with a quiet courage and, if they are balanced and in tune with their own needs, will often land in creative, yin-leaning careers. Finding relaxation in the exploration of the inner world, people with this constitution are often deep thinkers—hence the archetype of the Philosopher—and truth-seekers. They may even be slightly more introverted than the other constitutions (though not always). Highly imaginative and with a desire for deep understanding about our world and beyond, they are able to bring awareness to ideas, situations, and stories that are not readily apparent. As the Philosopher, their inner magical world can sometimes go unnoticed in our extremely yang environment. But make no mistake, people with a lot of Water in their constitution can be very present and highly intuitive.

EMOTION

The emotion of Water is fear. In many aspects of our lives, fear is a healthy response: a near-miss on the highway or a woman going into labor for the first time. These are natural and healthy fears that actually serve us in our survival and give us courage for

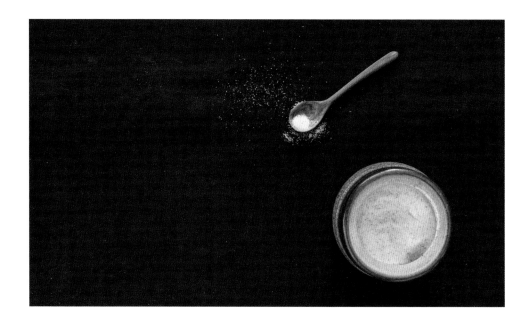

the many unexpected events in our lives. Fear is a forceful energy that is often chock-full of the hormones adrenaline and cortisol, both of which can fuel us with the energy to escape not only perceived, but also real, danger.

However, fear can sometimes get out of control and become a dominating emotion, leading to an unhealthy expression of this primal force. We may perceive danger everywhere when Water is out of balance. This is the experience of those with post-traumatic stress disorder (PTSD). Long after the danger is gone, they still see and feel it. On the opposite side of the coin, we may never perceive danger, which can be of equal cause for concern. Many of us dream of the day when we feel this fearless in our lives, but fearlessness is not a healthy state either, as it could quickly lead to taking risks that are too great. As with all things in life, finding our unique balance in this emotion is the key.

On a mental level, if you find yourself becoming fearful of anything and everything (phobias galore), then you know your Water element has gone out of balance. The same is true if you always see the world through the lens of fear first (even though you may subsequently pull through and decide to move toward the fearful thing anyway). When fear is primary, no matter the context, the Water element needs attention; the same is true if you are chronically fearless.

When the Water element goes out of balance, it is almost always due to depletion, most often in the kidneys and adrenal glands. Since the kidneys are the foundation of all yin and yang and therefore the root of all Fire and Water in the body, we could say that they are the most vital of organs to support. If they go out of balance, *everything* goes out of balance.

BATHING RITUALS

In many areas around the world, communal bathing is a rich part of the culture. In fact, dating as far back as the Neolithic Age, people would soak in hot pools they found as a way to warm up and release toxins. This practice continued in ancient Pakistan and Rome, and it is still very common in East Asia. If you don't have a natural hot spring nearby, you can deck out your bathtub with wonderful salts and still have a magical experience.

- Determination
- Courage
- Strong willpower
- Highly developed senses, especially hearing
- Deep imagination
- A thinker
- Use of fewer words with potent meaning
- Articulate
- "Wise beyond one's years"
- Calm, with calming energy
- Great boundaries
- Ability to act quickly when in danger
- Ability to endure great hardship
- Appropriately selective in partners
- High integrity
- Alone time required for balance

- Pervasive fear
- Anxiety
- Withdrawn personality (can be a loner)
- Severe phobias
- Absentmindedness
- Forgetfulness
- Difficulty setting boundaries
- Rigid beliefs
- Prone to exhaustion
- Fertility issues
- Stunted growth
- Scattered thinking
- Panic attacks
- Dogmatic beliefs (there is only one truth)
- Disheveled appearance
- Chronic lateness
- Low libido
- Impotence
- Lower back pain
- Blood pressure issues (high or low)
- Vertigo, dizziness, balance issues
- Urinary problems (chronic urinary tract infections [UTIs])
- Adrenal fatigue (hypothalamic-pituitary-adrenal [HPA] axis dysfunction)
- Edema
- Kidney stones
- Age-related brain disease (such as cognitive impairment, dementia, Alzheimer's disease, Parkinson's disease)

YOUR BODY IN WINTER

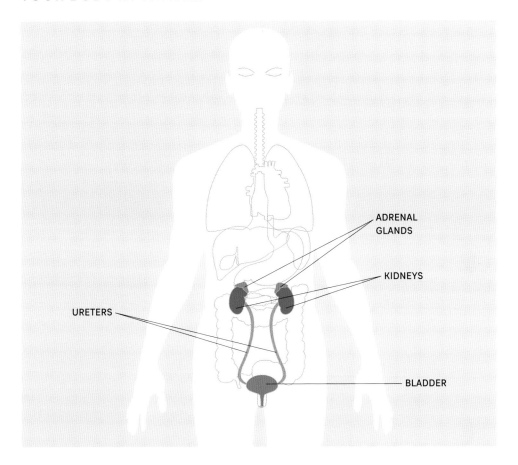

ADRENAL GLANDS

KIDNEYS

URETERS

BLADDER

The organs that help us process water both physically and energetically are the bladder and kidneys. On a physical level, when we drink water, it must pass through the digestive tract and into the kidneys to be filtered, then waste is carried on to the bladder to be excreted. Water that is retained by the kidneys and used in the body contains the vital minerals that we extract from it. This is why knowing where your water comes from is so important. These minerals are then used to create and infuse the bones and marrow—the two parts of the body governed by the Water element—with vital nutrients. In Chinese medicine, the brain is considered to be simply marrow and therefore is also governed by the Water element. (The ancient Chinese hierarchy of organs puts the heart at the top, not the brain. Imagine that!)

Kidneys

According to Chinese medicine, the kidneys serve as the root of our health throughout our lives. They are often referred to as the Palace of Fire and Water and the foundation of all yin and yang qualities in the body. We (most of us, anyhow) have two kidneys that reside close to the mid-lower back, tucked just under the lowest ribs. Each kidney is home to *millions* of tiny filters whose job is to keep the proper balance of blood, salt, and water in the body and make sure that these components are sent to the appropriate places. The kidneys also produce waste as a by-product of filtering, and that waste becomes the basis for urine. Urine is then carried to the bladder via the ureters.

OFFICIAL IN CHARGE OF THE WATERWAYS

In the ancient Chinese medicine texts, the character representing the kidneys translates as the "Official in Charge of the Waterways." On a physical level, the kidneys have so much responsibility in the processes of the body's water and blood supply. They are also a major meeting point between the ocean meridians and the river meridians. While we are constantly drawing from and replenishing the river meridians every day, we want to tap into the ocean meridians only when we need to. The kidneys are the same; think of them like a savings account. When we are going through a difficult time such as chronic illness, shock, or trauma, we need an extra boost to get us through.

Additionally, the kidneys are considered the home for our ancestral chi, also called jing qi. This is the energy we derived from our parents when we were born. In a perfect world, we would only tap into this reservoir of ancestral chi during times of great need so we will have enough to carry us through our lives and to pass on to our children, if we choose to have them. Ancestral chi is potent and strong and reason enough to care for our kidneys all year round. A big part of taking care of the kidneys is maintaining a nice balance between yin and yang and reducing unnecessary stress. The kidneys become depleted after constant exposure to even low-grade stress.

Not only is ancestral chi a source of energy, it is also a source of an "energetic imprint" with which we entered this world. Ancestral chi is the route for all physical, emotional, and spiritual inclinations that are passed down in a family's lineage as well as something known as *intergenerational trauma*. Intergenerational trauma is literally the imprint of trauma from a survivor that can be passed down to other generations.

→

Often this leaves the later generations with some form of post-traumatic stress that many will spend their lives trying to navigate consciously or unconsciously. We are just touching the tip of the iceberg when it comes to research on this topic in psychology, yet the ancient Chinese were well aware of these kinds of experiences being transferred from one generation to the next. This is something I have chosen to specialize in as part of my practice because it's clear to me that when we begin our healing journey, we have to take into consideration what we came into this world with. Not only that, but when we begin to heal, we must be aware that we are healing not just ourselves but also our families and lineages.

In a mother's womb, ancestral chi comes into the baby's body through the kidneys; it then meets and mixes with the spirit, which resides in the heart (also called *shen*, see page 173). This intertwining of Fire and Water energies and imprints is what creates who we become and sets us up with preferences and aversions, our unique personality, and ultimately our destiny. We can also call this the "blueprint for our lives," and this blueprint resides in our kidneys. The blueprint, like all things in Taoism, is not fixed. Rather, it is a guidebook for our lives, and we can listen to it or ignore it as much as we like; it will always be there regardless.

Adrenal Glands

Thanks, in part to our adrenal glands, we are built for survival. Our adrenal system has evolved in such a way that if we were to see a wooly mammoth coming around the corner, the combination of the activity in our brain and adrenal glands would allow us to move rapidly to ensure our safety and survival. Although they are of utmost importance, these glands are only about the size of grapes. They rest just on top of the kidneys and promote appropriate stress responses when we need them through hormones such as cortisol and aldosterone.

The problem is that many of us are living as though the wooly mammoth is just around the corner *all* the time. That means a constant low-level release of stress hormones in the system, which is why when life throws us curveballs, we sometimes find ourselves overreacting or just feeling overwhelmed and paralyzed. After many years of this constant low-level output of stress hormones, we become exhausted and depleted. This is also what happens with adrenal exhaustion and post-traumatic stress disorder (more on this in Part Three).

Bladder

The bladder is a sac located below the kidneys and closer to the front of the body, just above and behind the pubic bone. It can stretch and contract on a moment-to-moment basis. It requires emptying, and on average a hydrated person will feel the urge to urinate eight to ten times each day. That average goes up if you are taking certain herbs or medications that act as diuretics (which causes more frequent elimination).

Many of us are dehydrated at a core level, so when we start to really drink enough water, we may find ourselves running to the restroom constantly. This is because the bladder has gotten used to minimal water consumption and has shrunk. But if we give it a little time while we stay hydrated, the bladder will stretch back open (this takes longer the older we get because we lose elasticity in our tissues). This is similar to how the stomach works—stretching and shrinking depending on our food consumption.

OFFICIAL WHO CONTROLS THE STORAGE OF WATER

In Chinese characters, the bladder translates as the "Official Who Controls the Storage of Water." We can understand this translation on a physical level, but what about on a mental or spiritual one? Water is life-giving and vital for nearly every process in the body. Therefore, water is a major resource for us. When we have enough of it, our minds and spirits can rest easy, be in flow, develop strong will, and trust in the natural movement of our lives. The opposite is also true when our Water element becomes deficient. If the kidneys are like a savings account that we draw from only when necessary, think of the bladder as a checking account that we need to draw from each day for the basic functioning of our lives. It's important to replenish this checking account through the water we drink, the foods we eat, the love we give and receive from our families and community, the wisdom and connection we receive from our spiritual practices, and so on.

Bones

The bones are the keepers of the body's structure and movements, and they serve as a framework for all of the other organs and tissue. They are protective as well, such as the rib cage that surrounds the heart and lungs and the skull that protects the brain. There are approximately 206 bones in the human body, and if we are healthy, they don't break so easily. When they do break, if our Water element is full and strong, they heal properly and quickly. Bones also act as reservoirs of nutrients such as calcium, phosphorous, and the ever-so-vital bone marrow.

Bone Marrow

This vital substance lives inside the bones and serves as the production center for blood cells, fat, and cartilage, as well as the repair and maintenance of more bone. In Chinese medicine, the brain is referred to as the "Sea of Marrow." How different from the Western medical view of the brain. Bone marrow houses stem cells, which are a hot topic in the medical community. These cells can support the repair of nearly any tissue in the body; when they are injected into the body, they will turn into the very cells that are needed to heal damaged or diseased tissue. For instance, if someone has liver disease, doctors can inject stem cells that will then turn into liver cells and work to regenerate damaged liver tissue. Stem cells are quite miraculous!

Ears

The sense organs associated with the Water element and winter are the ears. The ears ironically mimic the shape of the kidneys and even grow at the same time the kidneys do in utero. In winter, our hearing can become heightened as everything in nature quiets down.

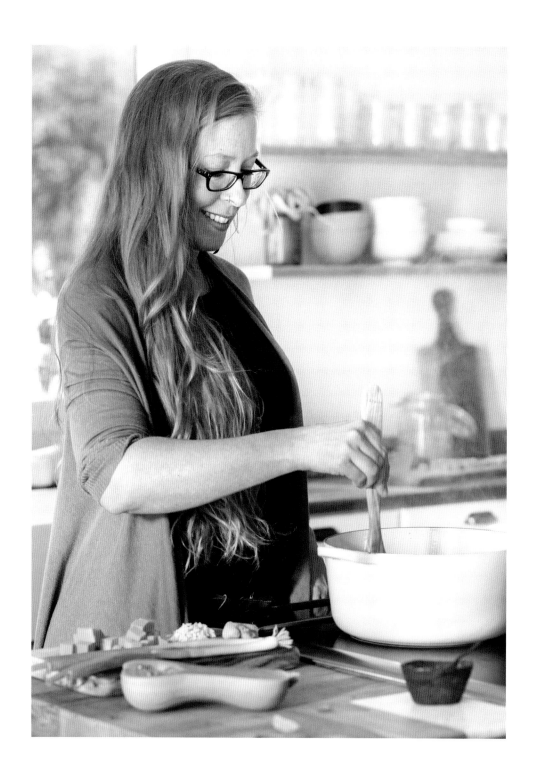

THE WINTER PANTRY

FEATURED RECIPES

The whole prerogative in winter is *restoration*. We need to allow time for our adrenal glands to rest from the many months of dishing out cortisol and adrenaline to manage our daily stressors. This is also a perfect time to allow our blood sugar to find homeostasis. Therefore, we don't need as many simple carbohydrate foods as we would in the summertime, and we especially don't need sugar-rich foods.

In winter, think *storage*—foods that not only store well but also provide energy that your body can store well. That means what you really need to focus on is fat and protein. Those are the most nourishing and stabilizing foods. When you eat them, your body will draw energy from them for a long time.

Here are the general principles of nutrition in winter:

- Cook everything (nothing should be eaten raw).
- Cook foods slowly, over a long period of time, and with less heat.
- Seek out salty flavors.
- Everything that enters the body must be warm in temperature.
- Focus on eating fats, proteins, and more complex carbohydrates (rather than the simple ones).
- Master the art of making nutrient-dense broths and drink them every day.
- Make sure not to go more than four hours without eating, except when sleeping.
- You can eat plenty of kidney-shaped foods like beans and seeds.
- Enjoy black and blue foods like blueberries, blackberries, black beans, and mulberries. (Since berries likely aren't in season in winter, rehydrating dried berries and cooking them would be most appropriate.)

Winter Staples

PROTEINS: Chicken, duck, goat, lamb, lobster, mussels, oysters, pork, salmon, shrimp, smoked fish, trout, tuna, venison

BONES: Chicken, cow, duck (the most nutrient-dense of all bones), fish, lamb

> NOTE: Be sure to always buy products involving animals that have been ethically raised and well cared for, grass-fed when applicable, and always organic. Since the bones serve as the foundation for an animal's life, you want to be sure you are extracting nutrients and minerals from them rather than stress hormones or antibiotics as with industrially farmed animals.

GRAINS: Buckwheat, corn, oats, quinoa

ROOT VEGETABLES: Artichoke, beets, carrots, celery root or celeriac, garlic, jicama, kohlrabi, onions, parsnips, radishes (daikon and red), rutabagas, sweet potatoes, turnips, yams, yucca

WINTER SQUASH: Acorn, butternut, delicata, hubbard, kabocha, spaghetti

ONION FAMILY: Chives, garlic, green onions, leeks, onions, shallots

FRUITS: Blackberries, blueberries, cherries, grapes, mulberries

SEEDS AND NUTS: Almonds, cashews, chestnuts, chia seeds, flaxseeds, hazelnuts, hemp seeds, macadamia nuts, peanuts, pecans, pistachios, pumpkin seeds, sesame seeds, sunflower seeds, walnuts

LEGUMES: Black beans, lentils

DAIRY: Avoid

HERBS AND SPICES: Basil, black pepper, cinnamon, cloves, garlic, ginger, horseradish, turmeric,

FOODS TO AVOID: Alcohol, citrus or tropical fruit juices, cold or cool temperature foods, ice water, liquids in excess, raw foods, sour milk products (yogurt, kefir), sugar

---

WINTERTIME FLAVOR: SALTY

- If you are **cold**, add in *pungent* (page 90) and *warming* foods (page 93).
- If you are **damp**, add in *bitter* (page 88), *pungent* (page 90), and *astringent* foods (page 95).
- If you are **dry**, add in *moistening* foods (page 94).

WINTER RECIPES FOR RESTORATION

The following recipes will serve you well in the winter by providing sustenance for the kidneys and bladder. They will also keep you warm and stabilize your blood sugar. When your blood sugar is stable, so is your energy and often your mood.

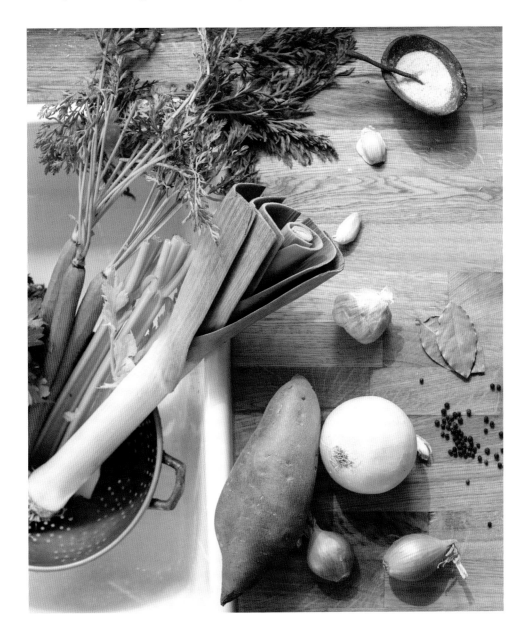

When it comes to making vegetable broth, I prefer to make more than I need and store what is left in the freezer. So, depending on how much you hope to end up with (a few days' worth or a few weeks' worth), you may need to modify this recipe a bit. Also, I have listed all of my favorite ingredients to put into a vegetable broth in order to reach maximum nutrient density. Feel free to mix and match some of these ingredients according to your own taste and needs. Onions, carrots, and celery are always a good base for any vegetable broth. From there, the modifications are all your own! If you are striving for a clear broth, leave out the sweet potato and the winter squash.

NOTE: Some vegetable broth recipes have you sauté a handful of vegetables first to increase the flavor of the broth. I recommend avoiding this, as cooking the vegetables first will kill off some of those nutrients you want to keep in the broth.

- 16 cups (4 quarts) water
- 1 to 3 large pieces kombu (seaweed)
- 1 thumb-size piece fresh ginger, skin removed and sliced (or 1 teaspoon ground ginger)
- 1 thumb-size piece fresh turmeric, skin removed and sliced (or 1 teaspoon ground turmeric)
- 1 teaspoon fine sea salt
- ¼ teaspoon black pepper
- 1 medium leek, sliced lengthwise and well cleaned (use white and light green parts)
- 2 medium carrots (save carrot tops)
- 3 stalks celery
- 4 to 6 whole cloves garlic, crushed
- 1 very small or ½ large sweet potato
- 1 cup winter squash (like butternut, acorn, delicata, kabocha, hubbard), cubed
- 1 cup fresh or ½ cup dried shiitake mushrooms
- ½ small bunch kale or chard (or a mixture of dark, leafy greens), leaves only
- 1 teaspoon ghee, butter, or olive oil, for serving

Add all the ingredients except for the greens and ghee to a stockpot or Crock-Pot with multiple heat settings. First, bring to a boil with the lid off, then set to low/slow simmer for a minimum of 2 hours with the lid on. Keep tasting to determine your ideal flavor strength—I like the broth to simmer for 4 to 5 hours. One hour before the stock is finished, add the greens, including the carrot tops, kale or chard, and any herbs you desire (see the box), and let simmer for the remaining hour. If you add herbs such as astragalus, burdock root, or reishi and plan to use the cooked vegetables after the broth is finished, consider tying the herbs into a cloth bag so they can be removed easily from the vegetables after cooking.

When finished cooking, strain the broth with a colander. Serve the broth with a teaspoon of butter, ghee, or olive oil on top. Once cooled, store the remaining broth in the refrigerator for up to one week.

You can let the strained vegetables go back to the earth as compost or use them to make a simple vegetable soup that will be a little heavier and higher calorie than the broth. If you would like to use the vegetables, pull out any skins (such as onion, garlic, or squash skins) and put the rest into a food processor. There will be some nutrients, mostly fibers, left in the vegetables, believe it or not! Blend the vegetables until smooth and add them to this broth or use them in another soup.

OPTIONAL MEDICINALS TO ADD TO STOCK OR BROTH

- For building energy and immunity: ¼ to ½ cup astragalus
- For adding moisture, building blood, and clearing heat: 1 large burdock root
- For building blood: ½ to 1 cup nettles
- For building blood and supporting the adrenal glands: ½ to 1 cup parsley
- For building energy and immunity: ¼ to ½ cup reishi

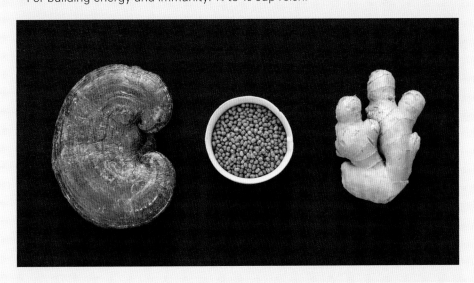

Having a nutritious and healing bone stock in your kitchen all winter long will keep you and your family healthy and your bones strong. The more collagen you have in your stock, the better! The collagen helps to repair any damage done to your intestines by a modern-day diet, which tends to be amplified around the holidays. Choose which bones you would like to make a stock with from the Winter Staples list on page 118. In general, you want to have 2 pounds of raw bones (cow, chicken, lamb, fish, or duck) per 1 gallon of stock. If possible, ask your butcher to cut the bones into 2- to 3-inch pieces.

Some bone stock recipes tell you to roast the bones first (the same as with sautéing vegetables before making broth). This is purely about flavor, as you will lose some of the nutrients in the roasting process. I suggest trying the stock without roasting the first time and then making modifications if you need to.

Additionally, if you choose to make a fish stock, be sure to include the heads, tails, and skins of the fish for added nutrients. If you prefer to make a seafood stock, save all those shrimp tails in the freezer and toss them into the stock. If you want beef stock, choose femurs and knuckles, as these will have the most marrow and collagen of all the bones.

2 pounds bones (cow, chicken, lamb, fish, or duck)

16 cups (4 quarts) water

2 chicken feet, for extra gelatin (optional)

2 tablespoons raw, unfiltered organic apple cider vinegar

OPTIONAL ADDITIONS

1 whole onion

2 carrots

2 celery stalks

2 to 6 cloves garlic

½ bunch parsley

Place the bones, water, chicken feet (if using), and vinegar in a large stockpot or Crock-Pot. Let sit for 30 minutes without any heat. This vinegar pretreatment helps the bones to release more of their nutrients once you start cooking.

Bring the stock to a boil with the lid off, then reduce the heat to a slow simmer (you should only see a bubble coming to the surface every 30 seconds or so). Cook according to the following guidelines:

Cow and lamb bones: 48 hours
Chicken and duck bones: 24 hours
Fish bones: 8 hours

Skim any foam (impurities coming out from the bones) off the top and discard.

If you choose any of the optional additions of vegetables or herbs for extra flavor or nutrients, do so about 2 to 4 hours before removing the pot from the stove (or turning off the Crock-Pot). When finished cooking using the times listed above, strain all the ingredients out of the stock with a colander. Once cool, transfer to the refrigerator. Enjoy a cup or more each day by itself or add as the base to other sauces or soups. Bone stock will keep in the refrigerator for about 5 days.

LEAVE NO WASTE

When it comes to making broths and stocks, think about compost. When you are cutting up vegetables throughout the week for different meals, consider saving some of the scraps for your broths rather than tossing them in the compost heap: carrot ends and tops, onions ends and peel, garlic peel, vegetable skins, and so on can all be used. You can keep them in the freezer until it's time to make broth or stock again, but use them within a year to get the most nutrients and flavor from your scraps.

Essentially any salad can be warmed. Granted, some of the lettuces, sprouts, and baby greens can become not just wilted but very soggy, very quickly. Some greens will change flavor once you cook them, getting sweeter or more bitter. So play with making warm salads during the cool winter months to find which greens you love.

1 pound rainbow carrots, sliced lengthwise and into 2-inch pieces

1 pound parsnips, sliced lengthwise and into 2-inch pieces

1 clove garlic, chopped

2 shallots, finely chopped

½ teaspoon chili powder

¼ cup olive oil

Salt and pepper to taste

2 large handfuls dark, leafy greens (such as spinach, kale, mustard greens, chard, or arugula)

Juice of 1 lemon

¼ bunch cilantro or ¼ cup basil leaves, chopped

FOR THE DRESSING

⅓ cup tahini (sesame seed paste)

¼ cup olive oil

¼ cup water

Juice of 1 lemon

1 clove garlic, chopped

Salt and pepper to taste

Preheat the oven to 400°F. On a sheet pan, toss the carrots, parsnips, garlic, shallots, and chili powder in the olive oil. Season with salt and pepper, and roast until tender (20 to 25 minutes).

On the stove, prepare a steamer basket or simply a pot with a lid and colander. When the water is boiling, flash steam the dark, leafy greens until they turn bright green, then remove.

For the dressing, place all ingredients in a food processor and blend until smooth. If the mixture is too runny, add a little more tahini. If it is too thick, add a little more water.

When the vegetables are finished roasting, toss them with the lemon juice and add the steamed greens and cilantro or basil. Top the salad with the dressing, and voilà!

TIPS • Feel free substitute other root vegetables and greens to make it taste like a completely different meal!

• I make this dressing often for other kinds of salads, roasted veggies, and as a dip for bread. Refrigerated, this dressing will last about one week.

This is a wonderful, nutrient-packed snack or addition to any meal! It is loaded with fats and proteins—two of the most important nutrients in winter—and will give your body fuel for hours. You can vary the kinds of seeds and nuts you use to vary the flavor and nutrients (pumpkin seeds are my favorite). You can also choose between the savory and sweet options, depending on what you need in your diet.

The key to making a good seed and nut pâté is soaking the seeds and nuts. Soaking helps to soften the outer layer, so we can digest them more easily and retrieve all the nutrients from them. Always be sure to rinse the soaked seeds and nuts after soaking as phytic acid is often released and can be difficult to digest.

1½ cups walnuts, sunflower seeds, or pumpkin seeds (You can also mix ½ cup of each)

3 cups water, at room temperature

1 teaspoon salt

SAVORY INGREDIENTS

1 clove garlic

2 sprigs cilantro, parsley, thyme, oregano, dill, or basil

2 tablespoons olive oil

Juice of ½ lemon

2 tablespoons miso paste

Salt and pepper to taste

SWEET INGREDIENTS

2 tablespoons maple syrup

1 teaspoon ground cinnamon

1 teaspoon ginger, chopped fresh or ground

½ cup dried raisins, goji berries, or blueberries

Put the seeds and/or nuts and the salt in the water and soak them overnight, or for at least an hour. When they are done, rinse and drain them.

Put the seeds and nuts and all savory or sweet ingredients into a blender and blend or pulse until you have a consistency that you like (I prefer smooth and creamy, but some prefer chunky). Transfer the mixture to a bowl and for the savory version, consider topping with chopped, roasted garlic, olive oil, parsley sprigs, or cracked black pepper. For the sweet version, consider topping with ground cinnamon, chopped dates, or fresh fruit.

Use the pâté as a dip for crackers, veggies, or bread. In the summertime, you can use the savory version rolled up in lettuce leaves with grated carrots for a nice appetizer. Or stuff the sweet version inside dates for a lovely dessert. The pâté will store well in the refrigerator for up to one week.

Congee is a grain porridge that has been eaten for centuries in traditional Chinese homes. It is often served for breakfast, and legend says it promotes good health and a long life! I believe this partly is because, in order for congee to become congee, it has to be cooked for a very long time. When it is well cooked, it is easy to extract all the nutrients from it (meaning it doesn't take much energy on our part to break it down), and it provides long-lasting energy for our bodies. Congee can jump-start sluggish digestion, strengthen the whole digestive system, and support a healthy metabolism.

Essentially any grain can become congee. If it's winter, I recommend using Winter grains that are slightly bitter or salty, such as amaranth, barley, millet, oats, quinoa, and rye. Congee is easy to make: it's one part grain to five parts water. Cooking it in a Crock-Pot is best, but the stovetop works too. You can go for either savory or sweet with this recipe. In Chinese homes, seafood congee is common and often includes shrimp, baby scallops, scallions, ginger, and garlic. What a great way to start the day!

1 cup grain (your choice)

5 cups water

Pinch of salt

SAVORY INGREDIENTS

1 cup proteins, such as shrimp or pork, cut into bite-size pieces or 4 scrambled eggs

1 to 3 cloves garlic, chopped

2 tablespoons scallions, chopped

1 tablespoon grated fresh ginger or 1 teaspoon ground ginger

1 cup sweet potato, carrots, winter squash, or pumpkin, cubed

2 handfuls spinach

SWEET INGREDIENTS

1 cup fresh or dried fruits (following the general guidelines for winter on page 117)

1 cup soaked pumpkin seeds, almonds, or walnuts

1 teaspoon ground cinnamon

½ teaspoon ground nutmeg

1 tablespoon grated fresh ginger or 1 teaspoon ground ginger

Honey, molasses, or maple syrup to taste

The best way to prepare congee is in a Crock-Pot, though you can also make this on the stovetop. If cooking in a Crock-Pot, add the base ingredients and either the savory or sweet ingredients to the Crock-Pot and cook for approximately 8 hours on low heat or 3 hours on high.

If cooking on the stovetop, put the base ingredients and either the savory or sweet ingredients in a covered stockpot and cook on very low heat for 8 hours. Check the congee once an hour and give it a stir to prevent the bottom of the pan from getting dry and burning the grain.

For either preparation, add more water if the mixture gets dry and begins to stick to the sides or bottom of the pot. The mixture should maintain a very creamy, oatmeal-like consistency, and you will know it's done when the vegetables are soft and cooked through.

THE WINTER MEDICINE CABINET

In wintertime, it's great to have staple herbs in the cabinet to gently support our daily lives during this very yin season. In places north of the equator, winter means it's the coldest and darkest that it will be all year long. Therefore, we are more vulnerable to becoming cold at this time. If we have spent more energy throughout the year than we have replenished, we will feel it now as exhaustion and/or Water imbalances in the body like edema, diarrhea, and UTIs.

HARAMAKI (KIDNEY WARMER)

Another thing to consider getting for wintertime is a *haramaki* (literally a "belly warmer"). This tube-like knitted item is worn just like a piece of clothing, often under the clothes, and is a kidney warmer. I find that it not only helps me stay present with my kidneys during this season (and therefore my energy throughout the day), but it also reminds me to keep my awareness at least somewhat in my own body (it's easy to stray). They have gotten so popular in Japan that you can now find them in designer prints.

Astragalus

PINYIN: Huang Qi

ORIGIN: China

PART USED: Root

ORGANS / SYSTEMS SUPPORTED: Immune system, central nervous system, liver, heart

USES: Exhaustion, weakened immune system, chronic and recurrent colds and flu, asthma, diarrhea, edema, also slows or prevents tumor growth, reduces allergic responses and reactions from food intolerances, supports a compromised immune system (as is with cancer or hepatitis treatments), shortens the duration of respiratory infections

PATTERNS SUPPORTED: Wei qi deficiency (see page 227), spleen yang deficiency, chi and blood deficiencies

FLAVORS: Sweet

TEMPERATURE: Slightly warming

ACTIONS: Moistening, tonifying, calming

CONTRAINDICATIONS: Not to be taken while on immunosuppressive drugs

BEST TAKEN: As a decoction (10 to 30 grams/day); simmer slices of the root in soups, stocks, and broths to add a slightly sweet taste and lots of healing power

Cinnamon

PINYIN: Rou Gui

ORIGIN: Sri Lanka, Bangladesh, Burma, India

PART USED: Bark

ORGANS / SYSTEMS SUPPORTED: Digestive system, blood, immune system, respiratory system, spleen, kidneys, heart

USES: Diarrhea, arthritis, insulin resistance, high blood sugar, sluggish digestive system, asthma, amenorrhea, dysmenorrhea

PATTERNS SUPPORTED: Kidney yang deficiency, spleen yang deficiency, chi and blood deficiencies, chi and blood stagnation

FLAVORS: Sweet, pungent

TEMPERATURE: Warming (hot)

ACTIONS: Astringent, tonifying

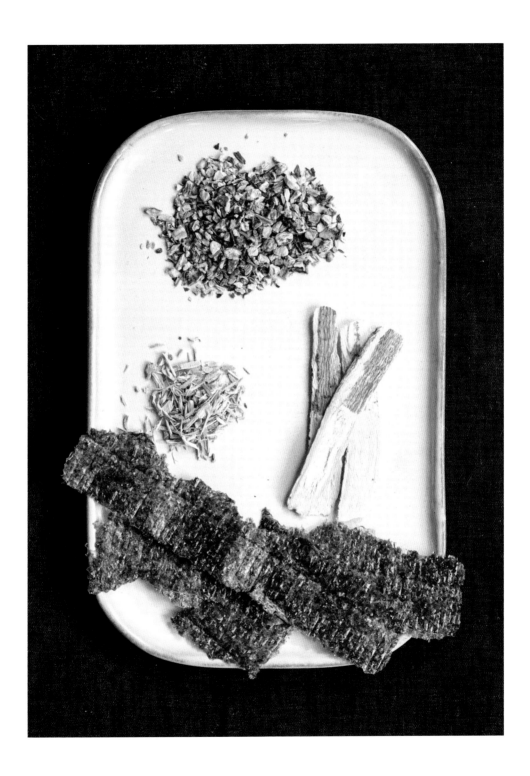

CONTRAINDICATIONS: Not to be taken (aside from culinary use) while on blood thinners; use caution with high doses during pregnancy as cinnamon is a stimulant

BEST TAKEN: Hot infusion (drink before each meal to stimulate digestion or between meals to regulate blood sugar and/or sugar cravings); decoction (1 to 6 grams/day)

Eleuthero (Siberian Ginseng)

PINYIN: Wu Jia Shen

ORIGIN: China, Japan, Korea, Russia

PART USED: Root

ORGANS / SYSTEMS SUPPORTED: Immune system, adrenals, central nervous system, heart, spleen, kidneys, endocrine system

USES: Stress, hypothyroidism, immune system imbalances, chronic and recurrent colds and flu, adrenal fatigue, chronic fatigue, infertility, polycystic ovary syndrome (PCOS), detoxification, pain and inflammation

PATTERNS SUPPORTED: Kidney yang deficiency, wei qi deficiency, spleen chi deficiency

FLAVORS: Pungent, slightly bitter

TEMPERATURE: Warming

ACTIONS: Tonifying, blood-building, calming (not a stimulant like its distant cousin, radix ginseng)

CONTRAINDICATIONS: None known

BEST TAKEN: Decoction (9 to 30 grams/day)

Polygonum (Fo Ti)

PINYIN: He Shou Wu

ORIGIN: China

PART USED: Root

ORGANS / SYSTEMS SUPPORTED: Immune system, respiratory system, liver, kidneys

USES: Immune system imbalances, anemia, high cholesterol, hardened arteries, infertility, erectile dysfunction, allergies and allergic skin rashes

PATTERNS SUPPORTED: Kidney yin and yang deficiency, liver blood deficiency, internal wind

FLAVORS: Bitter, sweet

TEMPERATURE: Slightly warm

ACTIONS: Astringent, blood-building, tonifying

CONTRAINDICATIONS: Use with caution in cases of stomach and spleen deficiency (may cause diarrhea, gastritis)

BEST TAKEN: Decoction (4 to 8 grams/day of processed polygonum)

Rehmannia

PINYIN: Shu Di Huang

ORIGIN: China

PART USED: Root

ORGANS / SYSTEMS SUPPORTED: Liver, kidneys, respiratory system

USES: PMS, heart palpitations, anxiety, insomnia, allergies, anemia, osteoporosis, chronic obstructive pulmonary disease (COPD) and other chronic lung imbalances

PATTERNS SUPPORTED: Liver blood deficiency, heart blood deficiency, kidney yin deficiency

FLAVORS: Sweet

TEMPERATURE: Slightly warm

ACTIONS: Blood-building, moistening, tonifying

CONTRAINDICATIONS: Not to be used in cases of dampness or phlegm

BEST TAKEN: Decoction (9 to 30 grams/day)

Wintertime Formulas

EIGHT TREASURE COMBINATION / WOMEN'S PRECIOUS (BA ZHEN TANG): Despite its name, this is a formula for everyone. Eight Treasure Combination Formula supports the building of chi and blood, providing respite from long-standing fatigue and frailty and recovery from blood loss such as with menstrual cycles, childbirth, and/or trauma. This nourishing formula is an excellent one to turn to for energy restoration.

KIDNEY QI PILLS FROM THE GOLDEN CABINET (JIN GUI SHEN QI WAN): This is a wonderful formula for wintertime when you feel exhausted and cold and are having symptoms of kidney deficiency, especially the yang type. This formula will warm you up and build your strength. It is useful in cases of excessive urination associated with kidney yang deficiency.

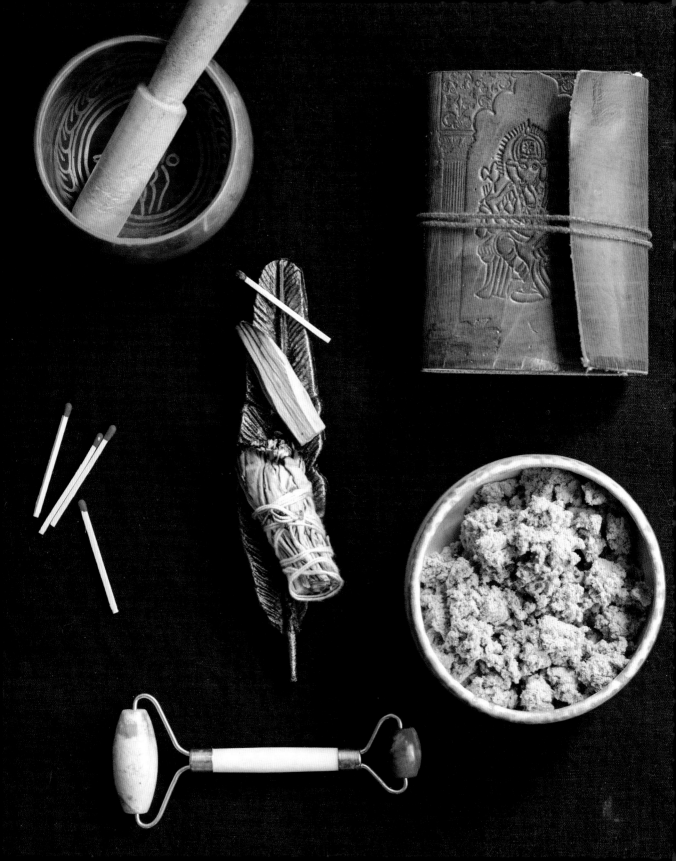

NOURISHING PRACTICES IN WINTER

Moving Your Body

While there is a natural slowing down of energy in winter, you do still need to move your body, to stretch and keep the joints lubricated and your blood moving. There is, however, one thing that changes how you do this in winter: you don't want to hike up your cortisol and adrenaline levels (remember you are trying to let your kidneys and adrenals rest and restore). This means exercises that bring up that kind of intensity and heart-pounding experience (running, intense weight-lifting, and so on) where you find yourself "pumped" should be kept to a minimum. Instead, try going for more mellow exercise so you can still move your body but not deplete yourself. Here are some of my favorite wintertime ways to exercise:

TAKING LONG, SLOW WALKS IN NATURE This allows you an opportunity to get outside and take your time. Go for a medium to slow pace rather than speed. Being outside this time of year allows you to sync up with the natural world. Hear the birds that stuck around and witness the naked trees.

PRACTICING YIN YOGA / RESTORATIVE YOGA This is a perfect winter practice, especially if you take it as a class in a studio, which allows you to be in community in a quiet and intentional way. (Sometimes it's nice to check in on the world in a soft way during winter.) Yin yoga is more than stretching on a mat—it is bringing consciousness into the body, moving slowly, and taking the time to really check in. Hot yoga, especially if you are feeling cold (but not depleted) much of the time can be a great addition. Donation-based and sliding-scale classes are offered in every major city, and there are plenty of free yoga classes to follow online.

SWIMMING This is an excellent wintertime activity because it allows you to actually be in water! Taking slow, methodical laps back and forth in the pool, focusing on your breathing, and making the most of your strokes will help to restore your nervous system while getting you some exercise. If you can't find natural hot pools of water, a visit to the local recreation center can work well too.

SNOWSHOEING / CROSS-COUNTRY SKIING As opposed to downhill skiing (which can be fun too), snowshoeing and cross-country skiing can be relaxing and mild on the nervous system while also getting you some time in nature. Here you can still move slowly through the natural world while getting good exercise.

Listening to Calming Sounds

It's important to protect yourself against noise pollution this time of year as the ears are governed by the kidneys. And I don't know about you, but my ears always yearn for quiet this time of year. Spend time in total silence or give your ears something lovely to enjoy each day during the winter. I love listening to the flute, singing bowls, and nature's plethora of sounds. Sound therapy, especially the magical sounds of singing bowls, has a wide range of healing benefits, including reducing cortisol (a stress hormone), lowering blood pressure, relieving pain and inflammation, and promoting deep relaxation.

Cleaning and Organizing Your Bathroom

Since your bathroom is the home of the Water element in the house, use winter as a time to clean it up, organize it, and give it a fresh new feel. Maybe add the colors of winter and the Water element: dark blue, purples, indigo, and black. Go through all your herbs and supplements and check the expiration dates on everything. Make it a sanctuary for your restorative bath time.

Scheduling Downtime

Winter is the time to have that annual check-in with yourself: "Who am I now?" "What has the last year taken with it, and what will the new year bring in?" I try to schedule several days off with myself each winter. I find that the first few days are filled with just catching up on life tasks, then I can settle more after that. I have about five days of really getting quiet with myself, cooking broths and drinking tea, then I spend the last two days preparing to return to my typical life.

Keeping a Journal

Since this is the most yin time of the year, spend a little time each day writing. This could be a journal entry or just a few stream-of-consciousness lines. But get some thoughts out and on paper. I have always loved Julia Cameron's Morning Pages exercise (from *The Artist's Way*). Here, she invites you to commit to three pages of anything each morning, including stream-of-consciousness. I find that it helps me to clean out anything I'm churning in my head, including dreams or residue from the last few days. Then I feel I can start my day more connected to myself and more present with others.

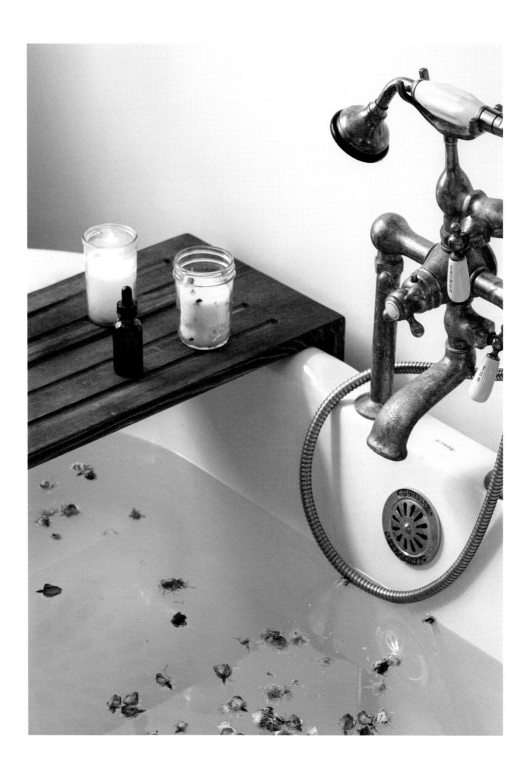

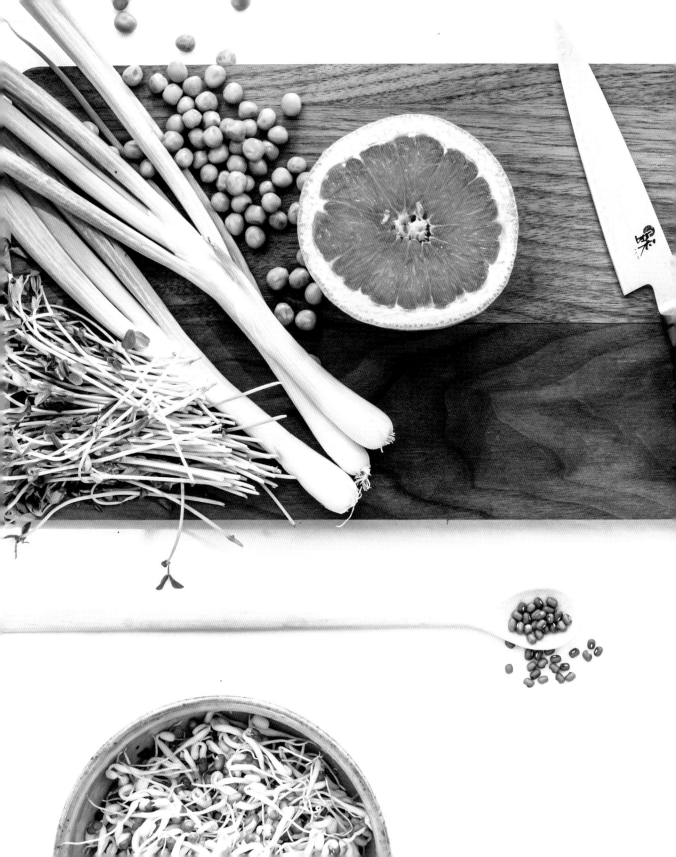

SPRING AND
THE WOOD ELEMENT

SPRING EQUINOX (MARCH 20)
THROUGH SUMMER SOLSTICE (JUNE 21)

What shape awaits in the seed of you to grow
and spread its branches against a future sky?
—DAVID WHYTE

— ◆ —

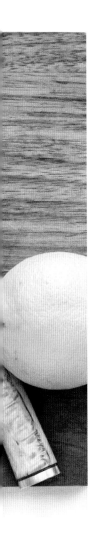

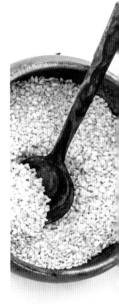

Like a breath of fresh air, spring follows winter, reminding us of brighter days and warmer weather to come. What is the vision you hold for your life? Where are you going from here? These are the questions that bubble up as the energy moves from the stillness and incubation of winter into the activity and hopefulness that comes in the spring. Spring is the time of year, after months of reflecting and restoring, when you begin to move a little bit more of your energy into activity, slowly increasing over the course of a few months. *Birth* and *growth* are the key themes of this season. All the little seeds you held during the cold winter months are now given the opportunity to shoot up toward the sun. Where are you going? What is the plan?

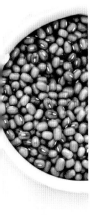

Since the energy of this season is all about birth and growth, we are provided with the opportunity to move toward our goals and dreams. When we look to nature, we can see that this is the time of year when the plants and animals all around us wake from their winter slumber and begin their irresistible, vertical ascent toward the sun. At the same time that growth moves upward toward light and warmth, plants are also securely rooting deep within the earth's soil. This journey takes knowing which direction to go and how much energy to put toward moving upward, balanced with how much energy to root downward. It requires steadiness and finesse.

A woman giving birth is a perfect example of this. While in utero, the baby is in the Water phase of life. But when the baby transitions and it's time to enter our world, Wood energy is precisely what is needed to push that baby through the birth canal. This energy, however, must be contained. If the mother pushes too fast, she risks tearing her body. If she pushes to slowly, she exhausts herself before the baby can make a grand entry. Balancing Wood energy is extremely necessary for this process.

With winter just before spring, we move from the most yin season toward increasing yang energy. This is why spring is considered to be a "yang season arising out of yin." As life emerges, we become hungry for movement. In the perfect conditions, sprouts can quadruple in size in a short period of time. It's easy to feel this energy and want to go from zero to one hundred with our own energy output. But to make the most of this season, we must find our yin and yang balance.

THE WOOD ELEMENT

Spring is the season when the element of Wood holds the most prominent energy. The Wood element is used to describe not only the physical wood found in trees, but also all plants and vegetation. Everything from the tender little sprouts that are the first to shoot up after winter to the oldest trees on earth.

It isn't just this physical manifestation that describes Wood; it's also the energy of birth and growth. This energy is vital for a little germinated seed, once it's received a bit of water and some warmth, to begin to crack open and move through the soil, stretching its way around obstacles and eventually stretching up to the sun. Wood energy provides the impetus that inspires the sprout to make it out of the soil and into the sunshine.

For anything to grow in our universe, there must first be a blueprint that will shape the vision for growth. For example, an oak tree has the blueprint for becoming an oak tree inside its original seed. The same is true for an aspen tree; it has the blueprint for becoming an aspen tree, and so on. That vision is only made manifest by Wood energy. Wood is what allows for growth that is congruent with the map of our destiny.

People who have a lot of Wood energy in their constitution are often very driven. They may even come off as a little pushy or loud because their energy is what is commonly behind the transformations we so need in our world. Wood energy allows us to have a vision that might look different than what others see. Martin Luther King, Jr., and other social change makers have certainly had a lot of this.

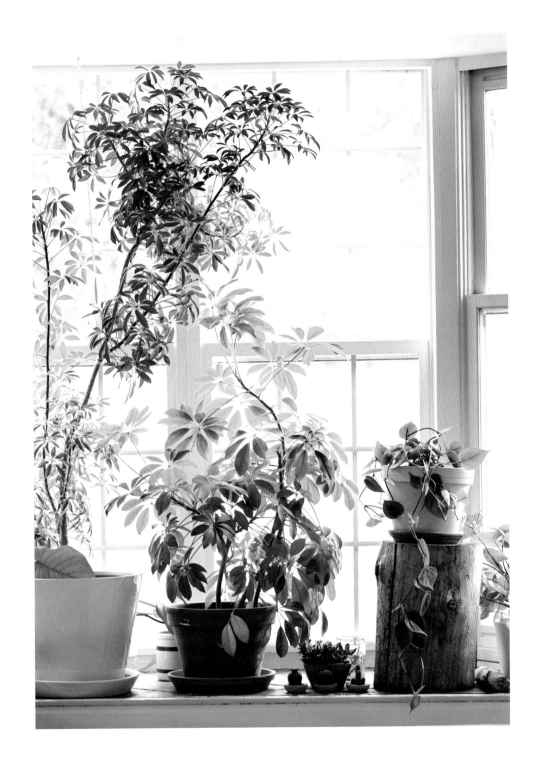

WOOD CONSTITUTION

ARCHETYPE: THE HERO

Those with Wood in their constitution are often true go-getters. They may have had visions from a very early age of all they wanted to accomplish in this lifetime, and then they just went for it. Because Wood energy is so driven, this often leads to a very accomplished person who has done a lot from a very young age. Since justice is so important to these people, they may find themselves at the front lines of various causes, possibly even lobbying for these causes. Individuals with a lot of Wood energy will always be searching for a better, faster, more just way to approach something. They have a contagious, strong spirit that, when balanced, can create a global movement for change. As with the Philosopher archetype, they are like pioneers, adventuring into often unknown territory to set things right in the world.

EMOTION

Anger is the emotion of Wood. I find that this emotion in particular can always use a little extra tending because anger gets a bad rap in Western culture. Most of us (especially women) are taught that anger indicates we are "out of control" and is not a welcome emotion to express. As children, many of us are encouraged to "go settle down" when we are angry before returning to the family or community. Yet anger is such a motivating and natural force of energy in our universe. I invite you to see anger a little bit differently with me right now.

When the ancient Taoists referred to anger, they were describing a quality of energy. Simply put, it is the energy of forward movement. Anger contains within it a sense of self-righteousness. When anger gets out of control, it can become one of the most destructive forces on the planet, and this I call rage. Rage is different from anger. The most important distinction we must make when discussing anger is to position it opposite rage, which is describing the out-of-control aspect of this energy that often equals destruction, not creativity. Anger in its own right is creative and constructive, and it can be fierce when we are fighting for something we believe in.

TRANSFORMING ANGER

Think about the last time you were angry. What were you fighting for? So often, there is a feeling of injustice underneath anger. Anger is the emotion that allows us to see clearly what we know could be different. What are you angry about in general right now in your life? If you could quit your job and dedicate your life to service, what would you want to see change in the world? As you think about this, feel the energy rise up in your body. That energy is the gift of the Wood element. Doesn't it fill you with an incredible sense of power and clarity? When skillfully used, this energy can lead to creative resolution in any arena.

When the Wood element goes out of balance, it is most often due to imbalances in the liver and, less often, the gallbladder, though the two organs really impact one another. Because the liver is responsible for the smooth flow of all chi in the body, when it goes out of balance, it is often very obvious. We can feel this imbalance every-where, including emotions, the digestive system, and even the musculoskeletal sys-tem. The expression of emotions of all kinds is what will keep our Wood element func-tioning optimally.

Wood element imbalances almost always lead to feelings of anger and resentment, because when the liver is depleted, it tends to get backed up with chi. This backup is both caused by and leads to repressed emotions. Interestingly, thousands of years ago when liver depletion was first described, it was significantly rarer than it is today. I can easily say that one in three people who come to my office are experiencing this imbalance. This is a sign of the times: many of us are not getting our deeper needs met.

Another challenge to the Wood element, and especially the liver, is that when we repress emotions, we naturally begin to look for ways to self-soothe. These ways often involve substances like caffeine, alcohol, marijuana, sugar, and prescription or other drugs. The consequence is that these substances end up taxing the liver even further. It's a vicious cycle brought on by the challenges of our time. The day-to-day pressures of finances, relationships, family, work/life balance, and so on are enough to challenge our very life force. Substance use is a way to make everything feel okay for now but only makes sense when we have no other tools to use to transform these difficult feelings.

BALANCED WOOD

- Clear vision and direction
- Goals that are important and practical
- Excellent planning and decision-making skills
- Expert in teamwork
- High energy
- Ability to focus
- Ability to rally others to action
- Natural leadership qualities
- Creativity
- Systems thinker
- Ability to find calm in the chaos
- Relaxation when there is structure
- Insight and intuitiveness
- Love of a challenge
- Ambition
- Competitiveness

OUT OF BALANCE WOOD

- Lack of direction in life, feelings of being stuck
- Anger, frustration, irritability
- Depression
- Repressed anger/experiences of rage
- Tendency toward addiction
- Bossiness, tendency to micromanage
- Isolation
- Grandiose ideas that aren't followed through
- Loud voice
- Exhibitions of temper
- Overly competitive/aggressive nature
- Clumsiness (bumping into things)
- Stubbornness
- Narrow-mindedness (can only see one way to do things)
- Resentment
- Sensation of oppression in the chest
- Nausea, vomiting, belching, sour regurgitation
- Bitter taste in the mouth
- Yellowing of sclera (jaundice)
- Dry, cracked, brittle nails
- Floaters in the eyes
- Dizziness, tinnitus
- Headaches, especially at the back of the head
- Bloodshot, painful, or burning eyes
- Sensation of a lump in the throat
- Muscle cramps, tremors
- PMS

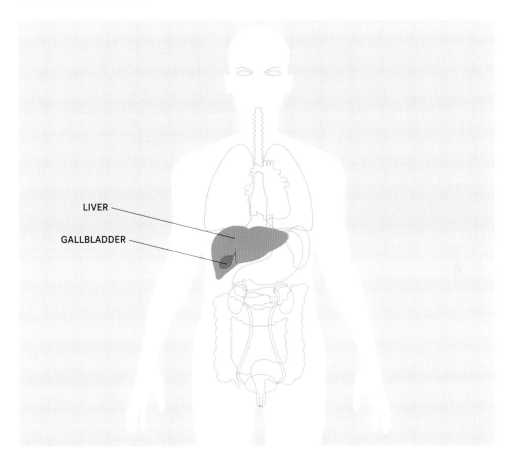

LIVER

GALLBLADDER

Liver

The liver is the largest internal organ in the body and is responsible for many processes, such as making proteins and blood-clotting factors, manufacturing triglycerides and cholesterol (fats), synthesizing glycogen (sugar), and producing bile. With all of these processes happening, the most important thing to remember is that the liver's primary job is detoxification. By passing all the blood in the body through its tissues, it is able to pull out toxins and help the body get rid of them. Even if someone is overloaded with toxins, the liver will actually hold on to them for a brief period so as not to inundate the body with them. Isn't that amazing? The liver also works as a storage facility for important vitamins such as folic acid; iron; and vitamins A, B_{12}, D, and K.

The production of bile is precisely what makes the liver both an organ and a gland. Since glands secrete chemicals, the liver functions to secrete bile.

OFFICIAL IN CHARGE OF PLANNING

In classical Chinese medicine the liver is referred to as the "Official in Charge of Planning." Its job, aside from the physical aspect of storing, filtering, and moving blood, is to assist us in planning for our lives. When healthy, balanced, and full of energy, the liver takes the blueprint from our kidneys and supports us in fulfilling that vision. Sometimes the liver is referred to as the "General" because when it is functioning optimally, it helps us to listen to our inner voice, to be clear about what our vision is for ourselves and our lives, and to create the necessary plans to carry out that vision. Sometimes this agenda can make us operate as a loving General, leading from our highest good, especially when we are fully tapped into body, mind, and spirit. However, if we don't have everything we need to fulfill our destiny, including ample liver energy, our agenda can become a blindfold instead of panoramic vision. We may start to become irritable and even give a little shout now and then. We may begin to see, instead of openings and opportunities, closures and impossibilities. When this narrowing of vision happens, we are at risk of becoming the General without an army to lead.

Gallbladder

The gallbladder is another organ governed by the Wood element. This organ sits just under the liver and is a sac that stores the bile produced by the liver. Its primary job is to release that bile into the small intestine each time we eat a meal to help us break down and absorb fats. Bile is made up of salts that assist in the breakdown of fats to help the small intestine absorb them. Interestingly, even if you don't have a gallbladder (because of surgery or were simply born without one), you still have the opportunity to carry the energy of this organ. In fact, the liver essentially takes on the gallbladder's job (though additional lifestyle changes and supplementation is often recommended).

Ligaments and Tendons

The Wood element controls the health of the ligaments and tendons throughout the body. Ligaments connect bone to bone, and tendons connect muscle to bone. When

In Chinese medicine the gallbladder is referred to as the "Official in Charge of Decision-Making and Judgment," and it works alongside the liver to assist in carrying out the plans needed to manifest our vision (from the smaller visions that make up each day to the larger vision of life). The gallbladder's job is to make sure that the decisions we make are in total alignment with the vision put forth by the liver, based on the blueprint from the kidneys. In the earlier example of a woman giving birth, in a perfect world, the kidneys would signal to her that she in fact wants to become a parent before she does. Then the liver would create the vision needed to manifest becoming a mother, and the gallbladder would assist in making the decisions necessary to support this vision and carry it through.

When the gallbladder isn't functioning well, however, decisions and judgment calls can become skewed. We may find ourselves making decisions that don't align with what we know we need or going into "analysis paralysis," where we have plenty of information but still can't make a decision about something. This is a sign the gallbladder needs support. On a physical level, when we have a gallbladder deficiency we might become clumsy, suddenly and repeatedly bumping into furniture that has been in the same position for years. This is because even our spatial awareness and proprioception (the ability to perceive where the body is in space without having to look) can become compromised when the gallbladder needs attention.

these tissues are nourished, we are strong yet flexible. If the ligaments and tendons are tight enough, they can hold a broken bone in place. But if they are either too tight or too loose, they can tear the bones apart. The health of the liver and gallbladder can be judged by the health of the ligaments and tendons. If you or someone you know is constantly tearing ligaments and tendons, that is a sign of a Wood element imbalance.

Eyes

The eyes are also governed by the Wood element. When bile backs up in your body, you get jaundice and this is visible first and foremost by the whites of your eyes turning yellow. Similarly, the eyes reflect much about the spirit, and when you are angry, your eyes are the first place it shows. The lids tend to open wider, and the eyes become fixated, developing a hardness.

Nails

The health of the fingernails is an excellent way to assess some aspects of Wood element health, most especially the liver. However, because the fingernails often take some time to grow, they won't be the first place to show an imbalance. Practitioners of Chinese medicine will often assess the health of your nails to check liver function and potential zinc deficiency. Strong, healthy nails with pink nail beds is what everyone wants. If you have white spots, ridges, or pale nail beds, it may be worth evaluating your liver with a practitioner.

WIND

There is a concept in Chinese Medicine called *wind* that can afflict someone on the outside or on the inside. In nature, wind tends to come around more in the spring and fall. However, springtime and the Wood element are often associated with this concept. Wind can be extremely aggravating for anyone, but especially so for someone with a Wood imbalance. Wind was considered primarily an external pathogen many years ago when most humans still lived outside and were especially vulnerable to the elements, bacteria, and viruses. Now that most people live indoors, external wind is less of an issue except in regard to pathogens. We do, however, still see quite a bit of what is called internal wind, which develops as a result of burning the candle at both ends and/or experiencing severe emotional stress. Both can create significant heat in the body which is most often the basis for internal wind. Internal wind pathology can be described this way:

1. Imbalances in which the symptoms move to different parts of the body (one day it's in the neck, the next it's in the shoulder, and so on)
2. Imbalances that cause excess movement of the body, such as tremors, epilepsy, Parkinson's disease, and dystonia
3. Imbalances that cause loss of movement, such as stroke, paralysis, tetany, and coma
4. Acute imbalances such as the common cold, flu, hay fever, sinus infections, itchy skin conditions, sore throats, coughs, dizziness, vertigo, and headaches

THE SPRING PANTRY
FEATURED RECIPES

Since most of what we see around us this time of year is birth and growth, the predominant theme of springtime is *renewal*. As such, this season is a perfect time to focus on building a good foundation for the rest of the year. This also means, by waking up the liver and gallbladder after their winter slumber, it's a great time of year to cleanse! Cleansing helps us to reset our systems so we can start fresh.

There are some things to consider during this transition from winter to spring, as it can be a fragile time of year, leaving us susceptible to illness if we aren't careful. This is partly due to the following:

- **We get moving too quickly.** Winter is supposed to be a time of slowness, and some of us get ants in our pants. Once we see that first spring bloom in our neighborhood, we grab our running shoes and out the door we go. We try to move from zero to one hundred in one fell swoop. That's going to get us sick. We must go slowly in those early weeks of spring. If you feel ready to get out and get moving, add more and more activity to each day to get up to where you would like to be.
- **We didn't winter well.** We may not have actually taken time to rest during the winter months. So while the mind may be ready for more sunlight, warmth, and movement, the body still wants to rest and restore.

Think of this transition as a gradual ascension of energy from the beginning to the end of spring. That means you incorporate springtime foods early in the season, and by the end you are eating mostly from this menu. This strategy will keep your energy moving and strong; prevent the colds that everyone else is getting this time of year; and sustain your body, mind, and spirit for the rest of the year.

Here are the general principles of springtime nutrition:

- Maintain the mostly cooked and warm principle of winter, especially in early spring.
- Cook foods at a slightly higher temperature for a slightly shorter time, leaving vegetables al dente.
- Begin introducing some raw foods into your diet early in the spring.
- Seek out sour flavors.
- Slowly increase the number of sour foods in your pantry over the course of the season.
- Reduce your intake of oily foods during these months.
- Eat lots of sprouts, shoots, and baby leaves.
- Master the art of sprouting seeds, nuts, and legumes.
- Avoid heavier foods such as dairy, fried foods, large amounts of protein, and nut butters.
- Eat all foods that are green in color.
- Drink one cup of warm lemon water every morning (juice of half a lemon).
- Enjoy fermented foods one or two times per day.

Springtime Staples

PROTEINS: Crab, crayfish, eggs, liver, lobster, mussels, oysters, pork, shrimp, squid, trout, venison, whitefish

GRAINS: Sprouted grains (if well tolerated)

VEGETABLES: Asparagus, baby greens, bamboo shoots, barley grass, beets, carrots, cruciferous vegetables (broccoli, cabbage, cauliflower, kohlrabi, and rutabaga), leafy greens (collard greens, kale, and Swiss chard), potatoes, spirulina, sprouts (all kinds), turnips, wheatgrass

FRUITS: Anything fresh and local, in moderation during the early stages of spring

LEGUMES: Mung beans, tempeh

NUTS AND SEEDS: Flaxseeds, pine nuts, sesame seeds

DAIRY: Goat's milk products (if well tolerated); avoid cow's milk products

HERBS TO COOK WITH: Apple cider vinegar, cayenne (avoid in cases of heat), chives, garlic, onions, parsley, turmeric

FOODS TO AVOID: Alcohol, caffeine, coffee, fried foods, greasy foods, spicy and hot foods, processed and refined foods, sugar

---

SPRINGTIME FLAVOR: SOUR

- If you are **cold**, add in *pungent* (page 90) and warming foods (page 93).
- If you are **lethargic**, add in *sweet* (page 89) and tonifying foods (page 95).
- If you are **dry**, add in *moistening* foods (page 94).

SPRING RECIPES FOR RENEWAL

The following recipes are ones that I find myself gravitating toward again and again during the spring. They provide that perfect edge of slight sweet-sourness in new baby greens and shoots. Each recipe serves to wake up the liver and gallbladder and to support their function of digestion of fats and detoxification.

Soaking and Sprouting

Since springtime is all about eating the new life popping up out of the ground, it is also about eating sprouts! Use this time of year to master sprouting; it greatly amplifies the nutrient density of beans, grains, seeds, and nuts. Sprouting also makes these foods significantly easier to digest; increases their availability of protein and minerals such as calcium, iron, and zinc, as well as vitamin B_{12}; and allows you to gain more available fiber from your food.[1] Sprouting is especially important if you have a more sensitive belly and don't tend to tolerate these foods raw.

So, what can you sprout? Just about everything! The only items that cannot be sprouted are heat-treated, processed, and roasted seeds, nuts, beans, and grains. For the most part, you can only do step 1 of the sprouting process (soaking) with nuts, as most of them won't actually sprout. Here is a list of some of my favorite things to sprout: almonds (soaking only), barley (unhulled), chickpeas, millet, mung beans, peas, and sunflower seeds.

The wonderful thing about soaking nuts is that they easily become nut milks after they have soaked. (Have a look at the Sweet Nut Milk recipe on page 211.) Additionally, nut butters, creamy sauces, cheese-like foods, and even gravies can be prepared from soaked nuts. The options are endless, but the nutrients are dense no matter what you choose.

Sprouting has two basic steps:

1. Soaking: This is the practice of putting seeds, nuts, grains, and legumes in water for a certain period of time (which differs depending on what you are using and for what purpose). Soaking softens the exterior coating of the seed, nut, grain, or legume and partially germinates it. This is the best process for digesting nuts since they do not sprout. Soaking must happen before the next step with all other items.

Choose a raw and unprocessed seed, nut, grain, or legume. Once you have selected what you want to soak, select a clean jar or bowl that will hold the amount you have plus several inches of water on top of it. After rinsing your seeds, nuts, grains, or legumes and discarding any debris, put them in the jar. Cover them with room temperature water that rises several inches above the top of what you are sprouting. Cover with a kitchen towel, and soak according to the time recommendations in the table on page 81. Strain and cover with fresh water every twelve hours while soaking.

After the soaking process is finished, put the product in the fridge and use within a few days. Or if you are sprouting the product, do that immediately after soaking.

2. Sprouting: This is the practice of fully germinating a seed, grain, or legume after soaking it. You'll know when it sprouts because the product will crack open, and a little shoot will reveal itself. Sprouts are far more nutrient-dense than foods that are simply soaked due to the increase in available nutrients.

Immediately after soaking, strain the product and place it in a shallow bowl on the countertop where it will be exposed to room temperature air. Keep it slightly damp as it is sprouting, either by spritzing with water or by sprinkling one or two tablespoons of water on top.

Sprouting time depends on the food you are working with. When you see sprouts, rinse them well, drain, and store them in the refrigerator for no longer than seven days. They are fragile and susceptible to mold, so they need to be rinsed with fresh water and drained every day they are in the fridge.

SPROUTED SAVORY MUNG BEAN PANCAKES
• MAKES 4 SERVINGS •

Hands down, this is one of my favorite Korean-inspired recipes to have either by itself or in combination with another side. Sprouted mung bean pancakes provide tons of nutrients and include all things spring, such as green onions, sprouts, and fermented foods! There are many variations of these pancakes, including vegetarian or not, and spicy or mild.

1 cup mung beans (turns into 2 cups once sprouted)

1 organic, cage-free egg or ¾ cup plain yogurt or full-fat coconut milk

1 tablespoon flour (rice or quinoa work well)

¾ to 1½ pounds organic pork loin, finely chopped

1 tablespoon sesame oil

1 tablespoon finely chopped fresh ginger

2 cloves garlic, finely chopped

½ teaspoon salt

¼ teaspoon black pepper

4 green onions, chopped

¼ cup cilantro, chopped

1½ cups kimchi, chopped

Butter, ghee, lard, or coconut oil for frying

FOR THE DIPPING SAUCE

¼ cup tamari

½ teaspoon sesame oil

2 teaspoons maple syrup

2 cloves garlic, minced

2 green onions, chopped

TIPS • Flour can be omitted entirely to accommodate grain-free diets.

• You can use tofu instead of the pork loin or omit the protein entirely.

Sprout the mung beans a day in advance following the guidelines on page 81.

To prepare the pancakes, combine the sprouted mung beans, egg or yogurt, and flour (if using) in a food processor or blender. Blend on medium-high until the mixture has the consistency of pancake batter. If it is too thick, add water, 1 tablespoon at a time, until it is the right consistency. Pour the batter into a large mixing bowl and add all the remaining ingredients except the butter. Reserve a tablespoon of cilantro for garnish.

Add 1 to 2 tablespoons of butter to a large frying pan or griddle and set to medium-high heat. When it is hot (but not smoking), pour in ¼ cup of the batter. Fry until the pancake is thoroughly cooked and browned, about 4 minutes on each side.

CONTINUES

While the pancakes are frying, make the dipping sauce by mixing all the ingredients together in a bowl.

Serve the pancakes with the sauce, and garnish with chopped cilantro, if desired. Leftover dipping sauce can be stored in the refrigerator for up to 10 days.

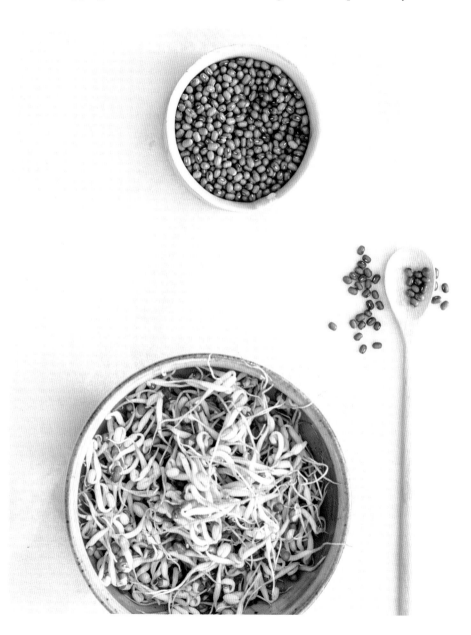

SPRINGTIME SALAD WITH GRILLED ASPARAGUS

This is one of my favorite salads to make in the spring because it is a mixture of bitter and sweet, cooked and raw, and it introduces healthy fats as well. Depending on where you live, asparagus may not be around until mid-April or May. But as soon as it hits the grocery stores, I invite you to begin finding a million ways to enjoy it. You can easily bake it in the oven and season it with olive oil, salt, and pepper for a simple treat. Or enjoy this fantastic liver-boosting recipe.

1 pound asparagus

¼ cup olive oil

Salt and pepper to taste

1 tablespoon fresh lemon juice

1 teaspoon Dijon mustard

1 medium shallot, minced

¼ cup organic plain yogurt (optional)

6 organic, cage-free eggs

6 cups organic arugula (can be baby arugula if matured is too spicy)

¾ cup freshly shaved Parmigiano Reggiano cheese (optional)

Heat a grill or grill pan. Brush the asparagus with 1 tablespoon of the olive oil and season with salt and pepper. Grill the asparagus over high heat until tender with a few charred spots, about 5 minutes. Keep warm in the oven. Instead of grilling, you can also preheat the oven to 450°F and bake the asparagus for about 5 minutes until crisp-tender, or broil for 3 minutes.

Make the lemon vinaigrette by whisking 3 tablespoons of the olive oil with the lemon juice, Dijon mustard, shallot, and yogurt (if using). Add salt and pepper to taste.

Bring a small pot of water to a boil, then gently add the eggs and boil for approximately 8 minutes. (This time gives you slightly runny yolks, so boil longer if you prefer them firm.) Remove the eggs and place them in a bowl of ice water for 2 minutes. Peel, cut into quarters, and season with salt and pepper.

In a large bowl, toss the arugula with the lemon vinaigrette, then transfer the salad to a large bowl or plate. Top with the asparagus, eggs, and cheese (if using). Enjoy right away!

It's more important to wake up the liver during this season than at any other time of year. So sticking to foods that make you pucker will continue to do that for you. This simple smoothie is something I drink a couple of mornings a week during spring. It's a quick and easy addition to breakfast.

½ grapefruit, peeled and cut in sections, leaving as much pith as possible

Juice of 1 lemon

2 tablespoons olive oil

1 clove garlic

Juice of 1 orange

Put all the ingredients in a blender and puree until smooth. Enjoy!

TIP · I highly recommend using fresh fruits for this recipe instead of simply the bottled juices. The reason is that many (if not most) of the nutrients you want from these fruits is found in the pulp and pith. Juice alone tends to just add sugar from the fruit.

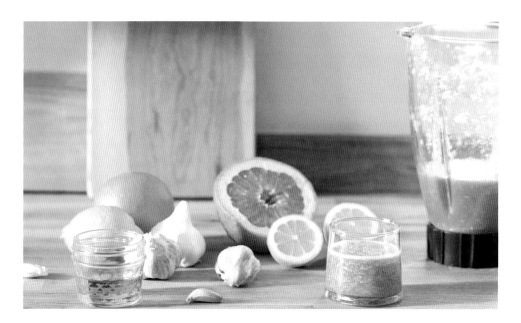

This tea is not to be consumed every day for an extended period. Consider drinking it daily for 14 days then taking at least 14 days off before starting again.

- 1 tablespoon dried dandelion root, chopped
- 1 tablespoon dried burdock root, chopped
- 2 tablespoons raw, unfiltered organic apple cider vinegar
- 2 tablespoons lemon juice
- ½ to 1 teaspoon ground ginger
- ½ to 1 teaspoon ground turmeric
- ¼ teaspoon ground cinnamon
- 1 dash cayenne powder
- 1 teaspoon raw local honey (optional)

TIPS • Omit the cinnamon if you have heat signs.
  • Add the cayenne powder only if you have cold hands and feet or sluggish digestion.

Bring 8 ounces of water to a boil, then pour over the dandelion root and burdock root. Steep for a minimum of 15 minutes or up to overnight and then strain and discard the roots. Add the dandelion and burdock root tea along with the rest of the ingredients to a cocktail shaker (if possible) or a large jar. Fill with 8 ounces of warm water and shake until thoroughly blended. Pour the tea into two glasses, and drink throughout the day.

CHRYSANTHEMUM TEA (JU HUA)

In China, this herb has legendary healing capabilities and its use can be traced as far back as 2695 B.C.E. The golden flowers of this plant are used to make a deliciously sweet and slightly bitter tea that is not only tasty but also serves to detoxify and cool the liver. Chrysanthemum tea is wonderful to enjoy all spring and summer, either hot or cool. However, if you are experiencing cold patterns (yang deficiency), this herb might be too cooling.

WARM GINGER LEMON TEA WITH MINT • MAKES 1 SERVING

Each morning, especially in the spring, I like to wake up and give my liver a little nourishment. The liver loves all things that make us pucker, so lemon water and lemon tea are the go-tos for drinks at this time of year. For simple lemon water, I recommend 1 cup of room temperature water with the juice of half a fresh lemon squeezed in. If you would like to add the balancing herbs of ginger (warming) and mint (cooling), they create a lovely synergistic tea that stimulates the brain, digestive system, and liver all at once.

Juice of ½ lemon

1 thumb-size piece of ginger, peeled and sliced lengthwise

3 to 5 sprigs of mint (spearmint, peppermint) or basil

1 cup hot but not boiling water

Steep the lemon, ginger, and mint sprigs in the water for 5 to 8 minutes. Strain before drinking.

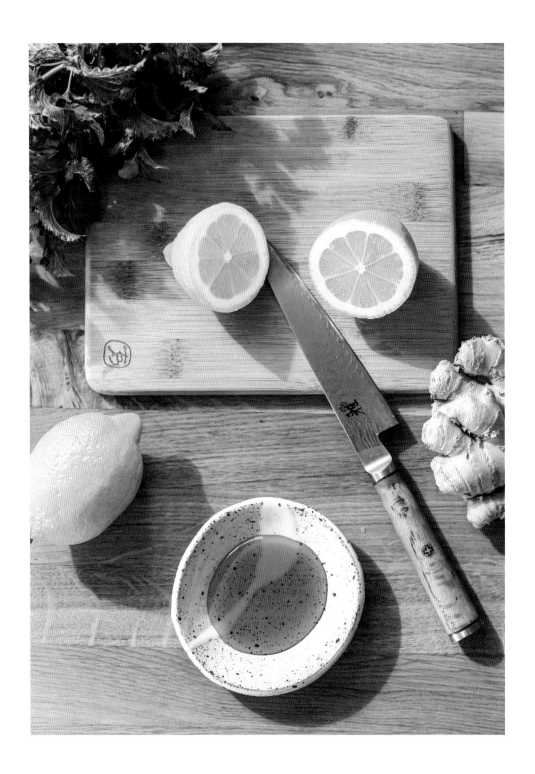

THE SPRING MEDICINE CABINET

This season reflects the movement from the most yin time of the year (winter) to the most yang time of year (summer). This season of transition can make you vulnerable to the changes in weather and energy storage versus energy output. It's a perfect time of year to ease into activity and slowly increase your energy for summer.

Since the liver and gallbladder are the primary organs in need of support this season, you will find that many of the herbs presented have a dual function of supporting the liver and gallbladder and of strengthening the immune system as you transition out of winter. To support the liver and gallbladder does not necessarily mean cleansing them. Sometimes the approach needs to be to nourish them instead. In fact, consuming cleansing herbs every day can wear out the liver over time. It's best to have a focused time for cleansing and then take breaks.

Bupleurum

PINYIN: Chai Hu

ORIGIN: China

PART USED: Root

ORGANS / SYSTEMS SUPPORTED: Liver, gallbladder, pericardium, stomach, triple burner, upper chest, uterus

USES: PMS (and virtually all menstrual irregularities), immune system imbalances, irritability, heaviness in the chest, dizziness/vertigo, emotional instability, bloating, gas, constipation, nausea, indigestion, hemorrhoids

PATTERNS SUPPORTED: Liver chi stagnation, spleen chi deficiency, wei qi deficiency

FLAVORS: Bitter, pungent

TEMPERATURE: Cool

ACTIONS: Tonifying, blood-building

CONTRAINDICATIONS: None known

BEST TAKEN: Decoction (3 to 12 grams/day)

Burdock

PINYIN: Niu Bang Zi

ORIGIN: Northern Asia and Europe

PARTS USED: Root (in the West); fruit/seeds (in the East)

ORGANS / SYSTEMS SUPPORTED: Digestive system, liver, lungs, stomach, blood, skin

USES: Recurrent colds and flu, weakened immune system, pneumonia, fever, cough, sore throat, hemorrhoids, skin conditions (eczema, acne, psoriasis), constipation

PATTERNS SUPPORTED: Liver chi stagnation, liver fire blazing, blood stagnation, wei qi deficiency (with fevers), damp heat in the large intestine, heat and dryness in the large intestine

FLAVORS: Bitter, pungent

TEMPERATURE: Cooling

ACTIONS: Tonifying, moistening

CONTRAINDICATIONS: Not to be consumed during pregnancy and lactation due to mild diuretic effect

BEST TAKEN: Decoction (6 to 9 grams/day)

Cyperus

PINYIN: Xiang Fu

ORIGIN: China

PART USED: Rhizome

ORGANS / SYSTEMS SUPPORTED: Liver, triple burner, spleen

USES: Digestive imbalances such as epigastric and abdominal pain, cramps associated with PMS, irregular menstruation, dysmenorrhea, emotional imbalances, breast swelling and tenderness (associated with PMS)

PATTERNS SUPPORTED: Liver chi stagnation, blood stagnation

FLAVORS: Pungent, slightly sweet, slightly bitter

TEMPERATURE: Slightly warm

ACTION: Tonifying

CONTRAINDICATIONS: For use only when chi or blood stagnation is present

BEST TAKEN: Decoction (6 to 12 grams/day)

Dandelion

PINYIN: Pu Gong Ying

ORIGIN: Asia and Europe

PARTS USED: Roots, leaves, occasionally flowers

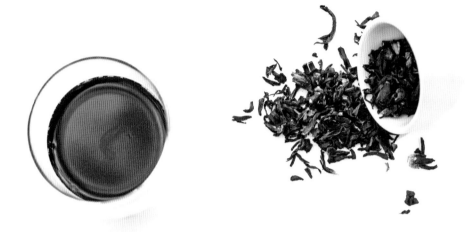
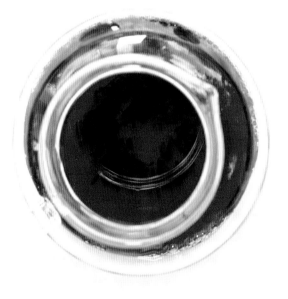

ORGANS / SYSTEMS SUPPORTED: Liver, stomach, kidneys, digestive system, skin, muscles

USES: High cholesterol, UTIs, irritability, fatigue, breast tumors, jaundice, urinary disorders, liver disease, loss of appetite, gallstones, constipation, eczema

PATTERNS SUPPORTED: Liver chi stagnation, blood stagnation, liver fire blazing

FLAVORS: Bitter, slightly sweet

TEMPERATURE: Cold

ACTIONS: Tonifying, astringent

CONTRAINDICATIONS: None known

BEST TAKEN: Decoction (3 to 5 grams/day)

Hibiscus

PINYIN: Mei Gui Qi

ORIGIN: North Africa and Southeast Asia

PART USED: Flowers

ORGANS / SYSTEMS SUPPORTED: Lungs, liver, digestive system, immune system, skin

USES: Cough, high blood pressure, gallstones (or other gallbladder issues), stubborn weight gain, high cholesterol, digestive problems (diarrhea and constipation), heart disease, diabetes, UTIs, menstrual disorders, fever, skin conditions with heat, chronic and recurrent colds and flu, anxiety

PATTERNS SUPPORTED: Liver fire blazing, wei qi deficiency, blood stagnation

FLAVORS: Sour, slightly sweet

TEMPERATURE: Slightly cooling

ACTIONS: Tonifying, mildly astringent, calming

CONTRAINDICATIONS: Caution required in cases of diabetes, as this potent liver cleanser may lower blood sugar

BEST TAKEN: Hot infusion (6 to 10 grams/day) or decoction (6 to 10 grams/day. Note that as these are flowers, they don't need to be cooked very long. So if you are preparing a decoction with other roots and barks, only add the hibiscus in for the last 5 minutes.)

Tangerine Peel

PINYIN: Chen Pi

ORIGIN: China

PART USED: Peel

ORGANS / SYSTEMS SUPPORTED: Respiratory system, digestive system, liver, gallbladder, spleen, stomach, large intestine

USES: Cough, congestion, loss of appetite, fatigue, loose stools

PATTERNS SUPPORTED: Spleen chi deficiency, liver chi stagnation

FLAVORS: Pungent, bitter

TEMPERATURE: Warm

ACTIONS: Tonifying, astringent

CONTRAINDICATIONS: None known

BEST TAKEN: Decoction (3 to 9 grams/day)

Springtime Formulas

MINOR BUPLEURUM DECOCTION (*PIN YIN XIAO CHAI HU TANG*): One of the most commonly used Chinese medicine formulas of the twenty-first century, this formula prevents illness and resets immune system imbalances. It supports the liver in all ways—detoxifying, treating hepatitis and jaundice—and eases inflammation in any of the organs.

FREE AND EASY WANDERER (*XIAO YAO SAN*): Hands down the most commonly prescribed Chinese medicine formula, this is used to treat liver chi stagnation, liver blood deficiency, symptoms of PMS, irritability, depression, and general moodiness. Fatigue, headaches, and dizziness are also often eased with this formula. Who wouldn't want to wander freely and easily?

NOURISHING PRACTICES IN SPRING

Moving Your Body

Coming out of winter and into spring is like a crescendo of energy coming into the landscape, into the wildlife, and into our bodies. Riding that wave means not simply jumping into high-intensity movement practices, but rather slowly increasing the intensity and frequency of our movements over the course of spring. Due to the liver's propensity to stagnate, it's vital that as the seasons change, we get moving a little bit every day. Some people, depending on their constitution, need exercise every day all year round and especially as spring emerges.

Taking Brisk Walks or a Short Run

This is soothing to the Wood element because both of these activities wake up the Liver and Gallbladder meridians that run along the inner and outer legs. A brisk walk will get your heart pounding and your lungs breathing hard; if it doesn't, perhaps a short run will do. In the spring I prefer interval running where you have moments of higher intensity followed by a moment of lower intensity (walk, run, walk, run, and so on). This type of exercise follows the energy pattern of the season quite well.

Practicing More Vigorous Yoga

You can begin increasing your yogic practice as well. Any Hatha Yoga classes and/or practices that you are drawn to this season will be great but avoid the hot yoga classes for now (unless you are coming out of winter feeling cold in your body). The challenge with hot yoga is that it can be depleting for some people and nourishing for others. Check your local studio for donation-based or sliding-scale classes if you need to, or take advantage of the many free classes online.

Growing Something—Anything

There is hardly anything more exciting and hopeful than watching a plant grow from a tiny seed into a beautiful flowering, fruiting being! So much of the theme of this season has to do with birth, growth, renewal, and hope. The emotions that stir in us, even as adults, when we watch a plant grow are hope and childlike wonder. Even if all you do is grow or nurture a flower pot or toss some seeds out by the front door, you are waking up that springtime energy and witnessing the manifestation of the Wood element in the natural world.

Doing Neti Pot Rinses

With all the plant activity of spring, many people can get sensitive sinuses or even seasonal allergies. The best way to work with this is to first, do a cleanse in the spring (see Appendix E), and second, do neti pot rinses one to three times each week using sea salt and warm water. This supports a good environment in your upper respiratory tract. Use only distilled, warm water and ¼ teaspoon of sea salt. Also, many people have forced air heat in their homes, which is challenging for the sinuses in the winter months. If you find that your sinuses tend to be dry, rubbing a little sesame oil in your nostrils after rinsing can be very hydrating and soothing. You can do this with a dropper and/or a cotton swab.

Creating a Vision Board

Since spring, and specifically the energy of the Wood element, is all about visioning and planning, what a perfect time of year to create a vision board. Try setting an intention by answering this question: "What would I like to call into my life this year?" Then grab a bunch of old magazines that you once loved and start flipping through them for the images, words, and letters that represent the answer to this question. Piece by piece, as you glue your board together, hold your intentions in your mind so that your vision board becomes a hanging reminder of what you are calling in until next spring.

Forest Bathing

John Muir wrote, "Thousands of tired, nerve-shaken, over-civilized people are beginning to find out that going to the mountains is going home; that wildness is a necessity." Forest bathing is this practice of "going home" by placing yourself in a natural environment without an agenda. Whereas hiking usually has a trail, a beginning, and an end, forest bathing is a meandering, with the only goals being to open your senses, follow your impulses, and go slowly. It's quite refreshing and much needed to balance those sometimes fast-paced, goal-saturated days.

Setting a Bedtime

The time when the Wood element has the most energy is from 11 P.M. to 3 A.M., and the classical texts advise that if you are not asleep by 11 P.M., you will likely feel falsely enlivened by your liver and gallbladder's energy as they wake up between those hours. You may find yourself getting a burst of creative energy or being loaded with thoughts if you don't make it to sleep before this window. You need the liver and gallbladder to do their work of cleansing and detoxing while you are asleep.

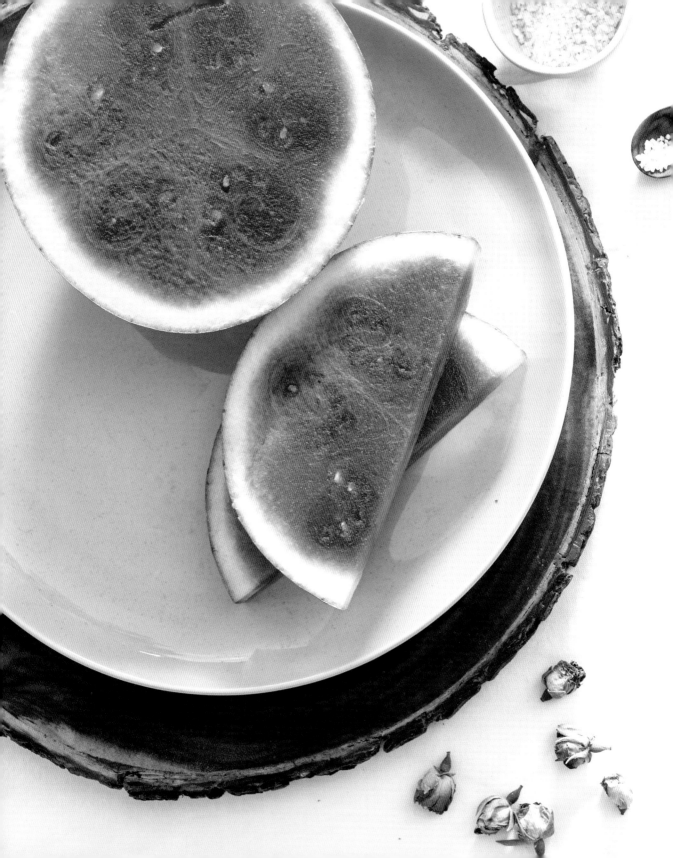

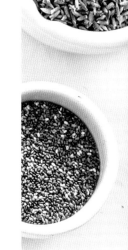

SUMMER AND THE FIRE ELEMENT

SUMMER SOLSTICE (JUNE 21) THROUGH MID-AUGUST

To be in harmony with the atmosphere of Summer,
awaken early in the morning and reach to the sun
for nourishment to flourish as the gardens do.
Work, play, travel, be joyful, and grow into selfless service.
The bounty of the outside world enters and enlivens us.

—PAUL PITCHFORD, in *Healing with Whole Foods*

— ◆ —

Following the significant birth and growth agenda of spring, summer holds within it a beautiful pause from the hard work of growing upward and instead begins to expand. This is also a time for some serious celebration. Summer is, after all, the most yang time of year. We may find ourselves naturally feeling lighter and more joyful. The weather changes to the warmest it will be all year, and that means it's time to play outside. It's time to enjoy ourselves now that we have worked so hard during winter and spring to get here.

The summer season is all about *expansion* and *activity*. This is the time of year when all the plants that have dared to germinate in winter and climb toward the sun in spring are going for their full capacity. The sun will be at its full strength for the longest time each day, creating the perfect conditions for this expansion. Therefore, this season provides the energy of taking up space by giving plants what they need to reach out to the farthest points possible. Most plants reach their full potential for the year during this season. The same is true for us too.

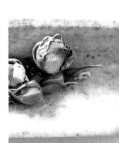

When the Fire is hot, we go play in the water, host parties, connect with friends, and plan travel. Summer is the time for being with people in a playful way and is a great time for connection.

Since Summer is the most yang season, we call it "Yang within Yang." This means that much of our energy can be spent in an extroverted manner relatively without consequence during this time (whatever yang means for our true selves). Nature will be doing the yang dance all around us—producing beautiful flowers with all the bright colors and putting smiles on our faces.

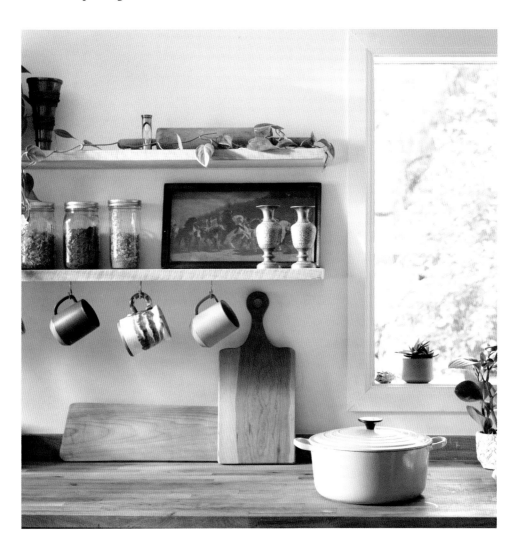

THE FIRE ELEMENT

Plain and simple, we all know the element of Fire. This could mean a hot, burning bonfire we sit around with our friends during the summer nights or the fiery ball in the sky we know as the sun. This element can represent the twinkling hot bed of coals at night under the stars or the gentle flame that ignites the gas to keep us warm or cook our food. Fire comes in many forms and represents a peak of energy, allowing everything to shine at its brightest, biggest, and boldest. Fire energy is about connecting deeply with those we enjoy and having a good time. It is about letting the inner child out to play and being filled with a sense of wonder no matter what our age. This is the energy of expansion and the most yang energy there is.

If we get too much sun, we can easily burn. But if we don't get enough, we can get really sick, so it's important to stay in sync with the Fire element. As we progress in an age of global warming, we are recognizing the extent of damage the modern industrial age has done to the atmosphere. The atmosphere's job is to provide a protective layer between us and the sun. Without it, the sun's rays are slowly becoming dangerous. Where we used to be lax about heading outside all day without sunscreen, we now know better.

If you have a lot of Fire in your constitution, you are probably very yang in nature. You are more playful, always wanting to plan an adventure and generally thinking big. While the Wood element can be fixated on generating the blueprint, the Fire element is all about getting creative with the plan and making sure it aligns with what makes you most passionate and excited about life.

FIRE CONSTITUTION

ARCHETYPE: THE MAGICIAN

People with a balanced Fire constitution tend to be very easygoing, social, and caring people. They listen well and often converse easily. They are the friends you call when you need a break from the stresses of life as they are more likely to get you out of the house and into some sort of adventure you might not have thought of on your own. In relationships, individuals with these constitutions (when in balance) are loyal because they themselves appreciate trust, transparency, and vulnerability. They may also laugh a lot and enjoy play as a way to lift the spirit. Similar to a magician, the Fire constitution type can be a bit theatrical but is also extremely attuned to others and naturally draws them in. When balanced, they are storytellers and entertainers, bringing life to all around them.

Joy is the dominant emotion of the Fire element, and it represents that crux of energy when two people share an intimacy. I'm not just talking about physical intimacy; it's also emotional intimacy or that moment when you see yourself in someone else. It is that excitement, curiosity, and pure delight of being with and truly seeing and being seen by another being. It is an energy of presence, as though nothing matters except for what is happening right here and right now. When we can bring this quality of energy and presence into our beings, our hearts naturally open, and love pours out of us. Everything that falls under our gaze when we are in a truly joyful state becomes beautiful and lovable.

Just like any emotion, even joy has its limits. In our culture we tend to think it's best to be joyful all the time, but that is not in balance with life. There are times for joy, of course. There is also time for sadness, grief, anger, fear, and a gentle contentment or peacefulness. To be joyful all the time can be exhausting. Have you ever been around someone who laughs a lot, and you don't get what's funny? Or the laughter simply isn't contagious? Maybe something feels off. That's a sign of an out of balance Fire element, at least on one end of the spectrum. In Chinese medicine, we sometimes refer to mania (one side of bipolar disorder) as a Fire imbalance.

If we have too much Fire, we may be overly loving (in an anxious way) or warm too quickly to a stranger and really hurt ourselves in the end. Whereas if we are exhausted and burned out and our Fire element is running low, we may feel flat, joyless, and sad.

The Fire element is most susceptible to burning out (depletion) and burning hot (excess heat), and due to the emphasis on connection and relationship at this time of year, we are more vulnerable to spirit imbalances as well. Often the first sign of a Fire imbalance is an emotional one. During summer, it's easy to get caught up in play, our social lives, and outdoor activities that we can sometimes forget to keep that yin around to maintain balance for our yang. Or the opposite can happen where we simply can't conjure up the energy for these kinds of things and find ourselves isolating or needing to modify our consciousness (like drinking a lot) to feel confident or have fun. The main organs that take the blow when our Fire loses balance are the yin organs: the heart and the pericardium.

BALANCED FIRE	OUT OF BALANCE FIRE
• Charismatic personality	• Anxiety
• Natural leadership ability	• Heart palpitations
• Highly social tendencies	• Restlessness
• Contagious laughter and sense of play	• Flatness
• Great sense of humor	• Disinterest in life
• "Life of the party"	• Chronic sadness
• Joyfulness/contentedness much of the time	• Sensitivity to heat
• High resilience	• Cravings for consciousness-altering substances
• People person	• Insomnia
• Trustworthiness and faith in others	• Depression
• Excellent speaker	• Propensity to stutter
• Optimistic outlook	• Inappropriate laughter
• Generosity	• Obsession with positivity (won't allow self to feel sadness or other emotions)
• Tendency to make friends easily	• Cold emotional behavior (or swings hot to cold)
• Many close friendships	• Bipolar disorder (manic to depressed or vice versa)
	• Canker or cold sores on mouth and tongue
	• Inability to trust
	• Hopelessness
	• Nervousness
	• Strong craving or aversion to intimacy, sex
	• Sense of dread
	• Vivid and/or disturbing dreams
	• Rapid or irregular heartbeat
	• Poor memory
	• Heart disease
	• Rapid and/or shortness of breath

YOUR BODY IN SUMMER

The Fire element is unique in that there are not two organs associated with it but four. They all work to keep the body warm or cool depending on what is needed, to sort through the pure from the impure, and to keep the blood moving.

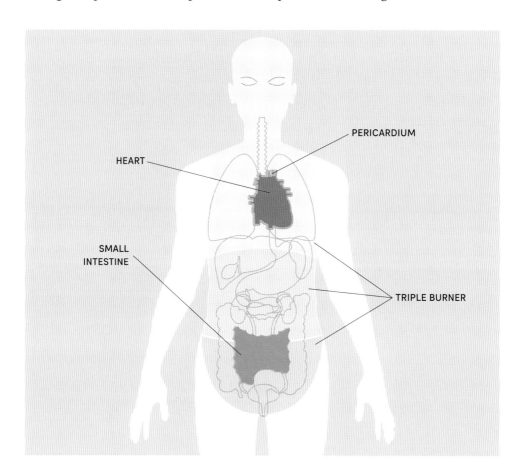

Heart

The heart is amazing. This single organ's job is to push five thousand gallons of blood throughout the entire body every twenty-four hours, ensuring that it receives oxygen and nutrients. The heart beats 100,000 times each day to make this happen, and it is only about the size of a fist. It sits in the chest, usually just a little off-center to the left. It houses multiple layers of muscles that protect its vital processes. Two upper chambers receive blood, and two lower chambers discharge it again. When the heart is functioning well, you feel fine and your body has access to good, oxygen-rich blood. When the heart is not functioning well, nothing in the rest of your body does either. The biggest strain on the heart at this point in human evolution is stress.

SUPREME CONTROLLER

In Chinese medicine, the heart is referred to as the "Supreme Controller" and is considered to be the empress or emperor presiding over the domain (meaning the rest of the body, mind, and spirit). As such, the heart is given respect as the leading force behind all aspects of life. When it comes to the importance of organs, the heart sits at the top of the hierarchy (rather than the brain as in Western science). The moment it stops functioning, you stop functioning. The heart is the ruler of everything and is therefore protected by all other organs in the system. They each have a unique relationship to the heart as they all serve different purposes in keeping it safe and in ensuring that the blueprint from the kidneys—intermingled with the spirit of the heart—is always being fulfilled.

Just as the kidneys are home to the ancestral chi, the heart is home to the spirit, or shen. The quality and vitality of your shen is reflected in your eyes and is therefore a wonderful way to assess how your spirit is doing. When you are spent, have struggled for a long time, or have experienced a trauma from which you are still recovering, the quality of your spirit as reflected through your eyes may look dull and lifeless. If you have ever looked into the eyes of an abused child, dog, or horse that was recently rescued, you will know exactly what I'm talking about. When you look into eyes like these, if your spirit is home and healthy, you can't help but feel compassion and tenderness.

Emotional health almost always comes back to the health of your heart and the strength of your spirit. Many mental and emotional health patterns can arise when this organ is not functioning well and therefore not creating the optimal home for your shen. Chinese medicine even has a diagnosis for this called "shen disturbance." This term indicates that the spirit of a person needs support and the number-one way to diagnose this is by looking into that person's eyes. Anxiety, depression, mania, hopelessness, inability to concentrate, insomnia, dream-disturbed sleep, heart palpitations, and being easily startled can also be signs of shen disturbance.

Small Intestine

The small intestine is about twenty feet long in an adult, and its job is to receive food from the stomach that has been churned and to process this food to sort out nutrients. Inside the lining of the small intestine are tiny, finger-like projections called villi. They even act like fingers combing through hair, pulling vital nutrients out of the chyme and sending them through the wall of the small intestine for absorption wherever they are most needed in the body. Ninety percent of the nutrients you need are absorbed in the small intestine! What's left is sent along to the large intestine. The small intestine is susceptible to certain kinds of bacterial overgrowth (called small intestine bacterial overgrowth, or SIBO) and to getting gummed up from eating gluten when there is sluggish digestion and especially gluten intolerance. Years of eating gluey gluten when your body doesn't process it well will flatten the villi, leading to less and less nutrient absorption.

SEPARATOR OF PURE FROM IMPURE

In Chinese medicine, the small intestine is called the "Separator of Pure from Impure." On a physical level, we can see this function as the villi literally separate what is useful to us from what is not. On an emotional and spiritual level, the small intestine's job is as a third (and final) line of defense against useless or harmful thoughts, information, and energy that could enter the heart. If the small intestine is doing its job, the mind feels free, our thoughts are clear, and our speech is both coherent and aligned with the true feelings of the heart.

Pericardium

The pericardium is a sac of muscle that surrounds the heart and functions as its protector. The pericardium ensures that the heart won't overfill with blood or overwork (literally by limiting its motion), lubricates the heart for smoother movement, and protects the heart from infection by being a physical barrier between the heart and the lungs (which are more prone to infection).

HEART PROTECTOR

The pericardium is referred to as the "Heart Protector" or the "Circulation-Sex Official" in classical Chinese medicine. Its job is essentially to take the blows from life and keep the heart out of the fray as much as possible. The Heart Protector is considered the second line of defense to protecting the heart from physical and emotional assaults. It also acts as an intimacy meter, helping us to ascertain whether or not a certain person or situation is "emotionally safe." To be emotionally safe means that we feel free to be who we are and express ourselves honestly (versus being physically safe, which has more to do with literal survival). When we get the thumbs-up, we then increase our emotional availability. When intimacy increases, the Heart Protector allows for more blood flow, an increase in circulation, and therefore an increase in sexual fluids. However, when we get a thumbs-down about a situation, the pericardium can restrict blood flow as well as our emotional availability.

When the Heart Protector is not well nourished, we may not be able to discern the emotional safety of a person or situation and walk right in with our hearts on our sleeves, placing trust long before it has been earned. Or in contrast, we may shut down, dissociate, and/or come off as aloof when it is really not what we mean to do.

Triple Burner

The triple burner (also called triple warmer, triple heater, *san jiao*, and three jiao) refers to the three major energy centers in the body and is not attributed to an organ at all but rather to a function. The triple burner's function is to manage the accumulated energy of each of the three energy centers: the low belly, midbelly, and upper chest. The triple burner's job is to maintain a steady, warm temperature throughout all three centers, hence its nickname: the "thermostat." The triple burner's function can be compared to the function of the hypothalamus, as it is responsible for regulating body temperature, blood pressure, heartbeat, fluid balance, appetite, digestion, and other basic autonomic functions.

The Three Burners

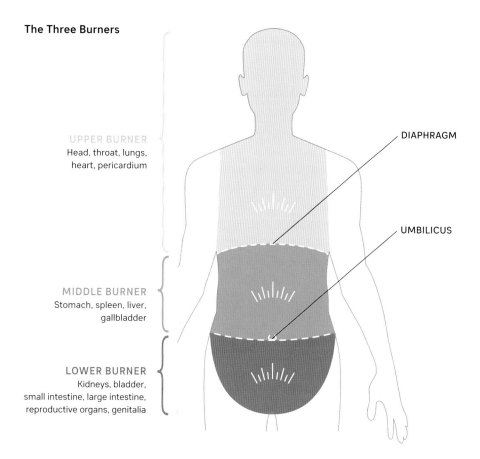

UPPER BURNER
Head, throat, lungs, heart, pericardium

DIAPHRAGM

UMBILICUS

MIDDLE BURNER
Stomach, spleen, liver, gallbladder

LOWER BURNER
Kidneys, bladder, small intestine, large intestine, reproductive organs, genitalia

OFFICIAL IN CHARGE OF THE THREE BURNING SPACES

The Chinese character for the triple burner is translated simply as the "Official in Charge of the Three Burning Spaces." And as this Fire function is our frontline of defense against physical, emotional, and spiritual assault, it regulates the physical and emotional warmth of the body, mind, and spirit. When we engage with our world, it is the triple burner that tells us to *move toward* the things that feel safe and nourishing or to *move away* from those that don't. You can see how this function can become challenged when the triple burner is not nourished. You might get cold or hot or switch back and forth in confusion over which physical or emotional temperature is most appropriate at the moment.

Blood

Blood is our everything! It carries inside it all the nutrients and moisture that keep each of our organs and every part of the body functioning optimally. Nutrients, oxygen, and waste removal are just a few of the blood's vital processes. As part of the Fire element, blood works synergistically with the heart, pericardium, small intestine, and triple burner. When the blood is lacking nutrients, oxygen, or volume or is unable to remove waste as needed, these three organs (and one function) cannot perform their jobs well. The opposite is also true: If any of the three organs and one function aren't doing their jobs properly, the blood won't have what it needs to nourish the rest of the body. Blood is often called the "mother of chi," as chi needs blood for nourishment, and blood provides a material basis for chi.

In Chinese medicine, blood is also responsible for nourishing the mind so that we feel grounded in ourselves and our thoughts, and we can remember things easily. We feel clear, sharp, and vital when the blood is nourished and strong. As such, it also helps us to sleep well and wake feeling rested. As you will see in Part Three, many mental health imbalances come back to the health of the blood. Since the heart is the home of the shen, and blood flows through the heart constantly, the blood is influenced by the state of the shen. If the shen is afraid and holding on to stories from the past, then the blood will carry this charge throughout the body. In Chinese medicine, it is said that when someone has a blood clot, it is the result of an emotional shock or betrayal of some sort.

Many times people will come to my office with what Chinese medicine calls liver blood deficiency, but nothing like anemia may have shown up in a Western medicine test. Partly this is because Chinese medicine works best by detecting imbalances before they cause problems (that is, before they would appear on a blood draw lab). Also, in Chinese medicine we look for so much more than the markers on a blood draw panel. We want to know if the blood is as nutrient-dense as it can possibly be. There are many indicators of this, such as the quality and color of the skin, hair, nails, and tongue, and the vibrancy of the eyes and face. Many emotional symptoms appear when blood is deficient, such as anxiety and dream-disturbed sleep.

Blood Vessels

The blood vessels are governed by the Fire element and are in charge of transporting the blood (and therefore chi). Healthy blood vessels are strong yet flexible. The types of blood vessels are veins, which carry blood into the heart; arteries, which carry blood away from the heart; and capillaries, which exchange nutrients between the blood and the various tissues. Since the face is home to a gazillion blood vessels, it is the place where we can assess the health of the heart and therefore the blood (a pale face = insufficient blood; a red face = heat in the blood).

Tongue

The tongue is governed by the Fire element and is also therefore used to assess the health of the heart (as well as several other organs in the body). A pale tongue indicates insufficient blood, whereas a purple tongue indicates blood stagnation. Speech impediments are often linked to an imbalance in the Fire element due to its relationship with the tongue.

THE SUMMER PANTRY
FEATURED RECIPES

The predominant themes in summertime are *expansion* and *activity*. Thinking about this in terms of energy, we want foods and beverages that not only nourish us but also increase and expand our energy, moving it upward and out. This movement of energy supports the heart, small intestine, pericardium, and triple burner by continuously moving the blood, reducing stagnation, and providing a lightness of spirit that will infuse us for the rest of the year. Since we all know this is the hottest time of year, several of these recipes are for drinks or lighter snacks to keep energy light and freed up.

As spring transitions to summer, be on the lookout for either too much heat or too much cold. Have you ever spent a summer getting too much sun and having way too much fun? Then at summer's end you felt exhausted and burned out. Your skin was dry and peeled, your eyes were bloodshot, and your cheeks were red. That's the heat we want to prevent. As such, we want to support your Fire element with nutrition by focusing on cooling foods.

But we don't want to get too cold. In the West we tend to live in air-conditioned homes when summer comes. This habituates us to a cooler body temperature, so when we step outside, it feels unbearably hot (perhaps hotter than it actually is). In response we start drinking ice water and eating ice cream. But when we have these cold foods and drinks, the stomach contracts, and this limits our ability to digest and to build nutrient-dense blood that will circulate everywhere it needs to go. So there is a fine balance depending on your constitution and where you live in regard to staying cool but not too cool during the summer.

That being said, because it is the most yang of all seasons, this is going to be the best time to eat more raw foods. The only caveat is that if your digestion is cold (cold hands and feet) or if your stool has undigested food particles in it, stick to warm and cooked foods until this evens out.

Here are the general principles of summertime nutrition:

- Slowly increase your raw food intake.
- Avoid iced/frozen foods except in small amounts.
- Seek out bitter flavors.
- Avoid large amounts of protein.
- Include digestive bitters with your meals.
- Cook foods on high heat, for shorter times.
- Reduce your intake of heavy foods like creams, gravies, and rich sauces.
- Eat foods that are red in color.
- Master the art of juicing.
- Eat lots of blood-building and blood-nourishing foods.
- Increase your intake of cooling foods when it's hot inside and out.
- Enjoy the most variety of foods you will have for the entire year.
- Consume less salt.

Summertime Staples

PROTEINS (LIMITED AMOUNTS): Abalone, anchovy, caviar, cuttlefish, eggs, shark

GRAINS: Amaranth, buckwheat, corn

VEGETABLES: Bamboo, beet, bitter gourd, bitter melon, carrots, cauliflower, celery, chicory, dandelion root and greens, endive, lettuce, lotus root, okra, red bell pepper, scallion, sweet potato, tomato, turnip, watercress

FRUITS: Apples, cherries, dragonfruit, figs, goji berries, grapefruit, kumquat, orange, persimmon, pineapple, rhubarb, strawberries, watermelon

LEGUMES: Adzuki beans, chickpeas, mung beans, peas, red beans, red lentils, soybeans, string beans

NUTS AND SEEDS: Pistachio, sunflower

DAIRY (LIMITED AMOUNTS): Goat, sheep

HERBS TO COOK WITH: Cayenne, chilies, jasmine, lavender, mint, rose, turmeric, white pepper

FOODS TO AVOID: Chocolate, dairy in large amounts, heavy or creamy sauces and gravies, iced or frozen foods, protein in large amounts, refined sugar

---

SUMMERTIME FLAVORS: BITTER

- If you are **hot**, add in *salty* (page 90) and *cooling* foods (page 93).
- If you are **restless**, add in *calming* foods (page 96).
- If you are **dry**, add in *moistening* foods (page 94).

SUMMERTIME RECIPES FOR EXPANSION AND ENERGY

Recipes we use this season will reflect a lightness, rather than the heavier creams and sauces of the colder months. Summertime recipes are about giving your body, mind, and spirit *more* energy for your long days.

Since bitter flavor goes straight to the heart, there is no better time than summer to master the art of making homemade bitters! In Chinese cultures, bitter is used just like the other four flavors of salty, sweet, pungent, and sour. However, in the West we rarely use anything that tastes bitter (or sour, for that matter). But bitter foods are incredible. We have receptors for these compounds scattered throughout the mouth, stomach, pancreas, liver, gallbladder, and intestines. When we consume bitter foods, these receptors wake up and trigger the secretion of digestive juices starting in the mouth, then the stomach secretes hydrochloric acid and pepsin, the pancreas secretes enzymes, and the liver secretes bile. This process happens anyway, but when food is bitter, the process is enhanced. The moral of the story? Bitters help us to digest our foods better (less inflammation, bloating, spasms, gas, cramping, and discomfort in general). In ancient China, bitters were served at every meal.

TIPS
- If you tend to experience cramping, bloating, or symptoms of irritable bowel syndrome (IBS), drink a 1-ounce glass of bitters *before* meals.
- If you tend to experience indigestion, heartburn, nausea, or an upset stomach, drink a 1-ounce glass of bitters *after* meals.
- Do not consume bitters if you have an active ulcer or are pregnant.

Peel of 1 orange

2 tablespoons dried dandelion root and leaves

1 tablespoon dried whole hibiscus flowers

¼ cup dried hawthorn berries

2 teaspoons grated ginger

4 dried whole star anise

6 cardamom pods

1 liter vodka or brandy

Raw local honey as needed for taste and immunity

OPTIONAL INGREDIENTS FOR WARMING

1 teaspoon ground cinnamon

1 teaspoon black pepper

OPTIONAL INGREDIENT FOR LIVER CLEANSING

½ grapefruit, chopped

SPECIAL EQUIPMENT

One 32-ounce Mason or Ball jar with lid

Small glass serving bottle

CONTINUES

◆

• If you would prefer to use a *nonalcoholic* base, substitute 1 liter raw, unfiltered, organic apple cider vinegar for the vodka or brandy.

Add all the fruit and herbs to the Mason jar. Fill the jar to the brim with vodka or brandy. Cover and shake well. Put a label on the jar and store it in a cool place away from sunlight. Remember to shake it every day.

Try your first taste two weeks after you close the jar. If it's the right amount of bitter flavor (note that if you aren't used to bitter foods, then even the slightest bitterness will taste strong), strain and pour into the small serving bottle. If you would prefer more bitterness, taste once a week for up to 6 weeks until you get your desired flavor. Add honey as needed to the serving bottle for taste and if your immune system needs a boost.

This mixture will last indefinitely (unless you added fresh grapefruit, in which case it will only last a couple of weeks). Serve with sparkling water if you want a little bubbly with your bitters.

COOLING WATERMELON MILK (OR JUICE) • MAKES 6 SERVINGS

If summer's heat is getting to you and you find yourself lethargic, uninterested in adventure, and generally rundown, consider adding some Watermelon Milk to your life. This special treat was used in tenth-century China, but it originates in northeast Africa and is well known in India. Since this fruit is 90 percent water, it is an excellent way to replenish electrolytes lost in the summer heat. Due to the sugar in melons, I recommend drinking this milk or juice away from meals as it can slow down your digestion.

3 pounds cubed seedless watermelon (no rind)	2 cups Sweet Nut Milk (page 211) or water	Mint sprigs for garnish

Blend the watermelon and milk or water in a blender or food processor. Serve with mint sprigs (but no ice). Store in the refrigerator for up to two days. Enjoy!

BLOOD-BUILDING SMOOTHIE • MAKES 1 SERVING

Because having good, nutrient-rich blood is excellent for all your organs, as well as your mind and spirits, you can build even more of this vital substance during the summer months to nourish yourself throughout the year. Aside from animal products like red meat, many vegetables and fruits contain high amounts of chlorophyll, also known as plant hemoglobin. These foods act as blood builders in your body while giving you energy for the hot summer days.

1 small beet, cubed

½ large carrot, chopped

½ cup chopped kale

½ cup chopped spinach

1 ounce chopped wheatgrass

½ cup cherries, pits removed

1 cup plain yogurt or nettle tea

Place all ingredients in a blender or food processor, and blend until smooth. Add more liquid as needed to make your perfect thickness. This smoothie will give you energy and stamina by building your blood and supporting your heart health.

TIP • Consider adding chlorophyll powder to give it even more of a blood-building boost.

Herbs not only support us when we are physically imbalanced, but they can also enhance our emotional health when our spirits are low or shaky. This recipe is an example of bringing in support for the mind and spirit, and it can even be used as prevention when you anticipate entering a challenging time of life.

¼ cup nettles

¼ cup lemon balm

¼ cup tulsi

⅛ cup reishi

10 cups water, boiled then cooled for 3 minutes, separated

2 tablespoons dried rose petals

1 tablespoon dried lavender flowers

SPECIAL EQUIPMENT

One 32-ounce Mason or Ball jar with lid

One 16-ounce glass jar with lid

Mix the nettles, lemon balm, tulsi, and reishi together in the Mason jar. Fill the jar to the base of the mouth with 8 cups of the boiled but slightly cooled water. Place the lid on tightly and leave the herb mixture to steep for at least 6 hours or overnight if possible. After steeping the herb mixture, make sure the lid on the Mason jar is tight, shake the jar to stir up the herbs, and then strain.

Put the rose and lavender in the 16-ounce jar and pour in the remaining 2 cups of boiled but slightly cooled water. Let the flower mixture steep for 3 minutes before tasting it (lavender can get bitter quite fast!); 3 to 5 minutes is usually enough. Strain the flower mixture and put it in the fridge. It will act as the flavoring for the herbal concoction.

To serve, pour a mugful of the herb mixture, add a splash (about 1 teaspoon) of the floral mixture, and drink cool. Both the tea and the rose and lavender mixture will store in the fridge for up to 1 week.

THE SUMMER MEDICINE CABINET

Since this is the most yang time of year and the heart and blood are at the peak of their energy, it's wonderful to stock your medicine cabinet with herbs to keep you feeling balanced, keep your blood flowing, and nourish your heart. Many of the herbs listed here can do that. Some, however, are also cooling, which can bring in the yin to balance the yang of the season. If you are feeling cool yourself (cold hands and feet), then avoid the cooling and cold herbs.

Angelica

PIN YIN: Dang Gui

ORIGIN: China

PART USED: Root

ORGANS / SYSTEMS SUPPORTED: Uterus, digestive system, blood, heart

USES: Anxiety, PMS, amenorrhea, dysmenorrhea, irregular menstruation, tinnitus, vision problems, women's reproductive health, abdominal pain, fibroids, PCOS, constipation, blood deficiency and blood stasis

PATTERNS SUPPORTED: Heart blood deficiency, liver blood deficiency, blood stagnation

FLAVORS: Sweet, bitter

TEMPERATURE: Warming

ACTIONS: Tonifying, blood-building, moistening

CONTRAINDICATIONS: Can cause photosensitivity when taken in high doses over a long period of time

BEST TAKEN: Decoction (4.5 to 15 grams/day)

Hawthorn

PIN YIN: Shan Zha

ORIGIN: Asia, Europe, North America

PART USED: Berries

ORGANS / SYSTEMS SUPPORTED: Heart, liver, digestive system, pericardium, blood/circulation

USES: Anxiety, insomnia, night sweats, high blood pressure, tachycardia, fatigue, paranoia, heart palpitations

NOTE: I often recommend that hawthorn be taken alongside prescription medications for high cholesterol, high blood pressure, and heart disease due to its heart-protective properties, but always check with your practitioner before taking herbs with prescription drugs.

PATTERNS SUPPORTED: Heart chi deficiency, heart yin deficiency, blood stagnation, liver chi stagnation, heart fire blazing, heart phlegm fire

FLAVORS: Sour, sweet

TEMPERATURES: Warming

ACTIONS: Astringent, calming

CONTRAINDICATIONS: Not to be used in conjunction with digoxin, a heart medication

BEST TAKEN: Decoction (9 to 15 grams/day)

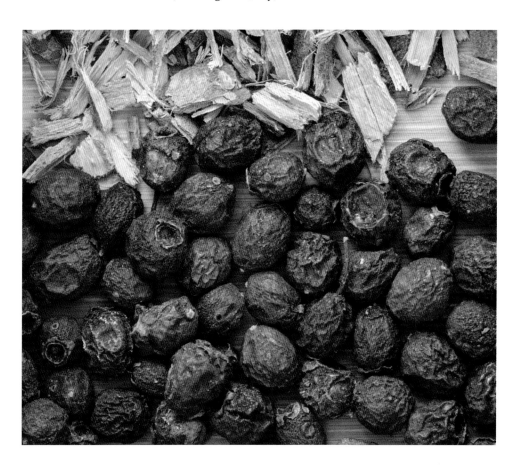

Jujube Seeds

PIN YIN: Suan Zao Ren

ORIGIN: China

PART USED: Seeds

ORGANS / SYSTEMS SUPPORTED: Heart, spleen, gallbladder, liver

USES: Anxiety, insomnia, agitation, restlessness, heart palpitations

PATTERNS SUPPORTED: Heart yin deficiency, heart blood deficiency, heart chi deficiency, liver chi stagnation

FLAVORS: Sour, sweet

TEMPERATURES: Neutral

ACTIONS: Calming, tonifying, mildly astringent

CONTRAINDICATIONS: None known

BEST TAKEN: Decoction (9 to 18 grams/day)

Motherwort

PIN YIN: Yi Mu Cao

ORIGIN: China

PARTS USED: Leaves, seeds

ORGANS / SYSTEMS SUPPORTED: Women's reproductive system, heart, liver, bladder

USES: Any reproductive system imbalances, anxiety, high blood pressure, skin conditions presenting with heat, infertility, PCOS, fibroids

PATTERNS SUPPORTED: Liver chi stagnation, blood stagnation, liver fire blazing

FLAVORS: Pungent, bitter

TEMPERATURES: Slightly cooling

ACTIONS: Tonifying, slightly astringent

CONTRAINDICATIONS: Consult with a practitioner before using during pregnancy

BEST TAKEN: Decoction (9 to 15 grams/day)

Reishi

PIN YIN: Ling Zhi

ORIGIN: China

PART USED: Whole mushroom

ORGANS / SYSTEMS SUPPORTED: Heart, lungs, respiratory system, liver

SPIRITUAL MUSHROOM

The Chinese character for *ling* can be translated as "spirit, soul, miraculous, sacred, divine, auspicious, and mysterious." The Chinese character for *zhi* can be translated as "mushroom of longevity or immortality." Therefore, the ancients spoke about this world-famous mushroom as a magical, spiritual mushroom with powers of longevity (and possibly even immortality).

USES: Anxiety, insomnia, nausea, high blood pressure, high cholesterol, detoxification, cancer, tumors, allergies, arthritis, asthma

PATTERNS SUPPORTED: Heart chi deficiency, lung chi deficiency, wei qi deficiency, heart yin deficiency, blood stagnation, spleen chi deficiency

FLAVORS: Bitter

TEMPERATURES: Slightly warming

ACTIONS: Calming, tonifying

CONTRAINDICATIONS: None known

BEST TAKEN: Decoction (3 to 15 grams/day)

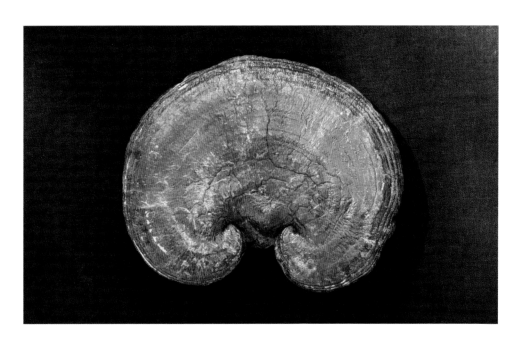

Summertime Formulas

PRESERVE HARMONY FORMULA (*BAO HE WAN*): This formula is excellent for that Summer heat that can build in your digestive system, often accompanied by dampness. This leads to food stagnation, feelings of heaviness, bloating, indigestion, diarrhea and/or constipation, nausea, vomiting, and loss of appetite. Between the hot days and the increase in sugar and alcohol, your digestive system can get a bit stifled at this time of year. Preserve Harmony Formula can dry up the dampness and cool down the heat, allowing your digestive system to return to its normal flow.

AGASTACHE QI CORRECTING FORMULA (*HUO XIANG ZHENG QI SAN*): With so much of your energy moving outward during this time of year, you can end up challenging your immune system and depleting your reserves. As such, dampness can build up in the systems, leaving you vulnerable to imbalances, especially in your immune system. Agastache Qi Correcting Formula is an excellent support for this experience. Acute summer colds, heat-related exhaustion, heat stroke, stomach flu, headaches, sinus pressure, and diarrhea all benefit from this formula.

NOURISHING PRACTICES IN SUMMER

Connecting with Community

The movement of energy as we move from spring into summer is like that of walking into a big outdoor festival: there is more activity, and people are out and about, some who we haven't seen for a long time. Music is playing, and it's as though we are celebrating something. We hear laughter and singing. This is the energy of summertime and is a welcome time to connect with friends without any particular agenda except to see each other and catch up.

Expressing Creativity

As summer provides the most amount of yang energy you will have all year long, it's a wonderful time to start a creative project. If there is a type of art you have always wanted to learn to do or something you have always wanted to learn to build, this is the time of year for learning new skills and finding new and authentic ways of expressing yourself. Learning to paint or play an instrument is a great way to use these energies. Whatever brings you joy in learning and practicing it will support and nourish your Fire element during these summer months.

Using Your Voice

Since the Fire element organs are all tied to the tongue and therefore to speech, what an excellent time of year to focus on using your voice. Paying attention to your speech, how you talk, and the kinds of things you talk about supports your heart in coming back to balance. In summer it's important to speak from your heart rather than hiding what you really think and feel or speaking carelessly. If you love someone, tell that person again and again. Find mantras, chants, or affirmations you can use to lift your spirits during summer.

Laughing

Laughter soothes the body, mind, and spirit. When you laugh, you experience a lightness of being that is both relaxing and uplifting. All the ways you can find to allow yourself to laugh moves Fire and specifically heart energy through your body.

Working Out

This means not only engaging in some exercise that increases your heart rate, but also working out with friends during this yang season. It's a wonderful way to connect with others while moving your body and blood. Go on walks or hikes that get you huffing and puffing a little so your heart can get flushed with fresh blood. And don't forget, the heart is a muscle, so the more you exercise it, the stronger it gets. A strong heart will serve you in maintaining/improving your physical and emotional health by becoming more resilient.

Practicing Forgiveness

Many heart studies have been conducted because of this organ's importance to our physical and emotional function and our questions as to how the heart and brain relate to each other. The HeartMath Institute says, "The heart is about 60 times stronger electrically and 5,000 times stronger magnetically than the brain." From the organization's extensive research we now know that when we experience positive emotions, the heart's amplitude increases even beyond that. One study revealed that when practicing forgiveness, the heart developed even stronger amplitude. And when experiencing resentment and anger, it actually contracted and beat irregularly.[2] Summer is the perfect time to practice forgiveness.

Being of Service

There is never any shortage in this world of ways to get involved and support those in need. Connecting with others or with a vision of change at this level, opens the heart like nothing else. From planting trees in an area devastated by a natural disaster to collecting donation items for your local shelter, you have the opportunity to contribute to a larger vision of the world and to develop greater compassion for people, animals, and ecosystems that suffer.

Waking with the Sun

With the sun coming up earlier and setting later, it's the perfect time of year to rise and sleep with the sun and reset any unusual sleep patterns you have developed over the last several months. Since the days are longer and hotter, don't feel shy about resting during the heat of the day. In the mornings you can feel the energy (much like a microcosm of the energy of the entire year) move from a fairly dormant energy of darkness to a high energy of light. I like to greet the morning sun with yoga Sun Salutations, starting slowly when the sun is just coming up (two to three breaths per posture) and increasing my pacing (one breath per posture) as the sun rises.

Cleaning and Beautifying Your Outdoor/Community Space

Since summer is especially important for turning up the energy and connecting with others, what a wonderful time to cleanse the spaces that bring people together. Whether it's a small balcony in a city apartment, a back porch, or a living room, add beautiful vibrant colors and decor to the space so that it becomes welcoming and a place to connect.

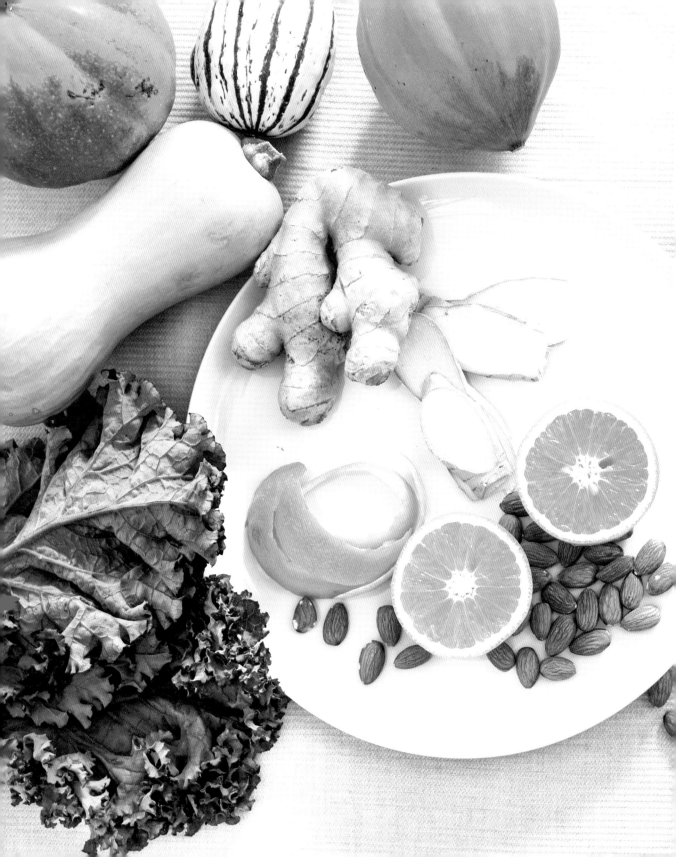

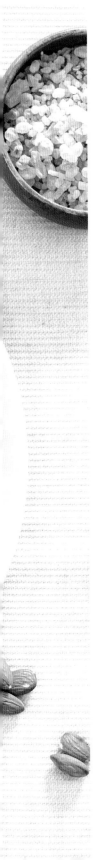

LATE SUMMER AND THE EARTH ELEMENT

MID-AUGUST THROUGH FALL EQUINOX (SEPTEMBER 22)

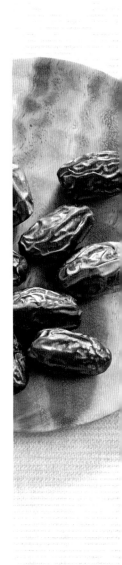

When it's over I want to say:
All my life I was a bride married to amazement.
I was the bridegroom taking the world into my arms.
—MARY OLIVER

— ◆ —

During summer, plants are busy taking advantage of the full, hot sun by growing as tall and wide as they possibly can. Yet when this season is coming to a close, they are no longer growing larger; instead their energy goes toward ripening their fruits. This time of year we begin to think about harvesting. This season is known as late summer, which is recognized as unique from summer and fall yet is sandwiched in between. This season is neither yin nor yang but a perfect pause and balance point of both. When in balance, this season brings with it a sense of nourishment, security (literally food security), and a resulting sense of relaxation.

The late summer season is all about *centering*, *grounding*, and finding *balance*. It's an excellent time to evaluate the harvest and abundance of our own bodies, minds, and spirits. Have we cultivated what we intended to over the summer? Is there plenty of nourishment for us to draw on for the months to come? Do our bodies, minds, and spirits feel nourished? Or do we feel depleted? Have we spent more energy than we had over the last year?

Late summer allows us a perfect window to reset whatever our unique yin-yang balance truly is. If we have depleted ourselves, or if we have overindulged over the last several months, we can now press pause and start over, setting ourselves up for a balanced rest of the year.

THE EARTH ELEMENT

The element of Earth literally refers to the planet we are on. More specifically, the Earth element refers to the soil that covers much of the land on this planet. The soil is made up of minerals, water, air, and organic matter such as dead plants and animals. It helps to guide rivers back into the ocean and gives plant and tree life something to root into, draw nutrients from, and lean on as they make their ascent to the sun. The quality of soil that we live near and extract our food from is directly linked to the nutrient density of our foods (and therefore our bodies), as well as the quality of the air we breathe and the water we drink.

When the fruits of plants and trees are ripening as they do now, they are essentially building sugar inside. The sugar, combined with the change in sunlight, allows the colors of the fruit to change and many of the leaves to begin to turn yellow. This is why the season is associated with the sweet taste and the color yellow. (It is also because the soil in the region of China where the classical texts were written is strikingly yellow due to the mineral content.)

People who have a lot of Earth in their constitution also often embody compassionate and care-giving energy. Think of the Great Mother archetype—someone who provides

SOIL DEPLETION

Our soil has been so depleted by the monocropping of the industrial era (growing the same, single crop year after year without diversifying or rotating the crop to different parcels of land). Nature never intended to grow only one crop on a large piece of land. In the natural world, if it is left to its own processes, many different species of plants grow in a single area because different plants extract different nutrients from the soil. Monocropping leads to significant nutrient depletion of the soil. When the soil is depleted, plants will stop growing; nature intends for us to move on and find another place to harvest while the soil naturally replenishes itself. Throughout most of history, humans were hunter-gatherers and that time was considered our most successful adaptation to the environment. In the industrial agricultural era, however, we have become stationary instead of nomadic. The lack of nutrients in the soil translates as a lack of nutrients in our bodies. Many of us are deficient in the most basic vitamins and minerals and are suffering because of it.

food and gatherings like potlucks or get-togethers for the family. We go to this person often to receive nourishment on all levels, whether we need someone to listen to us or just a little comfort and compassion. Like the soil, a healthy Earth element provides sustainable nourishment to all that grows in or around it.

EARTH CONSTITUTION

ARCHETYPE: THE PEACEKEEPER

Individuals with a lot of balanced Earth in their constitution exude a great sense of comfort. They tend to be very attuned to the needs of others and can provide nourishment in the form of words, physical touch, and of course food. A balanced Earth constitution means they are always able to think of more than just themselves. They tend to think of the greater good and meeting the needs of many. Often excellent chefs (or at least plugged into the nourishment of food), Earth constitutions know how to satisfy even the pickiest palettes and find a sense of joy in serving others. With the Peacekeeper as its archetype, this element's constitution is nurturing and stable but not self-depleting; Peacekeepers tend to become advocates for safety, food, and love for all, especially those who are most vulnerable.

EMOTION

Empathy/compassion is the emotion associated with the Earth element. It is best described by the energy between a mother and child: feelings of attunement, connection, tenderness, and awareness of the struggle that must happen for one to grow. Healthy protection and genuine compassion are attributes of this Earth energy—caring about all life on earth, regardless of differences, is a representation of this element. An Earth constitution provides all this amazing, healing energy, like the most perfect salve to any physical, mental, or emotional wound.

Empathy can get out of balance, as we can become overly empathetic. When this happens, we can have a difficult time seeing the difference between someone else's struggle and our own. We can grieve a loss almost as though it were ours. Extreme empathy can be unhealthy and exhausting. This is where healthy boundaries (the Water element) is vital to a healthy Earth element. On the other end of the spectrum, Earth can get out of balance and lead to a compassionless state in which we are unable to see ourselves in others. This often develops as a coping mechanism when we don't have the resources to manage our own feelings. If we are in this kind of struggle, we may appear to spend all our time and energy on ourselves (which is often deemed narcissistic).

The greatest challenge for the Earth element's emotion is that empathy can easily turn into worry, anxiety, and overthinking. This is why it is so important for the compassion to have something to do. Without a clear direction (set forth by the Wood element), Earth energy can just spin around with no point of reference. This leads to obsessive thoughts and behaviors, as well as incessant worry without action. For instance, if you are wondering about whether or not your spouse's parents actually approve of you, you could worry about it endlessly, create a bunch of stories in your head, and allow your anxiety to skyrocket. Or you could take all that energy and tell your partner you are worried about this; better yet, you could go straight to the source and say, "Hey, I feel worried that you don't think I'm a good fit for your son/daughter. Is that true?" Thought with action has a way of cutting through the stuck energy that Earth is prone to.

Having a healthy Earth element is vital for our basic survival and general sense of belonging and well-being. When we are hungry for something physical, mental, or emotional (and we can easily get confused about which is which), the stomach and spleen work together to help us figure it out, get this nourishment into the body, and do something satisfying with it. When we are confused about what is nourishment or mistake emotional nourishment for the physical kind, it's a sign that our Earth element is out of balance.

As Westerners many of us are taxing our Earth element, specifically the spleen. We have so many requirements when it comes to mental tasks (e-mail, snail mail, phone calls, text messages, studying, and so on), and many of us are tied to a computer all day. This burden eventually falls on the spleen and the digestive system. For our Earth element to stay balanced, we need to keep our activity balanced with rest. That means, for every two hours we spend sitting, we should spend some time walking and moving our bodies. For every hour we spend thinking, we should spend twenty minutes giving our minds a rest. With so much emphasis on our mental capabilities, many of us experience anxiety and worry. We are afraid we are forgetting things and feel an undercurrent of stress a lot of the time. Stress can lead to all kinds of nutritional deficiencies, because eating when we are stressed means we are not digesting our food well.

BALANCED EARTH ELEMENT

- Care of self and others
- Nurturing energy
- Good boundaries
- Compassion
- Understanding
- Empathy with others (no matter the differences)
- Good appetite
- Smooth digestion
- Healthy weight
- Toned, strong, and supportive muscles
- Good life rhythm
- Good life-work balance
- Ability to anticipate needs of self
- Ability to attune to others
- Ability to focus, study, and think clearly

OUT OF BALANCE EARTH ELEMENT

- Worry
- Anxiety
- Extreme empathy with others
- Lack of empathy for self or others
- Overwork or overextension to the point of depletion
- Insatiable appetite or no appetite
- Diarrhea or loose stools
- Weight that is over or under the ideal
- Cravings for or addiction to sugar
- Slow healing after injury
- Easy bruising
- Low energy
- Indigestion
- Food sensitivities and allergies
- Obsessive, circular thinking
- Unclear or muddled thinking
- Disconnection from own needs
- Guilt associated with having needs
- Ungrounded/uncentered quality
- Perpetual "caregiver" to others while own needs go unattended
- Digestive issues when stressed
- Stomachaches and pain
- Edema
- Cysts, nodules
- Irritable bowel syndrome

YOUR BODY IN LATE SUMMER

Digestion begins with the Earth element, which governs the appetite and desire for or lack of desire for food. Beyond that, the Earth element is in charge of the process all along the way: when we think of food and begin creating the necessary saliva to help us break it down, when we put food in our mouths and swallow, when we churn food up with the appropriate enzymes and hydrochloric acid in the stomach, and when we send it off to the small intestine (governed by the Fire element). This process requires that we first have an appetite, that we then know what is nourishing to our bodies, and finally that our bodies know what to do with this nourishment. All of this depends on the Earth element's health.

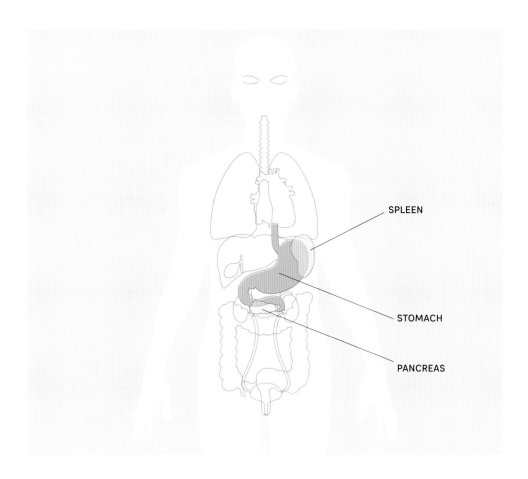

Stomach

The stomach is essentially a muscular sac responsible for receiving food from the esophagus (which is considered a part of the stomach in Chinese medicine) and secreting the appropriate amount of hydrochloric acid and enzymes needed to break the food down and churn it up until it is ready to be passed along to the small intestine. The stomach sits on the left side of the torso, just under the left rib cage. It has small ridges inside called rugae that further help to churn and break down food. Enzymes act as little puzzle pieces for the exact foods they help to break down.

When the stomach is healthy, the perfect (rather acidic) environment is ready and waiting to receive food. This environment allows for a healthy appetite, one that is in alignment with our individual constitution, lifestyle, and activity level. Usually an increased appetite comes with an increase in activity. When we experience little to no appetite, or a voracious appetite, we always look at the Earth element.

OFFICIAL IN CHARGE OF ROTTING AND RIPENING

The stomach is referred to as the "Official in Charge of Rotting and Ripening" in classical Chinese medicine. On a physical level, this function is literal, as the stomach is involved in this process with all the food and drink we take in. On an energetic level, the stomach is also responsible for knowing what nourishes us. When the stomach official is not functioning properly, our ideas of what could be nourishing may not be aligned with what we actually need (for instance, inviting friends over for a potluck only to discover that we are actually exhausted and could really use some rest). Or our ideas of nourishment may not actually be carried through, such as craving a warm vegetable stew on a cold winter day but eating ice cream instead. Worry, grief, anxiety, and any other unresolved emotional experiences can be particularly hard on the stomach official. Instead of processing those emotions, if the stomach isn't thriving, we might try to use food to soothe our emotions. The stomach, when well cared for, can help us root our physical, emotional, and spiritual nourishment, especially if we go slowly and learn to listen to the body's cues when we need something.

Pancreas

The pancreas is a glandular organ that lives in the abdomen, sitting behind the stomach. Its main function is to secrete enzymes in the junction where the stomach and small intestine meet to further assist in the breakdown of food. Additionally the pancreas is responsible for the regulation of blood sugar, or insulin. The purpose of insulin is to remove the sugar we eat from our blood and send it to the muscles and other tissues so we can use it as energy. If the pancreas does not produce enough enzymes, the whole body will suffer the consequences, because nutrients from food will not be extracted. The function of the pancreas is paired with that of the spleen (healthy spleen = healthy pancreas).

Spleen

The spleen is a small organ that sits in the upper left quadrant of the abdomen, often just to the left of and a little behind the stomach. The spleen's primary responsibility in Western science is its role with the blood and the manufacturing of white blood cells. It works to filter out old red blood cells and add in new platelets and white blood cells when needed. This activity makes it a key player in supporting the immune system.

OFFICIAL IN CHARGE OF TRANSFORMATION AND TRANSPORTATION

In Chinese medicine, the spleen is called the "Official in Charge of Transformation and Transportation" and is viewed differently than in Western medicine. While the stomach's job is to know *what to bring* in and prepare it for absorption, the spleen's role is to know *what to do with it* to use the nourishment. Rather than largely being involved in manufacturing white blood cells, the spleen is viewed as having an important role in transforming the food nutrients received from the stomach into chi and blood, then transporting the chi and nutrients via the blood to exactly where they need to go. In fact, the movement of all substances in the body (blood, urine, lymph, stool) begin with the functioning of the spleen. And since Chinese medicine always sees the holistic aspect of each organ and function, we are talking about not only physical nutrients, but emotional and spiritual nutrients too. The spleen is responsible for helping us process everything that comes into our bodies, minds, and spirits; know what to do with it and where it will be most valuable; and then send it there.

One way we are taxing our spleens in the modern world is with how fast everything moves. For example, when you are a student, you are required to learn a vast amount of information quickly and to be able to regurgitate it at a moment's notice. The way most educational institutions are set up don't allow for much time to process and integrate all that you are learning before moving on to the next subject. This is similar to eating a meal while also working, checking e-mails, scanning social media, driving, and so on. When we do all this, the spleen gets overworked and as a consequence, food will sit undigested in the stomach, or we might even find pieces of food in our stool (a sure sign of spleen chi deficiency). We need the spleen to stay nourished so that every tissue in the body and thought in the mind can receive nourishment at the pace that we are able to digest it and be nourished by it.

Muscle

The muscles are the body tissues governed by the Earth element. Healthy development of muscles is dependent on the proper nutrition in sync with proper activity and movement. The stomach receives the proper nutrition and is responsible for the first stages of breaking it down, and the spleen has the job of knowing where to transport these nutrients. When a person has weak or underdeveloped muscles, it is often the Earth element that needs the most support.

Mouth

The sensory organ related to the Earth element is the mouth (this includes the lips). The mouth is the first place from which we are able to receive physical nourishment, so if there are issues such as bleeding gums, bad breath, mouth ulcers, dry or cracked lips, or pale lips, it's important to look at the health of the Earth element.

THE MICROBIOME

We have all probably heard of microbiome by now and have some idea about how our gut health relates to our overall health. *Microbiome* is a word used to describe our personal ecosystems. You and I each have our own ecosystems that contain their own diversity and quantity of microbes. The health of the gut is extremely dependent on this personal ecosystem and its microbes.[3] Medical practitioners have always heard that the people in the Amazon (specifically Bolivia)[4] and Tanzania[5] don't have cancers and heart disease like we do in the West. The biggest difference between them and us is the quantity and diversity of microbes we carry inside and outside our bodies. People of the Amazon have lots more microbes in their guts than we do!

The more diversity, the better. Certain microbes provide greater health when they are present in large quantities, while others bring more benefit in smaller quantities. The reason it's important to have a strong microbiome is that it indicates superb digestion (excellent quality foods, extraction of nutrients, use of the nutrients, and elimination of waste products) and the presence of enough microbes to work and fight for us in case of illness or disease. This set-up creates a wonderful foundation, most importantly for the immune system. This is why having a healthy microbiome automatically equals having healthy wei qi, our protective chi.

Where we run into trouble in the West is primarily with our use of antibiotics. Not only do antibiotics wipe out bad bacteria, but they take the good along with it. If I have a patient with a very strong microbiome who needs to take a course of antibiotics, I usually see that patient recover in four to eight weeks, judging by pulses, the tongue, and digestive tolerance. If, on the other hand, I have a patient who already has a challenged microbiome, it can take more than a year to recover from even one course of antibiotics. For most of us, it takes time and diligence, which is something to consider before taking a round of antibiotics. We can speed our recovery time from antibiotics by supplementing our diet with diverse probiotics, prebiotics, and fermented foods and eating the skins on fresh fruits and veggies. In this case, a little dirt in the diet can actually enhance our health. In my practice, adults and children who were given antibiotics before the age of two and a half often seem to have lifelong immune system imbalances.

THE LATE SUMMER PANTRY
FEATURED RECIPES

Since late summer is all about the harvest (literally gathering all the foods we possibly can before they begin to rot and fall to the ground), the focus should be on creating nutrient-dense meals that are centering, grounding, and slightly sweet in nature. As this is a time when we pause somewhat between the yin and yang transition, the energy around food and cooking should be like that also—not too laborious but bringing people together to share in the nourishment.

More and more in Western science, we are learning of the great importance of the gut and digestive system. The digestive system serves as a foundation for health in all regards, including physical and mental health. The immune system is also established and either supported or challenged by the health of the gut. This is not just about digestion and whether or not we experience discomfort like gas, bloating, belching, acid reflux, and the like. Those symptoms are indicative of an underlying imbalance and must be given attention. But the health of the gut also has to do with whether or not we can break down our food well, absorb all the important nutrients, and eliminate the waste.

Here are the general principles of nutrition in late summer:

- Slowly increase your cooked food intake.
- Avoid cold foods and limit raw foods.
- Seek out sweet flavors.
- Master the art of stew-making.
- Eat foods that are orange or yellow in color.
- Use limited seasonings, keeping foods somewhat plain.
- Avoid complicated dishes with complicated combinations of foods.

- Share meals with others as much as possible.
- Spend a significant amount of time chewing and eating without distraction.
- Cook foods longer over medium to low heat.
- Reduce damp foods such as dairy, refined sugar, beer, and wheat.

Late Summer Staples

PROTEINS: Beef, carp, chicken, duck, eggs, goat, herring, lamb, mackerel, sardines, venison

GRAINS: Amaranth, brown rice, corn, sweet rice, teff

VEGETABLES: All cooked and some fermented vegetables (page 233), beets, cabbage, carrots, green onions, onions, parsnips, peas, radishes, string beans, sweet potatoes, turnips, yams

SQUASH: Acorn, butternut, delicata, hubbard, pumpkin, spaghetti

FRUITS: Apples, apricots, cantaloupe, dates, figs, grapes, papaya, peaches

LEGUMES: Adzuki beans, lentils, mung beans

SEEDS AND NUTS: Almonds, chestnuts, coconut, sesame seeds, sunflower seeds, walnuts

DAIRY: Avoid (If you have *any* difficulty digesting dairy products, I recommend avoiding dairy altogether but especially at this time of year. Since the focus is on supporting the spleen and stomach so you can reset your digestive system, going easy on these organs with dairy and other mucus-forming foods— alcohol, bananas, bread, cabbage, cereal, corn, eggs, pasta, potatoes, red meat, soy, and sugar—will be beneficial.)

HERBS AND SPICES: Coriander, cumin, garlic, ginger (Overall this season is about mild flavor, even blandness, so use sparingly.)

CONDIMENTS AND MORE: Vinegar (use sparingly)

OILS: Olive oil

SWEETENERS: Avoid if possible (only foods with a naturally sweet taste during this season)

FOODS TO AVOID: Cold foods and drinks, dairy, oily foods, overly spicy foods, raw foods, sugar and refined carbohydrates

LATE SUMMER FLAVOR: SWEET

- If you are **cold**, add in *warming* foods (page 93).
- If you are feeling **ungrounded**, add in *neutral* foods (page 93).
- If you are **damp**, add in *astringent* foods (page 95).

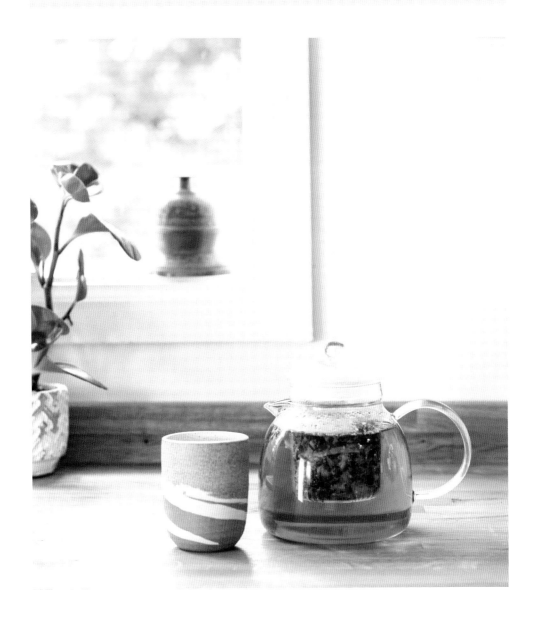

BASIC SOUP AND STEW • MAKES 16 CUPS

When I think of late summer, the first thing that comes to mind is a stew with orange-colored veggies. Either pumpkin, squash, or carrots make for a perfect, golden Late Summer season harvest and color. And since the goal is to nourish the digestive system without putting any extra strain on it, making soups or stews is the *perfect* way to do that. When we eat soups and stews, our bodies do not have to work so hard to extract the nourishment. This is because the ingredients are cooked at a low temperature for a long time. With this in mind, it's best to plan ahead or else consider using a Crock-Pot. Since we are following the Late Summer principles of eating by choosing foods that are sweet tasting and neutral in temperature, select items from the "Late Summer Staples" list in the preceding section.

Depending on where you live, late summer may still be quite hot. If that is the case, in addition to the sweet and neutral foods you use as the base of the soup, consider adding some cooling vegetables, herbs, or spices if you like.

MEAT: You can use any kind of meat that you feel drawn to (or none at all). Traditionally beef and lamb work very well and bring rich fats and flavor to the dish. Choose organic, free-range, wild-caught, and local (if possible) animal products to get those with the most nutrients and the least toxicity. Estimate about 6 ounces of meat per serving—a little more if you would like leftovers (and who doesn't like leftover stew?).

VEGETABLES: I like to choose at least one root vegetable and a few nonroot veggies, aiming for a total of about ½ cup per serving.

Root Vegetables: beet, parsnip, potato, rutabaga, sweet potato, turnip, yam

Vegetables: cabbage, carrots, eggplant, garlic, onion, mushrooms, string beans, Swiss chard

SPICES: Onions (½ onion per serving or 1 onion per pound of protein) and garlic (4-6 cloves) round out the flavors of the stew naturally. However, if you are foregoing the onions and garlic, consider simply using salt and pepper to taste. This supports the Late Summer principles of keeping things simple and somewhat bland. Otherwise, feel free to experiment with bay leaves, Chinese five spice (which contains all five of the flavors in Chinese medicine), cinnamon, dried chilies, orange zest, rosemary, or thyme.

LIQUID: Stews require ½ to 1 cup of liquid per serving, whereas soups require closer to 3 cups (or more if you are feeling particularly parched). I recommend choosing either water, Nourishing Bone Stock from page 122, or Medicinal Vegetable Broth from page 120 to serve as the base for your soup or stew. Additionally, consider switching out 2 to 4 cups of the base liquid for something flavorful such as apple cider vinegar, beer, red wine, or white wine.

OIL: A heat-stable oil such as coconut oil, butter, or lard for cooking.

TIP • If you would like to add a sweet twist to your stew, consider adding a seasonal fruit such as chopped apples, aiming for a total of about ⅛ cup per serving.

Cut the meat and vegetables into 1½- or 2-inch cubes. Season the meat generously with salt and pepper (if using). Prepare the liquid mixture of your choice.

DUTCH OVEN INSTRUCTIONS: Preheat the regular oven to 325°F. Add 1 teaspoon of oil to the Dutch oven and pan sear the meat on the stovetop until all sides are browned (about 3 to 5 minutes per side). Remove from the Dutch oven and set aside.

In the Dutch oven, add another tablespoon of oil and the onions and garlic (if using). Sauté over medium heat until translucent. Add in the liquid. Using a metal or wooden spatula, scrape the bits from the bottom of the Dutch oven (that's the good, flavorful stuff) to mix with the liquid, onions, and garlic. Stir in any additional spices and sauce and cook for 3 to 5 more minutes or until the mixture becomes fragrant.

Add the meat and make sure it is completely covered in liquid; add more liquid if needed. Cover with a lid and place in the oven. Cook for about 3 hours, checking every hour. Once the meat is fork-tender, add the vegetables and cook for an additional 45 to 60 minutes.

CROCK-POT INSTRUCTIONS: Set the Crock-Pot to low heat. Add 1 teaspoon of oil to a sauté pan and pan sear the meat on high heat until all sides are browned (about 3 to 5 minutes per side). Remove from the skillet and set aside.

In the same sauté pan, add another tablespoon of oil and the onions and garlic (if using). Sauté over medium heat until translucent. Add in the liquid. Using a metal

CONTINUES

or wooden spatula, scrape the bits from the bottom of the sauté pan (that's the good, flavorful stuff) to mix with the liquid, onions, and garlic. Stir in any additional spices and sauté for 3 to 5 more minutes or until the mixture becomes fragrant.

Place the meat and vegetables in the pot (yes, they go in at the same time) and pour over the liquid. Cover and simmer for 7 to 8 hours, or until the meat and vegetables are fork-tender.

Whether you are making a soup or a stew, the cooking times will be the same. Serve warm and enjoy!

SOUPS OR STEWS—WHAT'S THE DIFFERENCE?

Soups and stews are where it's at this time of year! The difference between the two is essentially the amount of liquid used to make the dish. A soup has more liquid than a stew. When it comes to Chinese medicine, you can decide which to make according to your constitutional and pattern needs. If you felt rather parched and dehydrated during the summer—which you can tell by your Chinese medicine pattern, the dryness of your skin, the brittleness of your hair, or the hardness of your stool—then a soup will be better suited to help you recover. On the other hand, if you felt waterlogged all summer because you were drinking so many fluids and had plenty of hydration, or if you feel your metabolism is rather fast, then perhaps a stew will strike your fancy this time of year. The best part about soups and stews is that they have endless combinations and are very flexible. You can bend this recipe to be vegetarian with a delicious vegetable broth or make a hearty stew with lamb and bone stock. It's up to you!

Lentils are a perfect Late Summer food as they are both sweet in taste and neutral in temperature. When cooked properly, they are easy on the digestive system and full of nutrients such as folate, manganese, iron, and about a gazillion other minerals. You can choose to go brown, red, or green (or even black) or use a nice mixture of them all. Green lentils tend to take longer to cook by about 10 to 15 minutes. Typically lentils do not need to be soaked as they break down much more easily than a traditional legume with regular cooking times. However, if you would like to reduce the time and support your digestion even more, you can soak them for 6 to 8 hours first, following the instructions on page 81.

2 cups lentils

5 cups water or home-
made broth/stock
(see pages 120 or 122)

2 tablespoons olive oil

2 medium onions, diced

4 cloves garlic

1 cup sliced fresh mush-
rooms (I prefer cremini
and/or shiitake)

2 teaspoons fresh or
dried rosemary, minced

2 teaspoons fresh or
dried thyme, minced

1 teaspoon fresh sage,
minced

1 teaspoon rice vinegar

1 tablespoon tamari or
soy sauce

2 tablespoons lemon juice

Salt and pepper to taste

TIP • For added richness and nutrients, consider adding ½ cup soaked walnuts to the mixture.

Add the lentils and water to a 3- to 4-quart pan and bring to a boil. Reduce the heat to medium-low, cover, and simmer for 20 minutes. Drain and set aside.

While the lentils are cooking, heat up a skillet on medium-high and add the olive oil. Once the oil is hot but not smoking, add the onions and garlic. Sauté for 1 to 2 minutes. Add the mushrooms and herbs, and sauté for another 3 to 4 minutes, until soft and fragrant. Transfer the mushroom mixture to a food processor; add the lentils, rice vinegar, tamari, and lemon juice. Process to a soft paste, and season with salt and pepper. (The pâté may need to be refrigerated for 30 to 60 minutes to firm up.)

Serve with flatbread or vegetable slices for a delicious snack or appetizer. Leftover pâté can be stored, covered in the refrigerator for up to one week.

Dates are an excellent way to get your sugar fix without turning to refined sugar products. I once had fresh dates from a date farm in Mexico, and they completely blew my mind. They were juicy, soft, sweet, and melted in my mouth. Eating them by themselves was a perfect way to enjoy them! Store-bought dates tend to be a bit drier but are delicious nonetheless.

- ½ cup nut butter of your choice
- 1 teaspoon ground cinnamon
- 1 teaspoon ground cardamom
- 1 teaspoon ground ginger (optional, for warmth)
- 1 tablespoon raw local honey
- 10 Medjool dates, sliced in half with the pits removed
- 2 tablespoons shredded coconut

Mix together the nut butter, cinnamon, cardamom, ginger (if using), and honey. Place a dollop of the nut butter inside each date half, sprinkle with coconut, and enjoy!

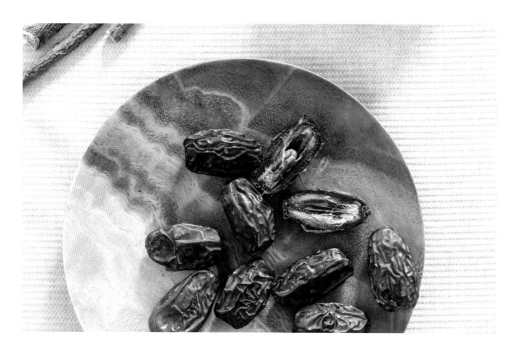

We make this weekly in our house because not only is it nutrient-dense, but it also serves as a substitute anytime there is a recipe that calls for milk or cream. We mix up the kinds of nuts we use to get a variety of nutrients and change up the flavor (especially useful if your family is picky). My favorite is the almond milk version. I like to make it in a 32-ounce Ball jar, as we tend to use that amount before it goes bad.

1 cup whole raw almonds, walnuts, pecans, or cashews

8 cups water (4 cups for soaking, 4 cups for making milk)

Pinch of salt

2 pitted dates

¼ teaspoon ground cinnamon

¼ teaspoon ground cardamom

¼ teaspoon ground nutmeg

SPECIAL EQUIPMENT

One 32-ounce Ball or Mason jar

Cheesecloth and strainer or nut milk bag

Put the nuts in the jar and fill to the brim with water. Soak overnight on the counter or at room temperature. In the morning, drain and rinse the nuts (which should be plump). Put the nuts in a food processor or blender along with 4 cups water and all the other ingredients. Blend well.

Set up a system to strain the milk. Rest a cheesecloth and strainer on top of a pot or large bowl. Once blended, pour the mixture into the cheesecloth and strainer, or alternatively, you can use a nut milk bag. Give the mixture ample time to strain (about 10 minutes). Squeeze the remaining blended nuts and spices into a ball to get the last bit of milk out. Transfer the milk to the Ball jar and store it with the lid tightly closed in the refrigerator for 3 to 4 days.

TIPS • If you are like me, you want to use every part of the foods you prepare. Save the leftover nut mixture and use it to make cookies or as a crust for a pie.

• If you prefer to make a plain nut milk, simply forego the dates and spices.

Once late summer arrives, many of us begin dreaming of an amazing Pumpkin Spice Latte (made famous by Starbucks but not nearly nutritious enough). I like to make a variation of this recipe that is both delicious and nutritious without hijacking my blood sugar. With this recipe, you can actually stabilize your blood sugar and nourish your spleen and stomach! This recipe only makes a cup of enjoyment, but you can make more if you get enthusiastic.

2 tablespoons pumpkin puree (homemade, canned, or store-bought)

1 cup Sweet Nut Milk (page 211)

¼ teaspoon vanilla extract

1 tablespoon full-fat coconut milk or heavy whipping cream

½ teaspoon Chaga Chai spice (page 235)

Sweetener to taste (Stevia, erythritol, maple syrup, and raw, local honey are my favorites)

TIP • If you like the coffee flavor in a traditional Pumpkin Spice Latte, add in 1 teaspoon instant ground coffee or a shot of espresso. Feel free to top with whipped cream for an added treat and/or sprinkle with extra spice. For additional warming, consider adding a slice of ginger to the brew.

Mix all ingredients together in a small saucepan and simmer for 5 minutes. Pour into your favorite mug and sip yourself into late summer bliss!

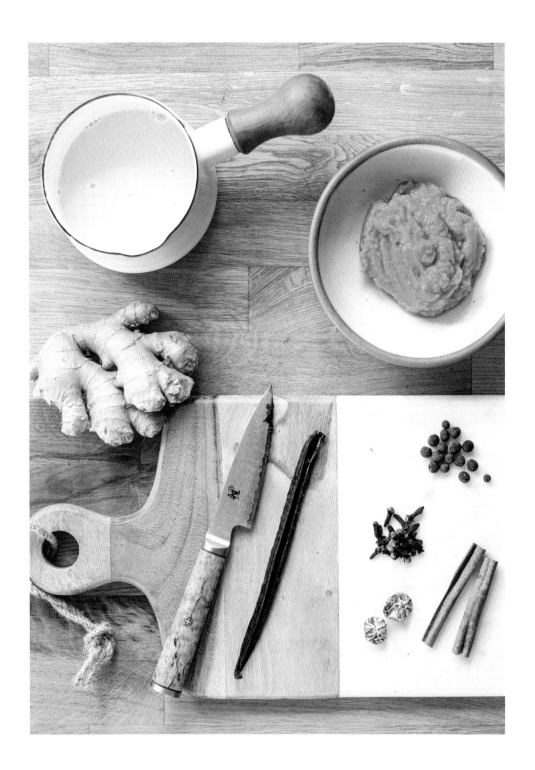

The important thing to remember about the transition from summer to late summer is that it's a wonderful window to begin thinking about supporting your overall system of health (and specifically targeting the digestive system) so you can face autumn and winter with ease. If you have any digestive issues now, it's a wonderful time to focus on and start healing them before the weather changes to a drier and cooler climate. If you are not having digestive issues per se, you can always focus on amplifying your gut's digestive abilities and growing your good bacteria. As far as supplements go, I highly recommend taking probiotics as a general rule of thumb to support not only your gut but your overall immune system for the rest of the year.

Agastache (Patchouli, Hyssop)

PINYIN: Huo Xiang

ORIGIN: China, India

PARTS USED: Leaves, flowers

ORGANS / SYSTEMS SUPPORTED: Lungs, spleen, stomach, digestive system

USES: Nausea (especially morning sickness), vomiting, summer colds and flu, stomachaches, diarrhea, bloating, headaches, sluggish digestion

PATTERNS SUPPORTED: Spleen chi deficiency, rebellious stomach chi, spleen yang deficiency

FLAVORS: Pungent

TEMPERATURE: Slightly warm

ACTIONS: Astringent, slightly tonifying

CONTRAINDICATIONS: None known

BEST TAKEN: Decoction (5 to 10 grams/day)

Atractylodes

PINYIN: Bai Zhu

ORIGIN: China

PARTS USED: Roots, rhizomes

ORGANS / SYSTEMS SUPPORTED: Digestive system, blood, urinary system, spleen, and stomach

USES: Diarrhea, abdominal distention, edema, dizziness, poor appetite, bloating, fatigue, nausea, vomiting, weakened immune system

PATTERNS SUPPORTED: Spleen chi deficiency, spleen yang deficiency, wei qi deficiency

FLAVORS: Bitter, sweet

TEMPERATURE: Warm

ACTIONS: Astringent, tonifying

CONTRAINDICATIONS: None known

BEST TAKEN: Decoction (5 to 15 grams/day)

Licorice ("The Grandfather of All Herbs")

PINYIN: Gan Cao

ORIGIN: Southern Europe, India, parts of Asia

PARTS USED: Roots, rhizomes

ORGANS / SYSTEMS SUPPORTED: Known to enter all twelve meridians; lungs, digestive system, central nervous system, kidneys, heart

USES: Blood sugar imbalances, immune system weakness, digestive system imbalances, sore throat, coughing, menstrual cramps, inflammation of the intestines and lungs

PATTERNS SUPPORTED: Spleen chi deficiency, stomach yin deficiency, lung chi deficiency, lung yin deficiency, heat and dryness in the large intestine, wei qi deficiency

FLAVORS: Sweet

TEMPERATURE: Neutral

ACTIONS: Tonifying, moistening

CONTRAINDICATIONS: None known

BEST TAKEN: Decoction (1.5 to 9 grams/day)

Mint (Chinese)

PINYIN: Bo He

ORIGIN: Mediterranean, western Asia

PARTS USED: Leaves, stems

ORGANS / SYSTEMS SUPPORTED: Lungs, liver, spleen, stomach, reproductive system, skin

USES: Fever, headaches, cough, sore throat, skin conditions that are hot and/or damp, moodiness, sluggish digestion, dampness in the digestive system

PATTERNS SUPPORTED: Spleen chi deficiency, stomach yin deficiency, liver chi stagnation

FLAVORS: Pungent

TEMPERATURE: Cooling

ACTIONS: Tonifying, astringent

CONTRAINDICATIONS: Too drying to be consumed by nursing mothers

BEST TAKEN: Hot infusion (1.5 to 6 grams/day); decoction (1.5 to 6 grams/day. Note that mint doesn't need to be cooked very long. So if you are preparing a decoction with other roots and barks, only add the mint in for the last 5 minutes.)

Poria

PINYIN: Fu Ling

ORIGIN: China

PARTS USED: Whole mushroom

ORGANS / SYSTEMS SUPPORTED: Stomach, central nervous system, digestive system, joints, lungs, liver, heart

USES: Edema, poor appetite, diarrhea, heart palpitations, insomnia, dizziness, anxiety

PATTERNS SUPPORTED: Spleen chi deficiency, spleen yang deficiency, heart chi deficiency

FLAVORS: Sweet

TEMPERATURE: Neutral

ACTIONS: Tonifying, astringent, calming

CONTRAINDICATIONS: Not recommended in larger doses for daily, long-term use

BEST TAKEN: Decoction (10 to 15 grams/day)

Seeds of Job's Tears

PINYIN: Yi Yi Ren

ORIGIN: China

PARTS USED: Seeds

ORGANS / SYSTEMS SUPPORTED: Spleen, lungs, kidneys

USES: Diarrhea, acne (or other damp skin conditions), arthritis, muscle spasms, edema, wet coughs

PATTERNS SUPPORTED: Spleen chi deficiency, stomach yin deficiency, spleen yang deficiency, damp heat in the large intestine, heat and dryness in the large intestine

FLAVORS: Sweet

TEMPERATURE: Slightly cold

ACTIONS: Astringent, tonifying

CONTRAINDICATIONS: None known

BEST TAKEN: Decoction (9 to 30 grams/day)

Formulas for Late Summer

CITRUS AND PINELLIA FORMULA (*ER CHEN TANG*): A formula that has been in use since the first and second centuries C.E., Citrus and Pinellia is considered possibly the most important formula for draining dampness and phlegm in the lungs, spleen, and stomach. Dampness leading to dizziness, nausea, gastritis, insomnia, and even depression can benefit from this formula. It is not to be used in cases of yin deficiency.

SIX GENTLEMAN FORMULA (*LIU JUN ZI TANG*): With six ingredients (radix ginseng, licorice, poria, atractylodes, tangerine peel, and pinellia), this formula has been documented in use since the sixteenth century. It primarily addresses deficiencies in the spleen and stomach, tonifying chi and drying dampness that has accumulated due to these deficiencies.

NOURISHING PRACTICES IN LATE SUMMER

Hosting a Potluck

To truly reap the rewards of the harvest, you must turn it into something that can be shared with your community. A healthy Earth element centers around community and nourishment, so bringing the two together in the form of a potluck is an amazing way to nurture this element during autumn. At our house, we host once-a-month

Sunday night community dinners, but during harvest time, we may host another and be invited to one or two more. It's a wonderful way to connect with others and explore different foods and cooking.

Cultivating Your Community

What is true community? It is a collection of people who connect regularly over a long period of time. They get to know each other either face-to-face or in some other manner (now that we have access to so much technology). The purpose of community is to know that you are not alone, to share your struggles and celebrations, and to know that you have more resources to draw on than just your own. May you build a stronger and stronger community during these challenging times. I recommend drawing a few concentric circles with yourself at the center like a bull's-eye. Begin listing the members of your community, from your closest friends (in the ring next to the bull's-eye, or you) to those out on the periphery of your group. Make a conscious goal to cultivate some or all of those relationships this season.

Cleaning Your Kitchen

What a perfect time of year to clean out the gathering place of your home, the kitchen. The pantry, refrigerator, all the cabinets—make it a free-for-all! Get rid of all those things you haven't used in more than a year and wipe down the ones you want to bring back out and use. Make sure you have easy access to all your best-loved appliances and gadgets and build yourself a beautiful centerpiece at your table or counter—wherever people sit together to share the bulk of your meals. Beautiful flowers in oranges and yellows really brighten up and bring earth-like energy into the home.

Assessing (and Reassessing) Your Life-Work Balance

Have you been feeling content regarding the balance of your career, hobbies, and personal life? If you are anything like most Westerners, you are struggling to find balance between work and your personal life. We really do get rewarded for becoming workaholics, and many of us are always living on the edge when it comes to finances. With these ever-present pressures, we can tend to take on too much. Some people have little choice in how much they work at any given moment, but overworking is very damaging to the spleen. So it's time to take a real hard look at what is really necessary for you. Are you living within your means? Are you working enough but not too much? Does anything need to shift to make you happier and make your energy more sustainable?

Developing Better Eating Habits

Most of us have learned to speed through meals. To chew just enough so that we can swallow and move on with our day (and an often-overwhelming number of responsibilities). The truth is, when we are stressed, we don't digest, we do not break down our food properly and can end up with all kinds of gas, bloating, indigestion, and other symptoms. Make it an intentional practice to prepare your meals, sit down, and focus only on eating; chew each bite thirty or more times before swallowing. You can eliminate many digestive problems by doing this practice each day.

Giving Thanks

Since this is a time where we are gathering foods that we have cultivated and tended all summer long, it's a wonderful time to be thankful for all the forces at play in this beautiful dance of creation. In our house we have collectively created a prayer of gratitude that we take turns saying before each meal. This not only allows us to express our gratitude for the food and all the components that are involved in getting the food to us, but it also helps us to center and ground before each meal.

Singing

While summer is all about expression and using your voice for clear and intentional speech, late summer is a time for singing, especially singing in a group! Singing used to be something that took place at most tribal gatherings hundreds of years ago. During all my travels around the world, I've seen that this is still happening. In fact, whenever I visit rural villages as part of my work, the local people always joyfully share their country's songs with me and want me to sing them "songs from my country." I used to have to explain that we don't really do that in America. But now, I've learned some songs and take them with me when I travel. Singing with others is a beautiful way to communicate and share an experience.

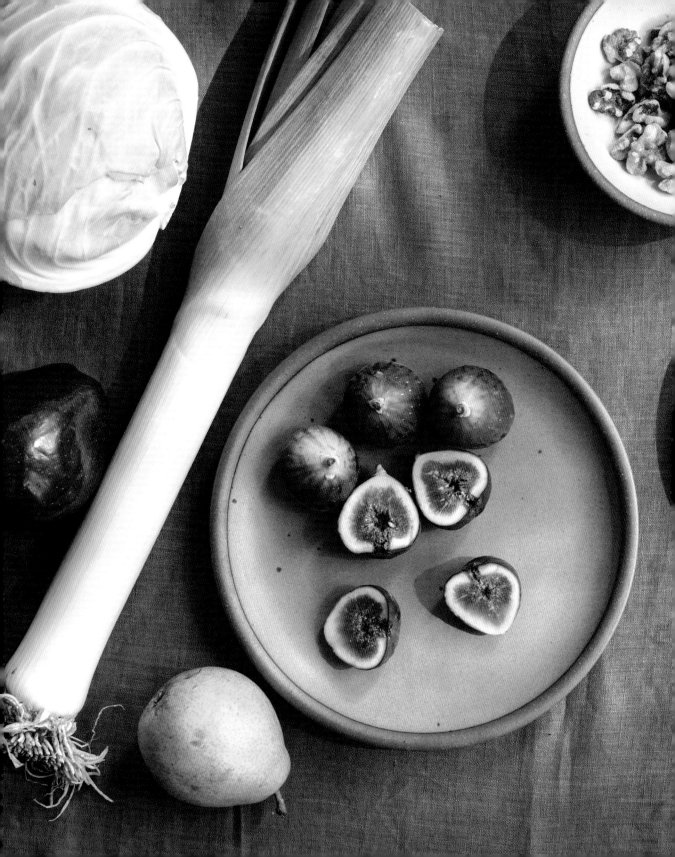

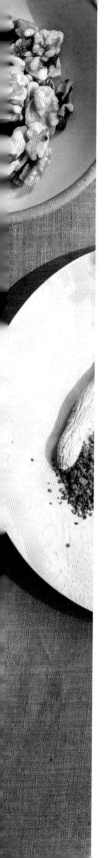
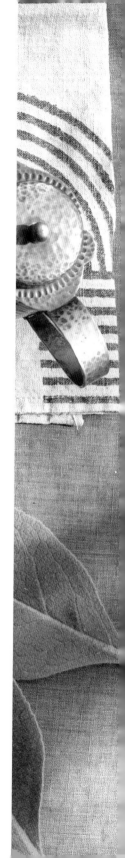

AUTUMN AND
THE METAL ELEMENT

AUTUMN EQUINOX (SEPTEMBER 22)
THROUGH WINTER SOLSTICE (DECEMBER 21)

Sometimes it's OK if the only thing you did today was breathe.
—YUMI SAKUGAWA

— ◆ —

Our internal and external energy is noticeably winding down this time of year, moving out of the total yang of summer and late summer but not yet descending into the total yin of winter. As such we call this season "yang within yin" to reflect that last burst of yang energy before the complete yin immersion in winter. Most people love this final burst as it reveals itself through the leaves changing color to the most beautiful bright reds and yellows. Where I live in Colorado, the aspen trees turn such an incredible gold color that it draws people from all over the world to witness their beauty.

The theme of this season is all about *letting go* and what I call *plugging back in*. All the fruit that didn't get collected during the main harvest will now become compost. Everything around us lets go and sheds what was once its bounty so it can begin to focus its energy internally (the way trees draw in their sap). We can mimic this in our own lives by looking around and letting go of that which no longer serves us. Sometimes during autumn we can hear the wind picking up. It's as though it is helping nature shed and let go of the last little bits of late summer's harvest. Know that this element (and in particular the lungs) are highly vulnerable to it.

Like the snake that sheds its skin, we can renew our values and sense of self by clearing away the things, thoughts, and activities that no longer make our hearts swell with joy. Many relationships end at this time of year, and there are more deaths than in any other season. It's as though the pressure of knowing winter is coming is enough for us to really have a deep check-in with ourselves. Heading into winter is like going into a cave: what do we need to take into the cave with us? This is not a time for frivolity.

When I use the term "plugging back in," imagine you have a cord attached to you. If you look to see where you've been sourcing your energy, you have been plugged into a power strip, and lots of other things are attached there too. So many, in fact, that you can hardly tell where your cord is plugged in. But what if you could take your cord and pull it out of the power strip and away from all the other activity? What if instead you could plug yourself directly into the outlet, one that you don't have to share with so many others? This is my analogy for autumn: it's a time for reconnecting more deeply with ourselves and to that which is greater than us. This can be called Spirit, God, Nature, Mother Earth—whatever works for you and brings that spark of mystery, joy, and wonderful feeling of being at home inside yourself.

THE METAL ELEMENT

During late summer, the fruit sweetened, and we harvested most of what we could. When fall comes, the fruit is becoming inedible; it has morphed from ripe and sweet to verging on rotten. The leaves and fruits themselves let go of the trees and fall to the ground to begin their journey of composting. As the leaves and rotten fruit deteriorate, they will make the soil beneath the plants and trees that much richer with nutrients and minerals for the next growing season. Plants and trees will suck up the minerals from the soil through their roots, and when we eat the resulting fruit, we will receive all that nourishment.

The Metal element in nature corresponds to this compost, which produces the minerals in our soil and then eventually turns into the rocks and stones that make up so much of our planet. What begins so humbly as compost on the forest floor or sea bed slowly, over hundreds of thousands of years, will crystalize and become the beautiful minerals and gemstones that we appreciate and adorn ourselves with today.

Many of us are unplugged from the preciousness, sacredness, and vulnerability of our lives on earth. The fact that we exist at all is quite extraordinary! Staying connected to this reality will keep us balanced even while we are engaged in the more mundane aspects of our lives (like paying bills and carting our kids around for various activities). In fact, studies show that people who have a spiritual connection and/or practice live longer and live better. At the end of the day, researchers found that it didn't matter what people believed in, but if they believed in something, they were happier at the end of their lives than those who had no spiritual view or practice.[6] This is perhaps the greatest antidote when we begin to feel burdened by our lives.

People who have a lot of Metal in their constitution tend to embody a strong sense of integrity, values, and purity and an undeniable connection to that which is greater than themselves. Think of the archetypal Priest or Priestess who spends much of his or her time communing with God, Goddess, Gaia, the Great Spirit, you name it. Note: Some traditions refer to the element of Air. The Metal element is most closely associated with the Air element.

METAL CONSTITUTION

ARCHETYPE: THE ALCHEMIST

People with a balanced Metal constitution are often very well kept and often adorned with beautiful jewelry or unique clothing or hairstyles. They are the type who pay attention to aesthetics, similar to a Japanese tea ceremony. There is a place for everything and a rhythm and method for how to steep the tea, how to pour it, how to hold the cup, and so on. Life can be like a Japanese tea ceremony for those with a Metal constitution. They appreciate the methodical aspects of their lives and live with integrity. Rules are very important because they set the stage of fairness and balance. With the archetype of the Alchemist, a Metal constitution can distill the essence of just about anything and find the true nuggets of wisdom.

EMOTION

Grief is the emotion associated with autumn and rightfully so. Grief is an emotional response to letting go and transformation (or change). Just like all the other emotions, grief is a natural movement of energy in our universe. We have the opportunity to experience grief many times throughout the day: the phone call we hoped to receive but didn't, the piece of china that was broken and could not be repaired, and even leaving our kids at day care while we go off to work. Then there are the greater losses that can bring up tremendous grief, such as the death of a loved one or the end of an important relationship. Grief draws us inward and has the impact of waking us up to our deeper values. Have you ever lost someone close to you and made some declarations about how your life was going to change moving forward? This is a common response, and it's because grief has the ability to unmask any "gunk" we have adopted that has clouded our true perception.

Grief, when not expressed, can get stored in the lungs. Asthma or respiratory ailments that won't heal are often indicative of harboring old losses that have never been properly grieved. In China (and some eastern Asian villages) when you go to a funeral, it's not unusual to find people jumping up and down while wailing in grief. They do this to prevent the grief from getting stuck in their lungs. To a Westerner, this looks very unusual, but from the perspective of energy, it only makes sense. Too often we "save face" and cry in private (or don't cry at all until many years later at some strange time). In Western culture we are shielded from death much more than those in other cultures where death is acknowledged by both grieving *and* celebration.

The Metal element is so closely tied to the lungs that anything significantly compromising the lungs becomes a Metal pattern of imbalance and impacts the body's immunity. In our daily lives we have many opportunities to degrade our immune systems. The chronic use of hand sanitizers and antibiotics deplete our body's microbiome, and we lose our defense system. A challenged immune system is the source of allergies, after all.

BALANCED METAL ELEMENT

- Strong immune system
- Connection to something/someone larger than self
- Identification with spirituality or religion
- Belief in fairness and equality
- Good organizational skills
- Self-discipline
- Conscientiousness
- Appreciation for structure and rules
- Deep inner strength
- Ability to grieve and let go when it's time
- Notice and enjoyment of beauty (can be brought to tears)
- Excellent sense of smell
- Liking for the finer things in life (and savors them)
- A wide perspective on things
- Comfort with being alone

OUT OF BALANCE METAL ELEMENT

- Overcritical of self and others
- Difficulty letting go
- Profound, long-standing grief
- Obsession with spiritual world
- Weakened immune system (asthma, allergies, frequent colds)
- Skin problems (eczema, rashes, psoriasis)
- Chronic constipation/bowel issues
- Feelings of self-importance, self-righteousness (I know the way)
- Aloofness, especially in relationships
- Negative outlook (talks trash)
- Appreciation for spaciousness but can be antisocial
- Low self-esteem
- Problems with authority
- Chronic lung issues (asthma, wheezing, COPD)
- Sensitivity to smells
- Perfectionist tendencies
- Nihilistic outlook
- Dismissiveness
- Arrogance, "high horse syndrome"
- A struggle with a sense of meaning, purpose
- Feelings of being cold and cut off from life
- Religious zealotry or complete atheism
- Fanaticism
- Allergies
- Aches, pains, or tightness in the upper chest, neck, or shoulders

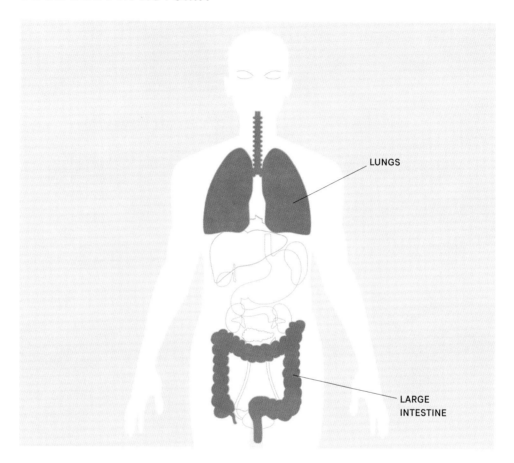

LUNGS

LARGE
INTESTINE

Lungs

The lungs are a pair of sponge-like, air-filled sacs that take up the majority of space in the rib cage. They are responsible for drawing in oxygen (emitted by plants and trees) and exhaling carbon dioxide (that the plants and trees use to make more oxygen). The lungs are part of the respiratory system, which begins with the nose and mouth and includes the sinus passages, trachea, bronchi, and bronchioles. Lungs are yin organs of the Metal element and are so vital that within minutes of their loss of function, we die.

OFFICIAL WHO RECEIVES THE PURE CHI FROM THE HEAVENS

Known as the "Official Who Receives the Pure Chi from the Heavens," the lungs are much more than sacs that move air in and out of the body. They bring us into relationship with that which is greater than the self and are responsible for giving us inspiration and self-respect. When they are functioning well, we see the value not only in our favorable qualities but also our shadow qualities. We can see all the aspects of our beings and lives as if from a bird's-eye view, able to touch on the preciousness of our (and all others') existence. When challenged, the lung official can cause us to question our sense of belonging and connectedness in a big way and can even lead us to become nihilistic and deeply insecure.

The lungs set the stage for the immune system since they are the front line of defense against the world (constantly taking in the air around us). The energy produced by lung activity is responsible for building what Chinese medicine calls *wei qi* (pronounced "way chee"). This term is used to describe the state of our immune system and the development (or lack) of a protective energy field that surrounds our bodies, extending about as wide as our outstretched arms and legs. In Western science, something called the "microbiome cloud" has been discovered, which is a field similar to that of wei qi. The microbiome cloud is a collection of diverse microbes that surround us like a cloud. The more diverse this collection of microbes is, the more protected we are from sickness and vice versa.

Wei qi, translated as "defensive or protective chi," was described thousands of years ago in a similar way. It serves as our personal, unique guard against unhealthy bacteria or even unhealthy energies that come our way. The stronger our wei qi, the less susceptible we are to getting sick. When I hear someone say, "I catch every cold that comes through town," I know that person's wei qi is down. If your wei qi is particularly challenged, you may find yourself having trouble sloughing off the energy of others, letting things get to you that at other times would have slid right by. Building strong wei qi happens when we care for our lungs. Those who smoke (anything), use steroid inhalers (or take steroids for any other reason), or are under high stress tend to have challenged wei qi. Root canals can also be a culprit for diminishing wei qi as they can house bacteria that the body subtly fights for a long time.

Large Intestine

Connected to the small intestine is a similar tube-like organ, though it is wider in diameter, thicker walled, and only about five feet long compared to the small intestine's twenty feet. The large intestine's primary jobs are to absorb water, gather the last few minerals from food that the small intestine missed, and eliminate what is not usable as waste. It's important to eliminate waste daily.

GREAT ELIMINATOR

In Chinese medicine, the large intestine is referred to as the "Great Eliminator" because its sole focus is to move stool out of the body. However, there is a similar function on an emotional and spiritual level: find the gems, the most important nuggets of wisdom and love, and let go of the rest. When we learn to let go appropriately, we find becoming present a much easier task than when we were holding on to too much of our history. Emotional backing up leads to physical backing up and vice versa.

Skin

In Chinese medicine, the skin is referred to as the "third lung" because it moves secretions in and out of the pores. Coincidentally, when someone tends toward having dry stools, that person also often tends to have dry skin. Additionally, when there are imbalances in the lungs or large intestine, the skin will sometimes show symptoms. An example of this is how eczema often accompanies asthma. Chinese medicine says this is because of a wei qi deficiency, possibly due to food allergies. The skin is also a vital part of our detoxification system, purging chemicals that don't belong in the body.

Nose

The Large Intestine meridian opens to the nose and is therefore responsible for our sense of smell. Unlike all other senses, the sense of smell is directly tied to the limbic system. This is the brain's processing center of memory and emotions, which is why a smell can easily trigger a memory. In fact, some say smell is the quickest way to remember something.

THE AUTUMN PANTRY
FEATURED RECIPES

Since this season is about letting go and recharging (supporting us into getting back to what is most important to our bodies, minds, and spirits), our diets can help us to physically clear out the rubbish in our systems and shore up our health for the coming winter months. Autumn is an excellent time of year to focus on the immune system and support the lungs for health the entire rest of the year.

Here are the general principles of nutrition in autumn:

• Returning to mostly cooked and warm foods.

• Avoiding cold and raw foods.

• Seek out pungent flavors.

• Master the art of soup-making and fermenting.

• Eat foods that are dark in color (like lots of dark leafy greens).

• Add light to medium spice to foods where enjoyed (unless you are too warm already).

• Add small amounts of salt to your meals.

• Use allium family plants as much as possible: onions, garlic, leeks, shallots, etc.

• Cook foods longer and over low heat.

• Steam and boil foods where possible.

Autumn Staples

PROTEINS: Clams, eggs, oysters, pork

GRAINS: Congee (page 126), rice

VEGETABLES: Asparagus, beets, broccoli, cabbage, celery, cucumbers, leeks, mushrooms, mustard greens, onions, parsnips, potatoes, radishes, sweet potatoes, watercress

FRUITS: Apples, apricots, bananas, figs, grapefruit, grapes, lemons, limes, pears, plums, pumpkin

LEGUMES: Navy beans, soybeans

SEEDS AND NUTS: Almonds, walnuts

HERBS AND SPICES: Black pepper, cardamom, chilies, cinnamon, garlic, ginger

CONDIMENTS AND MORE: Miso, olives, pickles, sauerkraut, vinegar

DAIRY: Cow or goat cheese, yogurt (if well tolerated)

FOODS TO AVOID: Cold foods and drinks, hot peppers (if you are experiencing wind or dryness), melons, raw foods

THE MYTH OF FLU SEASON

Autumn sometimes gets a bad rap as being a time of year when everyone starts getting sick. As if all of a sudden there is this new bacteria or virus floating around that starts infiltrating our homes and work environments! That isn't the case. In fact, the change often happens *within us*. We might have spent a little more energy than we had over the summer and late summer months, and when the weather changed in autumn, we became more vulnerable because we didn't have the energy to spare. Stress is also a major contributing factor to illness in general, but especially now. Many of us settle back into jobs with which we don't feel truly aligned, the kids go back to school, and the routines start up again whether we like them or not. This can lead to disappointment, which can also make us feel vulnerable to imbalances. Sugar intake also begins to increase this time of year, starting around Halloween. With sugar's ability to tank our immune system, we can participate in setting the stage for illness by overindulging. Remember, the pathogen is nothing; the host is everything.

AUTUMN RECIPES FOR LETTING GO, RECHARGING, AND STRENGTHENING THE IMMUNE SYSTEM

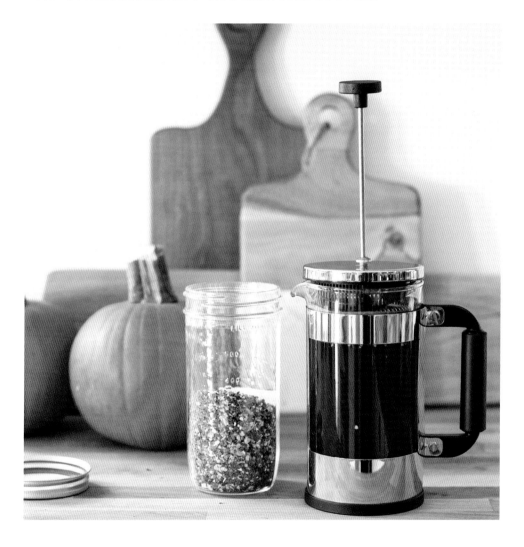

With the changing of seasons from moist and warm to dry and cool, it's important to take care of your immune system and keep from drying out and getting cold before winter comes. One of my favorite recipes to make is my Immunity Stock; I drink it like I would hot tea throughout the day. Allium family vegetables and herbs are plentiful in this recipe as they set the foundation for a balanced immune system in autumn.

1 tablespoon olive oil, butter, or ghee

2 large white onions, quartered

6 to 7 scallions or spring onions, white and green parts, whites thinly sliced, greens left whole

2 to 3 leeks, white and green parts, thinly sliced

2 large shallots, thinly sliced

2 carrots, thinly sliced

2 heads garlic

Any onion peels or allium greens you have around

3 celery stalks, thinly sliced into half moons

2 tablespoons white wine vinegar (or fermented veggie juice, kimchi, or sauerkraut)

15 black peppercorns

4 cloves

2 bay leaves

16 cups water

Salt to taste

TIP   • To amplify this soup's immune system power, consider adding medicinal mushrooms. I recommend 8 to 10 fresh or dried shiitake or reishi, or 2 to 3 maitake. Put them in the stock with the rest of the ingredients before bringing to a boil.

Put the oil in a stockpot over medium heat. Once it is hot but not smoking, add the onions, leeks, scallions, shallots, and carrots. (You can include the skin from the onions, shallots, and garlic as well.) Sauté until the vegetables are softened and the onions are translucent. Add the rest of the ingredients and bring to a boil, skimming any foam from the top. Once the stock is boiling, reduce the heat to a simmer (you should see a bubble come from the bottom of the pan every couple of seconds) and cook for 2 hours or until the stock has reduced (become concentrated) by about 40 percent. Taste and remove from heat when you enjoy the flavor; if it gets too strong, add more water. Strain the stock. Season with salt to taste. Enjoy at least a cup a day or freeze some to save for soups! This will keep in the refrigerator for up to one week.

Not only is there a ton of extra life (good bacteria) in fermented veggies to support the immune system, but these vegetables are also pungent and sour, so they support the liver by clearing fats and mucus from the detox pathways. Fermented veggies can be enjoyed with every meal as a small side dish, and the juice adds a good immune system boost to any soup, sauce, or salad dressing. This is a basic recipe for fermenting your own veggies in a week's time (4 to 10 days, depending on which vegetables you use and your taste preferences).

Enough sliced, diced, or chopped veggies to fill a 1-quart jar (cabbage, carrots, broccoli, radishes, parsnip, beets, cucumbers, onions, or a medley)

Seasonings of your choice (such as peppercorns, garlic, dill, thyme, basil, bay leaf)

2 cups room temperature water

1½ tablespoons salt

You will need a 1-quart, wide-mouthed Ball or Mason jar with a lid. (If you find you enjoy the fermenting process, you will need to buy replacement metal lids, as the metal lids corrode easily, or you might consider getting plastic lids instead. You can also place a piece of parchment or waxed paper between the top of the jar and the lid.)

Fill the jar to the bottom of the neck (1 inch from the top) with the vegetables and seasonings. In a bowl, stir together the water and salt until dissolved. Pour the water over the veggies until they are completely submerged. If you want to follow the traditional method for this recipe, put a cabbage leaf on top of the vegetables and push them down even farther to ensure that no food is sticking out of the water and to get rid of any air bubbles (where unwanted bacteria can grow). Screw the lid tightly on the jar and store it in a dark place at a moderate temperature (between 68°F and 75°F).

Check the veggies after 48 hours; you should be able to see little gas bubbles forming. Holding the jar over a sink, open the lid just enough to let the air out, and then screw the lid on tight again. We call this "burping." Do this every day until the veggies are exactly to your taste. Once you open the lid completely, keep the jar stored in the fridge with the lid tightly sealed. The veggies will keep for a couple of months.

FIRE CIDER IMMUNE SYSTEM TONIC • MAKES 3 CUPS (SEE NOTE)

This wonderful blend captures all the things I love about autumn in a single tonic! This drink/syrup starts out fermented, then you use honey to sweeten it like an aperitif when you are feeling run down or vulnerable to sickness. Depending on the pattern you are experiencing, you can add or take away some of these herbs and spices.

1 thumb-size piece of horseradish, peeled and chopped

1 thumb-size piece of ginger, peeled and chopped

1 thumb-size piece of turmeric, peeled and chopped

6 whole cloves garlic, peeled and chopped

1 red onion, peeled and quartered

1 teaspoon cayenne

1 lemon, quartered

1 tablespoon black peppercorns

3¼ cups raw, unfiltered organic apple cider vinegar

¼ cup raw local honey

SPECIAL EQUIPMENT

1-quart wide-mouthed Ball or Mason jar and lid

Square of parchment paper large enough to cover the jar opening

Put the vegetables and spices in the jar and fill it with vinegar to the bottom of the neck (1 inch from the top). Make sure all the ingredients are under the liquid and there are no air bubbles. If you see air bubbles, tap the jar on countertop until they rise and disappear. Place a square of parchment paper on top of the jar, close the lid over the paper, and seal tightly. Shake vigorously, then store in a dark place at a moderate temperature (between 68°F and 75°F).

Let sit for 3 to 6 weeks, shaking daily and burping (see page 233) as needed. I recommend starting your tasting around 3 weeks and continue to taste once or twice each week. Once the tonic has achieved your desired flavor, strain out the herbs and spices. Mix the honey into the tonic. Store the jar in the fridge and use within six months. I like to have a jar of this tonic always fermenting from about August to May as it is such a potent immune system support.

NOTE: You will end up with a total of 3 cups of tonic that can be used in a number of ways. You can take a smaller dose (½ to 1 ounce) daily as a preventative or you can use it during times of stress. If you start feeling under the weather, you can take a larger dose more frequently (1 to 2 ounces, 1 to 5 times per day).

CHAGA CHAI • MAKES 8 CUPS

Hands down one of my favorite parts about autumn is that it becomes suddenly hip to have a warm beverage in your hand at all times. Store-bought chai beverages are often oversweetened and brewed with black tea, which you shouldn't have too late in the day if you want a good night's rest. That being said, I love enjoying chai well into the evening, so I make it without black tea or refined sugar. I also like to add chaga mushrooms with their antiviral and antibacterial properties to support a healthy immune system. When I make this recipe, I make extra chai spice so I can store it and make a cup anytime I want. This recipe will make multiple servings, depending on how strong you like your brew.

½ cup dried chaga mushrooms (not freeze-dried)

1½ teaspoons ground cinnamon

1½ teaspoons ginger, ground or fresh chopped (fresh is spicier)

1 teaspoon ground cardamom

½ teaspoon ground cloves

Pinch of salt

Pinch of black pepper

Water

Milk (preferably homemade nut milk, see page 211)

Sweetener (optional)

Put the chaga mushrooms in a coffee grinder and blend until powdered. Add the chaga powder and all the spices, salt, and pepper to a small jar and shake thoroughly to mix. Store the jar at room temperature in your spice cupboard.

To brew a cup, begin with 1 heaping teaspoon chaga chai spice and a 1:1 ratio of water to milk. Whisk together in a small saucepan over low heat. When the mixture is steaming but not boiling, cover and let it simmer for 10 minutes. Strain using a small colander, pour the mixture into your mug of choice, and enjoy immediately.

CONTINUES

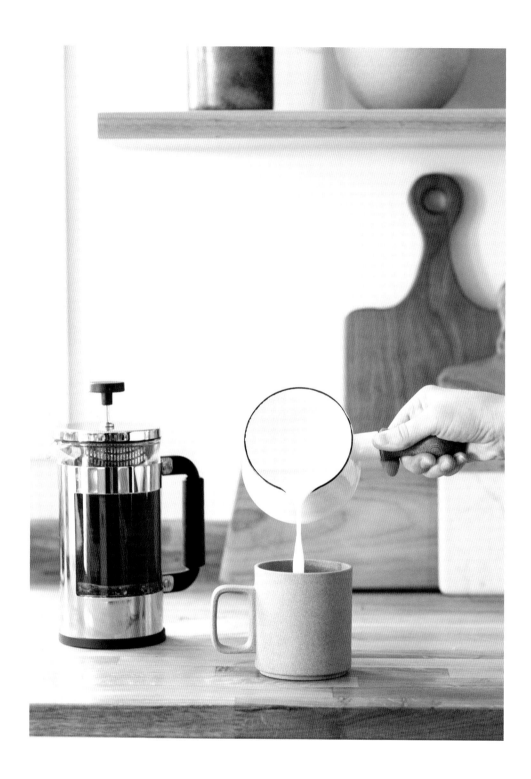

If you prefer your chai stronger, you can play with the amount of chaga chai spice you put in your milk-water mix. If I feel particularly run down, have cold hands and feet, or feel sluggish in my digestive system, I will use 3 or 4 heaping teaspoons of the spice mix!

Feel free to add additional herbs to mix up this drink such as reishi (to increase the immune system support), powdered chicory and burdock root to support the kidneys and adrenals, or powdered dandelion root to add support for the liver. One or two additional teaspoons added to the saucepan usually does the trick.

THE AUTUMN MEDICINE CABINET

The transition from late summer to autumn can bring about feelings of beauty, awe, and wonder as we watch the world change color all around us. For some it may be a time of mourning or sadness about leaving the fun of summer behind. The lungs and therefore the immune system can become more vulnerable now, due not only to stressors but also to the changes in climate and emotion. Grieve your losses if you feel that is important, but also boost your immune system in preparation for the dryness of autumn and prepare for the utmost yin of winter.

Cordyceps

PINYIN: Dong Chong Xia Cao

ORIGIN: China, Tibet

PART USED: Whole mushroom

ORGANS / SYSTEMS SUPPORTED: Lungs, kidneys, liver

USES: Fatigue (acute and chronic), immune system imbalances, cough, bronchitis, asthma, infertility, erectile dysfunction, Crohn's disease, altitude sickness, lupus

PATTERNS SUPPORTED: Lung chi deficiency, wei qi deficiency, kidney yang deficiency

FLAVORS: Sweet

TEMPERATURES: Warming

ACTIONS: Tonifying, slightly astringent

CONTRAINDICATIONS: None known

BEST TAKEN: Decoction (3 to 10 grams/day)

Elecampane

PINYIN: Tu Mu Xiang (Root)

ORIGIN: Europe

PARTS USED: Roots, flowers

ORGANS / SYSTEMS SUPPORTED: Lungs, spleen, liver

USES: Exhaustion, irritability, sporadic sweating, chronic cough, bronchitis, asthma, whooping cough, diarrhea, wet cough, nausea, physical PMS symptoms, constipation, autoimmune conditions

PATTERNS SUPPORTED: Lung chi deficiency, kidney yang deficiency, spleen yang deficiency

FLAVORS: Bitter, pungent

TEMPERATURES: Warm

ACTIONS: Astringent

CONTRAINDICATIONS: Not for use while pregnant or nursing

BEST TAKEN: Decoction (3 to 9 grams/day)

Ginger

PINYIN: Sheng Jiang

ORIGIN: China

PART USED: Rhizome

ORGANS / SYSTEMS SUPPORTED: Lung, spleen, stomach, digestive system, sinuses

USES: Nausea, colds, flu, immune system imbalances, bronchitis, wet cough, vomiting, diarrhea, morning sickness, sluggish digestion, constipation

PATTERNS SUPPORTED: Lung chi deficiency, wei qi deficiency, spleen qi deficiency

FLAVORS: Pungent, slightly sweet

TEMPERATURES: Warming

ACTIONS: Astringent, tonifying

CONTRAINDICATIONS: Not to be used when there is heat in the stomach

BEST TAKEN: Decoction (3 to 9 grams/day)

Radix Ginseng

PINYIN: Ren Shen

ORIGIN: China

PART USED: Roots

ORGANS / SYSTEMS SUPPORTED: Lungs, spleen, respiratory

USES: Chronic illness, fatigue (acute and chronic), stress, insomnia, restlessness, asthma, wheezing, shortness of breath, infertility

PATTERNS SUPPORTED: Lung chi deficiency, spleen chi deficiency, heart chi deficiency, blood deficiency, spleen yang deficiency, kidney yang deficiency

FLAVORS: Sweet, slightly bitter

TEMPERATURES: Slightly warm

ACTIONS: *Strongly* tonifying

CONTRAINDICATIONS: Use caution in cases of high blood pressure; consult with a practitioner if you are taking warfarin or phenelzine

BEST TAKEN: Decoction (3 to 9 grams/day)

THE MAGIC OF GINSENG

More than two thousand years ago, the famous Chinese herbalist Shen Nong said, "Ginseng is a tonic to the five viscera [major organs], quieting animal spirits, stabilizing the soul, preventing fear, expelling vicious [negative] energy, brightening the eyes and improving vision, opening the heart, benefitting understanding [comprehension], and if taken for some time will invigorate the body and prolong life."

Schisandra

PINYIN: Wu Wei Zi

ORIGIN: China

PART USED: Fruit

ORGANS / SYSTEMS SUPPORTED: Lung, heart, kidneys, liver, spleen, respiratory system, central nervous system, endocrine system

USES: Stress, anxiety, low libido, chronic cough, diarrhea, irritability, night sweats, insomnia, dream-disturbed sleep, allergies, skin conditions (especially weeping rashes)

PATTERNS SUPPORTED: Lung chi deficiency, kidney yin deficiency, liver chi stagnation

FLAVORS: Sour, sweet, salty, bitter, pungent

TEMPERATURES: Warming

ACTIONS: Calming, tonifying, astringent

CONTRAINDICATIONS: None known

BEST TAKEN: Decoction (1.5 to 15 grams/day)

Autumn Formulas

HONEYSUCKLE AND FORSYTHIA FORMULA (*YIN QIAO SAN*): One of the best formulas to use *the moment* you begin to feel like you could be catching a cold, presenting with the early stage symptoms of fever (with slight or no chills), cough, sore throat, headache, and thirst. This formula is best known for its use in acute colds, tonsillitis, or bronchitis, as it strongly supports the wei qi. The key is to take it as soon as you have a fever coming on, even if it's slight.

JADE WINDSCREEN FORMULA (*YU PING FENG WAN*): With its use recorded more than eight hundred years ago, this formula is excellent when you find yourself catching every cold that goes around. Jade Windscreen is not for the acute cold sufferer, but rather for someone who has been deficient for a long time and has compromised wei qi. Colds, sinus infections, allergies (to both food and the environment), and chronic fatigue are the perfect reasons to look to this formula. Jade Windscreen can be taken preventively during times when you know your defenses are down.

ROSE HIP TEA

Nature's single most potent source of vitamin C, rose hip tea, is an excellent addition to any seasonal medicine cabinet to support the immune system. Rose hips are the very sour and slightly astringent fruit of the rose plant. They grow after the bush sheds its flowers and look like small pink, red, and orange berries. Rose hip tea can be consumed anytime, day or night, and can be especially useful in cases of excessive mucus production and wet coughing.

NOURISHING PRACTICES IN AUTUMN

Taking an Early Morning Walk

Since lung and large intestine time is early in the morning (lungs, 3 A.M. to 5 A.M.; large intestine, 5 A.M. to 7 A.M.), it's a perfect time of day to have intentional time with yourself while getting some exercise. Early morning is so precious, especially if you can get a glimpse of it before everyone else begins to stir. The birds are out singing their songs, and the energy is otherwise very still. Monks all over the world start their meditation at around 4 A.M. Chinese medicine says that the time between three and five in the morning provides a window where "we are closer to the heavens" and are therefore more likely to have spiritual, awakening, or enlightening experiences at this hour.

Letting Go of Everything You Don't Love

Nature begins to let go all around us. The plants and trees shed the last of their fruit and leaves, and the birds and animals prepare for their departure from our environment (through either migration or hibernation). This activity can remind us to shed our own "stuff" that we no longer need in order to prepare for our own version of a winter hibernation. Open your closet, your kitchen cabinets, and all the spaces where things get stored in your house and start peeling through the layers. What is important to you at this point in your life? Have you worn or used these items in the last twelve months? One of my favorite questions to ask as I am preparing to head into winter is "What do I want to take into the cave with me?"

Building or Cleaning Your Altar

In honor of this seasonal transition, consider building yourself an altar or cleaning/recharging an existing one. Even if you don't consider yourself a religious or spiritual person, an altar can serve as the place in your home (or yard) where you collect items of significance and beauty. You can display all those seashells you brought home from the beach last summer or cover it with pictures of your family members, including those who have passed away. The opposite side of the coin from the vision board you made in spring, which held your intentions for what you wanted to bring in, you can build an altar that holds all of the items that remind you of who you are, where you have come from, the people who have influenced you the most, and anything else that brings you into your heart. Be sure to spend time with your altar each day during the autumn months. Lighting a candle or burning incense will open your senses and change the energy around your altar, recharging it if it you haven't tended it in a while.

Skin Brushing

Skin, the third lung, is a wonderful vehicle for moving lymph and supporting healthy wei qi. Lymph is a rich fluid that runs through the entire body (twice as much as blood), and it is full of white blood cells, making it one of our greatest front lines of defense against bacteria as well as the body's big detoxifier. While the lymph fluid itself is governed by the spleen and therefore the Earth element, the healthy function of the lymph supports not only the spleen, but also the liver and the immune system.

Skin brushing is a great way to stimulate lymph flow. Choose a skin brush made with natural bristle and a long wooden handle. One of the best ways to do it is on dry skin just before a shower or alternatively after a bath or shower. Dry brush in sweeping motions from head to toe in gentle strokes, always going toward your heart. Brush with about as much pressure as you would brush your hair on your head, brushing several times in each area or until you see a nice pink skin color. After your shower, replenish your skin with an oil or lotion you love, or try one of the following:

BREAST CARE

Women readers are going to think I'm crazy when I say don't be afraid to skin brush your breasts. I know they are sensitive and it sounds uncomfortable, but so much lymph flows through our breasts, and (despite our torturous underwires and other contraptions we use to suspend our breasts all day) we need that lymph to flow so we can have healthy breasts. Start off small, as your breast tissue will be sensitive at first, and then slowly increase the number of strokes and the pressure over time. Do not brush your nipples, as they *will* be sensitive. As a side note, I recommend doing away completely with underwire bras or any bras that are so tight that they leave indentation anywhere on your body—these bras impede the flow and drainage of lymph, and don't allow your body to get rid of toxins as efficiently. It is time we start curbing the often harmful, aesthetic-based habits we've adopted and re-route them toward health.

- **Jojoba Oil:** Neutral, great for all skin types
- **Almond:** Neutral, lighter oil, great for all skin types
- **Sesame Oil:** Warming, great for dry skin
- **Coconut Oil:** Cooling, great for sensitive skin

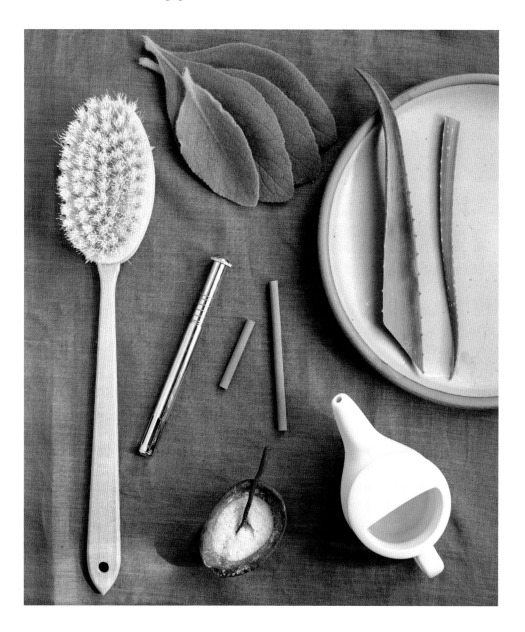

Square Breathing

All it takes is sixteen seconds to radically change your brain waves from a state of chaos to a state of relaxation. Square Breathing is a technique I recommend for spending time focused on your lungs, amplifying your lung capacity, and supporting you in managing stressful feelings. Picture a square in your mind's eye. Take a breath in, stretching it out for four seconds; pause for four seconds, then stretch out your exhalation for four seconds and pause for four seconds. Imagine each part of this exercise as a side of the square in your mind; you are moving around the sides of the square as you breathe. Repeat as many times as you are able. You may find that when you first start Square Breathing, you can't quite get to four seconds, and that's okay. Keep practicing and you will find it easier over time.

Finding Time for Contemplation, Meditation, and Prayer

These three terms, though they each carry their own charge, are all used to describe essentially the same thing: spending time with an intention in your heart and mind. So whichever practice stands out to you, whether it is using a mantra, singing a song, focusing on your breathing, or inviting something into your world, choose one to practice every day during the autumn season. These practices are important for bringing your awareness into the present moment, focusing your attention, and quieting the sometimes overwhelming "monkey mind" that can have you at its mercy. Without contemplation, meditation, or prayer, you can spend your entire day trapped in thoughts of the past, present, and future without ever being fully present with yourself, your family, or your community.

Earthing

The practice of Earthing is literally to place your bare feet on the ground in order to discharge any negative energies you may have picked up in your day-to-day life, and to reboot your system with energy directly from the earth. Many of us often wear shoes that do not conduct energy (like rubber soles) and walk on floors that create even more of a barrier between us and the earth. Walking directly on the earth is as natural as drinking water and can be just as restorative. It's like "plugging in" to an outlet that has the perfect vibration that brings you home to yourself.

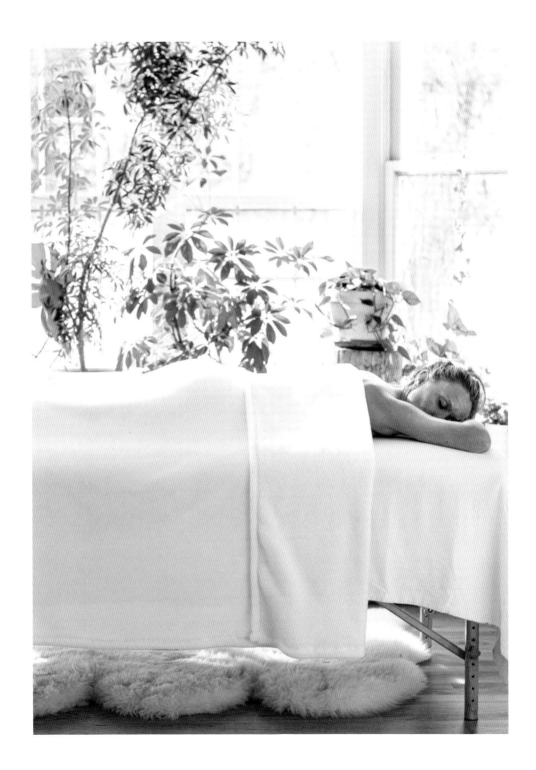

— ◆ —

PART THREE

ADDRESSING EVERYDAY IMBALANCES

— ◆ —

EVERYDAY IMBALANCES are a natural part of life, even when we are feeling healthy and in tune with our bodies, minds, and spirits. I use the term *imbalances* to indicate the transient nature of our experience of disharmony. Often we adopt a Western medical diagnosis as though it is who we are, and contrary to that way of thinking, Chinese medicine doesn't view health and/or the experience of symptoms in such a finite way. Rather, it sees them as an experience we are having.

The goal is not to completely avoid imbalances, as that would be impossible. Rather, it is to identify that we are having an imbalance; understand how it came about and how it affects us in body, mind, and spirit; and then do what we can to find balance again. For many of us, balance may mean uncovering our sense of peace, even with the continuation of symptoms. For instance, if you were to fall down and break your arm, your body would naturally attempt to heal from the fall. Your arm might develop scar tissue, and the bone that was broken might never be the same. Does this mean you would forever be in a state of imbalance? No. As a highly adaptable creature, you would find a new homeostasis, even without a complete return to your pre-fall state. The key is to understand all the implications of the imbalance and to do what you can to support your return to healing and homeostasis.

Part Three introduces you to the most common everyday imbalances. These chapters certainly do not cover the width and breadth of all the ways you can struggle with your health, but they will provide a snapshot of those I find most common and therefore most useful to understand. For each of the imbalances presented, you will be given the Chinese medicine interpretation of the imbalance and, for some, the Western medical interpretation as well. I find it helpful to understand both interpretations so that if you choose to take an integrative approach (using Chinese and Western medicine), you can make sense out of the treatment options stemming from each system. Additionally, I will present the most commonly prescribed diets, lifestyle considerations, herbs, formulas, and nutritional supplements for each imbalance. As always, I recommend seeking the support of a qualified practitioner to guide you through making any changes.

If you are having multiple symptoms that seem to relate to several different patterns of imbalances, it can feel overwhelming to see all the information and protocols to consider. Instead of just doing everything and taking every herbal medicine and supplement, *begin with your diet first.*

1. Clean out your pantry.
2. Ensure that you are drinking enough water (see page 75).
3. Clean up your diet (consider doing phases 1 and 2 of the cleanse, see Appendix E).
4. Follow an elimination diet (if you are still having symptoms, see page 285).
5. Restore your microbiome (see page 202).

Once you have taken these steps, check in again with any symptoms you are still experiencing. If you are still seeing multiple patterns of imbalance, then find a practitioner to work with who can guide you on your healing journey.

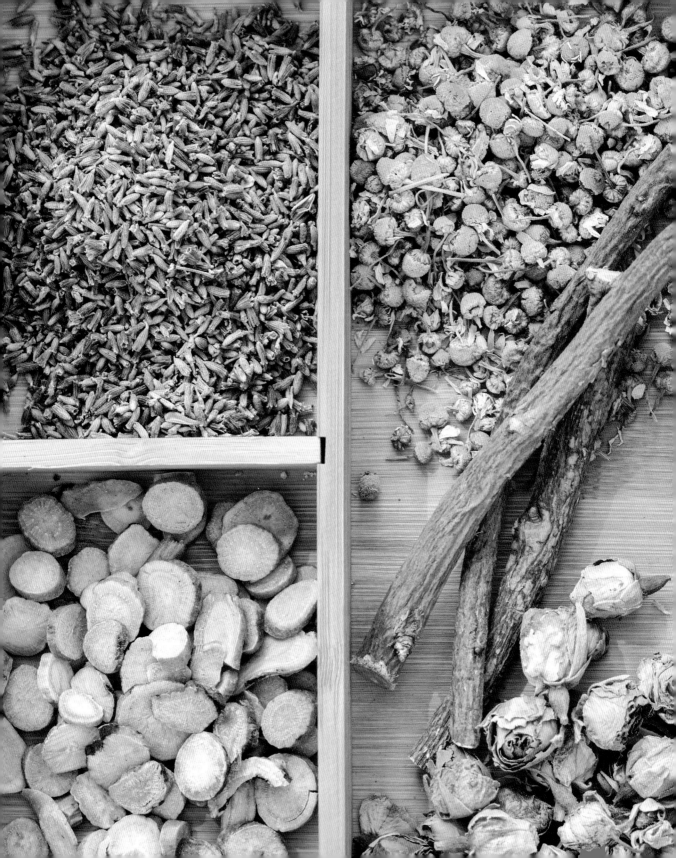

EMOTIONAL IMBALANCES

Emotional imbalances are becoming quite common in our modern world. An estimated one in five adults in the United States experience mental health problems.[1] There are many reasons for this, including nutritional imbalances, unrealistic career and family demands, nervous system imbalances, almost constant exposure to stimulation, and issues of self-worth.

These imbalances are severely exacerbated by our society, which teaches us that our value is tied to our performance and accomplishments. This is a message worth examining, as it creates unnecessary suffering and leaves us in an unending race to find our worth in outside sources. The unrelenting effort to live up to unrealistic expectations leaves us in a constant state of fight-or-flight. It's important to note that people who struggle to get their basic needs met (food, shelter, and so on) are two to three times more likely to develop emotional imbalances.[2]

Any emotional imbalances you feel must be examined for potential truth. Anxiety might be showing up to tell you something is off. Maybe you have taken a job that doesn't feel right or bought a house you can't actually afford. Maybe you are in a relationship that is not satisfying you, or maybe you just drank too much coffee this morning. Regardless, you can use these feelings to identify your core needs. Constantly keeping up with the societal standards of who you should become or what it should look like isn't all there is. Maybe it's time to blaze your own trail.

In addition to self-worth, many emotional imbalances stem from digestive imbalances. If you are in a constant state of fight-or-flight, you will not be able to digest properly and absorb the nutrients from your food. Improper nutrition, feeling stressed while eating, or eating quickly also impacts your ability to digest. Digestive imbalances almost always lead to deficiencies in vitamins, minerals, and amino acids—the building blocks of important neurotransmitters like serotonin and dopamine that support feelings of self-worth.

SUPPORTING EMOTIONAL IMBALANCES WITH DIET: Eat nourishing, seasonal, easy-to-digest foods (warm and cooked, nothing raw or cold). Focus on increasing your intake of healthy fats and anti-inflammatory foods while eliminating food additives, preservatives, and refined sugar. Adequate protein is important when it comes to building the necessary neurotransmitters to support emotional health.

LIFESTYLE CONSIDERATIONS FOR EMOTIONAL IMBALANCES: Move your body daily in a way that brings you joy. Aerobic exercise, weight training, yoga, and tai chi are all wonderful physical practices to include in your day-to-day routine. Increase community connections by joining a Meetup group, attending a class for something you'd like to learn, or practicing meditation to calm your mind and spirit.

ADDITIONAL TESTING TO CONSIDER: Salivary hormone, neurotransmitters, heavy metals, GI health panel, food sensitivity, complete blood count, comprehensive metabolic panel, nutritional deficiencies, salivary cortisol, genetic testing (For more information, see the "Resources for Delving Deeper" section at the end of this book.)

STRESS

Stress is an everyday imbalance that affects most people on the planet right now. Whether you are struggling to make ends meet or are agonizing over a presentation you have to give at your next work meeting, stress will find you. Stress is a response to life circumstances and *not* a disease process in itself.

Stress isn't all bad; in fact, it can be the motivating factor to help you accomplish things and build confidence in yourself and your abilities. If there is too little stress in your life, then you can wind up bored and unmotivated, feeling directionless. Whereas if there is too much stress, you can unravel and feel emotionally (and sometimes physically) paralyzed. Finding that sweet spot is the key to balance.

Most of us are not living in our sweet spot—we have moved way beyond the motivating mark and into the unravelling and near-paralysis place. When stress becomes too much, you challenge all of your systems, including the immune, digestive, and endocrine systems. Cortisol, the hormone that floods your body when you are under stress, may give you a little boost of energy in the short term, but chronic, long-term exposure to it will lower the body's immunity, and you may find yourself with recurring colds, among other imbalances.

Additionally, your system only operates in one response or the other: it's either *rest* or *run like heck*. Cortisol tells the body to run, so if you are trying to eat a meal with cortisol in your systems (while you are feeling any kind of stress), your body won't put out the appropriate digestive enzymes to break down the food. Instead, it is busy sending all the important signals to help you survive this perceived life threat (even though the perceived threat might be that rent is due tomorrow and you are barely scraping it together).

The wonderful thing about a stress response is that it has ensured human survival for many years. Stress switches your brain into survival mode when you are under threat. Your body releases all the appropriate hormones and chemicals to help you get out of the dangerous situation. Then once you are back to safety, your body can return to a normal homeostasis and a state of wakeful relaxation.

The trouble that I see most frequently with the stress response is that nowadays it doesn't just present itself when things are and *should be* stressful. Instead, it lingers. When this happens, the stress hormones linger in your system also and store in your tissues. Stress hormones create an acidic environment in the body, leading to pain and inflammation. Chronic exposure to cortisol (the major stress hormone) can actually degenerate tissues in the digestive system, joints, and even the brain. Chronic stress can keep you in a state of mild survival mode 100 percent of the time versus 100 percent survival mode on the rare occasions that you need it.

The body wasn't built for this day-in and day-out, insidious, low-grade stress response. The chemical reactions that happen in response to stress wear on your body, mind, and spirit. In fact, the National Institute of Health has publicly recognized that "Emotional stress is a major contributing factor to the six leading causes of death in the United States: cancer, coronary heart disease, accidental injuries, respiratory disorders, cirrhosis of the liver, and suicide."[3]

If you feel you are stuck in a stress response, know that your health depends on you unwinding that pattern and returning to balance. Don't get me wrong: life will have stressful periods, but you need to be certain that you come back down to a calm state of being. I'm not suggesting that, to be healthy, you need to remain calm and peaceful all the time. But being under rampant, chronic stress is no way to live. To begin chipping away at stressors, take a look at the source of your stress and make a realistic evaluation of what is changeable and what is not. Begin making those changes right away. In addition, consider the following:

1. Determine your natural yin/yang balance. Assess your life through this lens. Make any necessary changes.
2. Determine your constitution (take the quiz on page 52) and make the necessary lifestyle changes, incorporate the practices, and add in the nourishing foods for that element.
3. Assess your work-life balance. Do you really need to be working as much or with such intensity?
4. Learn stress management techniques, such as Square Breathing (see page 244), meditation, being in nature (even a quick walk outside), spending time with loved ones, and scheduling time off in advance.
5. Understand how stress shows up for you. (Common stress reaction patterns and the elements are described in the next section.)

Stress and the Elements

STRESSED WOOD: Those with a lot of Wood in their constitution tend to react to stress by getting very physical and/or working out more (I sometimes call this "work-out-aholism"). Over time, because they rely on a healthy Wood element, ligaments and tendons may experience tears and strains. Wood constitutions process stress in the liver. Since the liver (in conjunction with the kidneys) has the most difficult time dealing with stress (hence, the rampant Chinese medicine diagnosis of liver chi stagnation), addiction can be more prevalent.

STRESSED FIRE: Those with a lot of Fire in their constitution tend to react to stress (seemingly better than the other elements) by turning to play and adventure. However, they can get into trouble if this play and adventure becomes an act of dissociation and avoidance. A common theme is "I know the problem is there, but right now I don't want to deal with it. I just want to play." That's okay in the moment, but if years have gone by and the piles of things they have been avoiding has just grown higher and higher, they are going to be faced with much more stress! This element also tends to see more manic symptoms. Fire constitutions process stress in the pericardium and heart, which is where the heart palpitations and anxiety come from.

STRESSED EARTH: Those with a lot of Earth in their constitution tend to react to stress by developing unhealthy relationships with food. Considering the yin and yang aspect of Earth, if they are stressed out, they may turn to food to soothe the underlying feelings (yang) or turn away from food and deprive themselves (yin). Additionally, boundaries can become difficult to maintain, and Earth constitutions can easily overdo just about anything (compassion fatigue, caring for everyone, and so on). Either way, stress on the Earth element will change weight and muscle mass and may even interfere with the enjoyment of food. Earth constitutions process stress in the upper digestive tract, which can cause stomachaches, diarrhea, gas, and bloating.

STRESSED METAL: Those with a lot of Metal in their constitution tend to react to stress by becoming overly competent workaholics (to manage the increase in desire for perfectionism) and/or dissociating into the spiritual realm. Stress can make Metal become more rigid. This rigidity can show up in creating more rules, having inflexible boundaries, and often adding more pressure to the already stressed-out system. Metal constitutions process stress in the large intestine, typically by becoming constipated, and in the respiratory system, with recurrent colds, sinus infections, and asthma.

STRESSED WATER: Those with a lot of Water in their constitution tend to react to stress by isolating and/or shutting down. Stress is extremely hard on Water because the kidneys are home to the adrenal glands. Stress causes the brain to signal the adrenals constantly and forces them to put out adrenaline and cortisol (both stress hormones) to help manage the stress. Because stress can become so overwhelming to a mostly yin person, collapse or the desire for isolation is common. Water constitutions process stress in the kidneys and adrenal glands, which can lead to HPA Axis Dysfunction (also know as adrenal fatigue syndrome).

In addition to addressing your stressors on the outside, I urge you to work on the inside as well. Stress is a response after all, and you are in charge of your responses—more so than you would think. In addition to the supportive recommendations already discussed, look into herbs known as *adaptogens*. They negate the effects of cortisol and other stress hormones on the body without making you sleepy or sedated. Here is a list of my favorite adaptogenic herbs: ashwagandha, astragalus, bacopa, eleuthero, lemon balm, licorice, rhodiola, reishi, schisandra, and tulsi.

ADDICTION

Chinese Medicine Interpretation

All addiction begins with the same desire: to fill a void. Behaviors or substances that fill that void vary, but regardless, the seeking is essentially the same—to uplift the shen, or spirit. After repeated use (and consequent abuse), we begin experiencing a restless spirit, known in Chinese medicine as shen disturbance (see page 173). In my practice, I'm not so concerned with the specific behavior or substance to which a client is addicted. I ascertain the energy *around* the substance or the behavior. How intense is the energy of the substance when we talk about it? What happens if the client thinks about quitting the substance or behavior? Those questions guide us in determining whether this is an imbalance worth looking into. Most of us know when we are addicts and may even try to hide or normalize it, even as adults. This is because addiction is painful and carries a significant amount of shame with it. Depending on the particular substance being used, different patterns may arise.

Special Considerations

Addiction is the thought or behavior that arises out of a vulnerable nervous system. These vulnerabilities most often find their roots in a challenging childhood where the primary attachment figure wasn't available to meet the needs of the child. If a child repeatedly goes to a parent looking for nourishment and doesn't find it, that child will eventually learn to look to outside sources for nourishment. This is a common precursor for addiction, as it sets the stage for deep insecurity. If parents are addicts themselves, then the child is twice as likely to be drawn to using substances.[4]

Another common underlying theme for addiction is trauma. Trauma destabilizes the nervous system, creating vulnerability that can then lead to addiction. The third most common cause for addiction that I see is nutritional deficiencies. These can leave us searching for nutrients, albeit not in the best places, such as alcohol and drugs. For instance, when clients tell me they are addicted to alcohol, I can't help but wonder if they are getting enough dopamine from their diet, since alcohol gives us a dopamine high (though not without consequence).

In my opinion, we are all addicts, whether it is to work, coffee, perfectionism, marijuana, video games, Netflix, stimulation, or anything else. A nervous system that struggles with overstimulation is often drawn to addictive substances that are more sedating, whereas a nervous system that struggles with understimulation (like depression) will likely be drawn to substances that are more stimulating. With as much pressure as we are under, it's important to learn coping strategies for managing stress that do not rely on outside sources. In addition, to truly address addiction, we must begin to heal our nervous systems through practicing awareness, meditation, therapy, somatic experiencing, and other modalities. I recommend receiving the National Acupuncture Detoxification Association (NADA) protocol of ear acupuncture from a licensed acupuncturist and/or registered NADA practitioner. There are NADA clinics in every major city. (For more information, see the "Resources for Delving Deeper" section at the end of this book.)

ADDICTION	
Symptoms	Engaging in a destructive behavior or consuming a substance without being able to stop Having withdrawal when the behavior or substance is discontinued Experiencing insomnia Having changes in appetite (increase or decrease) and digestion Experiencing anger, especially when confronted Continuing substance use/behavior despite health problems Making social and/or recreational sacrifices Maintaining a good supply of a substance Taking risks Justifying behavior or substance use to "deal with problems" Exhibiting obsession, secrecy, solitude, and denial
Chinese Medicine Patterns	Heart fire blazing Liver chi stagnation **If left unaddressed in the short term can lead to:** Liver overacting on stomach Liver overacting on spleen Heart chi deficiency Lung chi deficiency (from smoking) **If left unaddressed in the long term can lead to:** Heart yin deficiency Kidney yin deficiency Kidney yang deficiency Lung yin deficiency (from smoking)
Chinese Herbal Formulas	Free and Easy Wanderer (*xiao yao san*) Free and Easy Wanderer Plus (when heat signs are present)(*jia wei xiao yao san*) Great Stabilizer (*chai hu long gu mu li tang*) →

Chinese Herbs	Licorice	Hawthorn
	Schisandra	Skullcap
	Ashwagandha	Burdock root
	Bupleurum	
Other Herbs	**To cleanse the liver and kidneys:**	**To curb nicotine cravings:**
	Dandelion root	Lobelia
	Burdock root	
	Milk thistle	**To curb caffeine cravings:**
	Fumitory	Tyrosine
	Echinacea	Chamomile
	Oatstraw	Feverfew
	To soothe the nerves:	
	Valerian	
	St. John's wort	
	Vervain	
	Kava kava	
	Lemon balm	
Nutritional Supplements	B-complex (including B_2, B_3, B_5, B_6, and B_{12})	Gamma-aminobutyric acid (GABA)
		N-Acetylcysteine
	Vitamin C	Glutathione
	Milk thistle	L-Carnitine
	Magnesium	
	Calcium	**For sugar and alcohol cravings:**
	Potassium	Good Earth original tea
	Selenium	Chromium
	Zinc	L-Glutamine
	Vitamin E	
Acupressure Points	Conception Vessel 17	
	Liver 3, 13, and 14	
	Large Intestine 4	
	Governing Vessel 19 and 20	

◆

ANXIETY

Chinese Medicine Interpretation

Second to concerns about stress, anxiety affects practically everyone who enters my office or signs up for my courses. Whether it is anxiety about bills or social situations, it impacts people from all walks of life. Anxiety often brings about all kinds of phobias, including social ones. Chinese medicine views anxiety as energy getting trapped in the head (often due to spleen chi deficiency) or around the heart (often due to heart chi deficiency). When this happens, we feel ungrounded and uncomfortable inside our own skin, our minds often run amok with worry, and our hearts feel like they could beat right out of our chests.

Special Considerations

Anxiety and depression can be viewed as two sides of the same coin, depression being the more yin aspect of this imbalance, and anxiety being the more yang aspect. Whereas depression is often an "under-arousal" (parasympathetic) response from the nervous system, anxiety is often an "over-arousal" (sympathetic) response. If there has been a rise in intense emotions, thoughts, or feelings and the nervous system has reached its capacity, we become overwhelmed because we can't integrate the emotions, thoughts, or feelings at the rate they are coming in. In psychology we call this "emotional flooding," and it can cause significant anxiety and even panic attacks.

On occasion I have seen a physical presentation of anxiety due to energy being stuck in the abdomen, creating limited space for circulation and breath to move. Adhesions (internal scar tissue) can also develop around the diaphragm, restricting the full capacity of the lungs. In this case, bodywork with someone skilled in working at this level of physicality and emotions is valuable.

If there is any self-worth issue wrapped up in your anxiety (which there usually is), addressing it is going to be par for the course. Learning breathing techniques (such as Square Breathing, page 244) and how to stimulate your parasympathetic nervous system can support you in coming out of a state of arousal. Also, learning to call a time-out so that you can catch up with your own body and emotions is helpful.

ANXIETY

Symptoms	Panic, fear, and uneasiness Sleep problems Inability to stay calm and still Cold, sweaty, numb, or tingling hands or feet Shortness of breath	Heart palpitations Dry mouth Nausea Tense muscles Dizziness Obsessive-compulsive disorder
Chinese Medicine Patterns	Spleen chi deficiency: Liver blood deficiency Heart yin deficiency	**If left unaddressed can lead to:** Heart fire blazing
Chinese Herbal Formulas	Calm the Shen and Supplement the Heart (*an shen bu xin wan*) Eight Treasure Combination (*ba zhen tang*) Great Stabilizer (*chai hu long gu mu li tang*) Serene Spirit (*gan mai da zao tang*)	
Chinese Herbs	Angelica Licorice Hawthorn Reishi	Eleuthero Jujube seed Polygonum Ashwagandha
Other Herbs	Lemon balm Kava kava Tulsi	Valerian Passionflower St. John's wort
Nutritional Supplements	L-Theanine B-complex (methylated forms) Vitamin C 5-hydroxytryptophan (5-HTP) or tryptophan	GABA Magnesium Calcium
Acupressure Points	Pericardium 6 Stomach 36 Large Intestine 4 Liver 3 Spleen 4 and 6	Yin Tang Bladder 15 Gallbladder 39 Conception Vessel 12

DEPRESSION

Chinese Medicine Interpretation

Depression is a painful emotional imbalance experienced by many people, with symptoms ranging from a feeling of dullness or lack of interest in life to no longer wanting to be alive. When you experience depression, it can be difficult to get out of bed in the morning or to find joy in anything. The saddest part about it is the shame that often accompanies this condition. Shame adds yet another layer to the imbalance and can sometimes be more painful than the depression itself. One consideration for chronic depression is the lungs and grief. Unprocessed grief can lead to symptoms of depression. (If you feel this might be related to your pattern, see page 224.)

Over these last few years, I have noticed more of a type of depression that I call "hyperfunctioning depression," where instead of the classic lethargy and lack of interest evident in a more typical presentation of depression, there is higher energy and the drive to "do it all." This may also look like workaholism. Hyperfunctioning behavior is tricky in our society because we often don't catch it for a long time, and when we do, it comes as a surprise because we have usually been rewarded for our hard work, keeping it together so well, and so on. But it can be just as harmful a behavior as almost any other.

Special Considerations

The most common form of depression I see in my office is due to liver chi stagnation; however, there are other patterns that follow closely. There are many reasons for depression, but modern research is telling us there aren't as many neurotransmitter imbalances leading to this condition as we once thought. (For more information, see the "Resources for Delving Deeper" section at the end of this book.)

DEPRESSION		
Symptoms	Feelings of helplessness and hopelessness	Loss of energy
	Loss of interest in daily activities	Self-loathing
	Appetite or weight change	Reckless behavior
	Sleep changes	Concentration problems
	Anger or irritability	Unexplained aches and pains

DEPRESSION		
Chinese Medicine Patterns	Liver chi stagnation Spleen chi and heart chi deficiency	Kidney yang deficiency Liver blood deficiency
Chinese Herbal Formulas	Free and Easy Wanderer (*xiao yao san*) Restore the Spleen Decoction (*gui pi tang*) Serene Spirit (*gan mai da zao tang*) Bupleurum Soothe the Liver Formula (*chai hu shu gan wan*) Free and Easy Wanderer Plus (when heat signs are present) (*jia wei xiao yao san*) Decoction to Drain Liver Fire (*long dan xie gan tang*) Pinellia and Magnolia Bark Decoction (*ban xin hou po tang*) Preserve Harmony (*bao he wan*)	
Chinese Herbs	Rhodiola Radix Ginseng	
Other Herbs	St. John's wort Milk thistle	Dandelion root Oatstraw
Nutritional Supplements	B-complex Eicosapentaenoic acid (EPA)/docosahexaenoic acid (DHA) 5-hydroxytryptophan (5-HTP) or tryptophan Melatonin Probiotics	
Acupressure Points	Liver 3, 5, and 14 Kidney 3 and 24 Governing Vessel 12 and 20	Conception Vessel 6 Bladder 15 Heart 5

BIPOLAR DISORDER (MANIC-DEPRESSION)
Chinese Medicine Interpretation

In Chinese medicine bipolar disorder is considered an imbalance between Fire and Wood (heart and liver, to be more precise). I mostly see the pattern beginning in the liver, either through excesses (such as drinking or drugs) or through deficiencies such as repressed emotions (trauma being the cause of many imbalances). When this liver pattern goes on too long, it begins to create stagnation and, consequently, heat in the body; that begins to irritate and heat up the heart. When the heart is inflamed, we end up with feelings of mania, not to mention our spirit becomes deeply troubled (shen disturbance). The intensity of emotional imbalances is increased when phlegm is present. One of the most notable symptoms of bipolar disorder is not the highs but rather the lows on either side of them. After the internal Fire burns hot for some time, it will eventually burn out, which leads back to the symptoms of depression. Remember to treat the depressive pattern when you are experiencing the depressive symptoms and the mania pattern when you have mania symptoms.

Special Considerations

This diagnosis is becoming more and more prevalent. This condition seems to comprise bouncing back and forth between yin and yang with no real middle ground or homeostasis in between. This can be very uncomfortable to experience. Bipolar disorder often brings a sense of a loss of control and groundlessness. It becomes difficult to make plans because you never know how you are going to feel when the day or time comes. So there is often a loss of community associated; you feel very alone. Finding a support group is important not only to heal but also to grow an understanding community.

BIPOLAR DISORDER (MANIC-DEPRESSION)		
Symptoms	Manic phase: Heightened sense of self-importance Exaggerated positive outlook Significantly decreased need for sleep Poor appetite and weight loss Racing speech, impulsiveness Ideas that move quickly from one subject to the next Poor concentration, easily distracted Increased activity level Excessive involvement in pleasurable activities Poor financial choices, rash spending habits Excessive irritability, aggressive behavior	Depressed phase: Feelings of sadness or hopelessness Loss of interest in pleasurable or usual activities Difficulty sleeping; early morning awakening Loss of energy and constant lethargy Sense of guilt or low self-esteem Poor concentration Negative thoughts about the future Weight gain or weight loss Talk of suicide or death →

BIPOLAR DISORDER (MANIC-DEPRESSION)

Chinese Medicine Patterns	**Manic phase:** Liver fire blazing Heart fire blazing Heart phlegm fire Blood stagnation or stasis **Depressed phase:** Liver chi stagnation (sometimes with phlegm accumulation) Spleen chi deficiency Liver blood deficiency Heart chi deficiency (sometimes also with gallbladder deficiency)
Chinese Herbal Formulas	**Manic phase:** See guidelines in Anxiety table and consider adding in Peaceful Sleep Formula (*an mian pian*) Heavenly Heart Formula (*bai zi yang xin tang*) Serene Spirit (*gan mai da zao wan*) Great Stabilizer (*chai hu long gu mu li tang*) **Depressed phase:** See guidelines listed in Depression table
Chinese Herbs	Schisandra Ashwagandha Reishi Hawthorn
Other Herbs	Lemon balm Nettles Tulsi Kava kava
Nutritional Supplements	Probiotics GABA EPA/DHA
Acupressure Points	Stomach 40 and 41 Bladder 17 Large Intestine 5

TRAUMA AND POST-TRAUMATIC STRESS DISORDER

Chinese Medicine Interpretation

In Chinese medicine, trauma is said to induce a state of shock in the nervous system and body (similar to what we think of as shock in Western medicine). However, PTSD occurs when that experience of shock never clears. It's as if the nervous system's response of fight-or-flight gets frozen in time. Until we can reset the system and rewire the connections in the brain, we will stay in a loop of shock. The goal in Chinese medicine is to treat the underlying pattern of disharmony, and the earlier we can catch it, the better.

Special Considerations

Sadly, the opportunities to experience trauma are everywhere. However, what determines whether or not an experience will be labeled as traumatic depends on a few different things: your personal bandwidth, your strength of spirit, and the abundance (or lack) of your personal resources (such as close friendships, self-care practices).

We each have our own capacity to tolerate shock and trauma, which I refer to as our "personal bandwidth." This is based on (1) our upbringing and whether or not we had a close relationship with a healthy attachment figure, and (2) previous experiences of suffering that were manageable and integrated. Children who are shielded from any and all suffering become adults with a smaller bandwidth, yet children who have little protection and are exposed to significant suffering become adults with vulnerable nervous systems. There is a sweet spot in the middle that builds bandwidth and confidence through experiences that we are able to integrate, given our age and maturity.

A strong spirit will give you added resilience (hence Chinese medicine's focus on strengthening the spirit in all cases of imbalance), because it infuses you with a heartier connection to the bigger picture and a stronger connection with yourself. Having a strong spirit can carry you through significant turmoil. Two women once joined my practice who were each diagnosed with stage 4 metastatic breast cancer and were in their early sixties. They didn't know each other, though they had a similar trajectory of decline and prognosis according to Western medicine. The first client, after her diagnosis, started making her bucket list right away and began checking things off as quickly as she could. She was also interested in trying a few alternative treatments to support her energy while the cancer was growing. This client outlived her prognosis by more than four years and was able to cross all but two items off her list.

The second client, on the other hand, was very down about her diagnosis, and it took her into a deep, dark depression. Despite support from her husband and many family members, she was resistant to trying new approaches to healing that could have supported her energy, her immune system, and her spirits, saying, "What's the point? I'm dying." She scoffed at the idea of a bucket list and argued with her family almost daily. This woman didn't even make it to her prognosis date, passing away six months before.

Of course, there were many differences between these two women, but the biggest difference was their *strength of spirit*. While the first client's spirit was clearly strong and supported her through her difficult times, the second client's spirit was challenged. This is where Chinese medicine and acupuncture can really shine.

Personal resources are another big determining factor in the experience of trauma. Supports like beloved people and places, practices, practitioners, pets, herbs, and supplements can provide a deep level of nourishment. The more we can develop our personal resources throughout our lives, the more capable we will be of healing from trauma.

In a tribe or clan, if one person experienced trauma, the whole group would respond and provide support for that person to return to health and balance. The way our lives are set up now, we often suffer alone or with the support of one or two other people. The larger we can grow our network of support, the quicker we will heal. Finding ways to reach out and seek support (even in some small way) may put an end to the painful and isolating symptoms.

In addition to these recommendations, consider using some of the treatments for PTSD, such as emotional freedom technique (EFT), eye movement desensitization reprocessing (EMDR), neurofeedback, and somatic experiencing.

TRAUMA AND POST-TRAUMATIC STRESS DISORDER

Symptoms	Easily startled Flashbacks to a traumatic event Irrational fears Severe anxiety and mistrust Loss of interest or pleasure in activities Guilt, shame Loneliness, social isolation Agitation, irritability, hostility Hypervigilance Self-destructive behavior Insomnia and/or nightmares Distress for more than a month following a traumatic event	
Chinese Medicine Patterns	Acute stage of trauma: Heart fire blazing Liver fire blazing Heart phlegm fire	If left unaddressed, can enter the chronic/PTSD stage: Liver chi stagnation (with heat signs) Liver blood deficiency and spleen chi deficiency
Chinese Herbal Formulas	Peaceful Spirit (*yang xin ning shen wan*) Calm Spirit (*ding xin wan*) Great Stabilizer (*chai hu long gu mu li tang*) Emperor's Heart Yin (*tian wan bu xin dan*) Free and Easy Wanderer Plus (when heat signs are present) (*jia wei xiao yao san*)	
Chinese Herbs	Reishi Ashwagandha Codonopsis Jujube seed	Tangerine peel Salvia Skullcap Poria
Other Herbs	Tulsi Kava kava	Dandelion root Milk thistle
Nutritional Supplements	Vitamin B_{12} B-complex Vitamin C	EPA/DHA L-Theanine Bovine adrenal glandulars
Acupressure Points	Pericardium 6 Kidney 3 and 24 Liver 3 Large Intestine 4	Spleen 6 Stomach 36 Heart 7

DIGESTIVE IMBALANCES

Digestive health as the foundation of overall health is a blind spot in Western medicine and leads to considerable, unnecessary suffering. According to Chinese medicine, digestive imbalances could easily be the root of almost *all* imbalances because they lead to poor nutrient absorption, nutritional deficiencies, and a weakened microbiome. I can't emphasize this enough: with a weakened microbiome, it's difficult to develop a strong immune system; healthy tissue; and a clear, calm mind. When digestive health is disturbed, you wind up developing digestive imbalances that are no fun. They can leave you tied to the toilet or unable to enjoy the pleasures of food. Chronic use of nonsteroidal anti-inflammatory drugs (NSAIDs), antacids, and antibiotics and limited strategies for managing stress are major contributors to digestive imbalances.

These imbalances have a common thread of inflammation. This is why it's vital that you look into removing the trigger of the inflammation (getting to the root cause) so you can begin healing. Sometimes the trigger is food-related, perhaps an allergy or intolerance to certain foods. Allergies aren't always what you think. You can recognize a major allergy because it causes obvious symptoms like hives and even anaphylaxis. However, some allergies are more insidious and can develop internal symptoms that you are unaware of for some time. I call these "intolerances" because the body becomes intolerant and dishes out a bunch of inflammatory responses and stress hormones to deal with them.

Other times the trigger for digestive imbalances is emotional—often feeling overwhelmed with chronic exposure to stress, self-criticism, and otherwise repressed emotions. Facing and doing your best to begin healing your wounds, old and new, is critical so you can heal your digestive system. The overall focus here is on reducing the stress response, decreasing inflammation, repairing any injured tissue, and rebuilding the microbiome and digestive system.

SUPPORTING DIGESTIVE IMBALANCES WITH DIET: Eat nourishing, easy-to-digest foods (warm and cooked, nothing raw or cold). Focus on increasing your intake of healthy fats, fermented foods, and anti-inflammatory foods; eliminate food additives, preservatives, and refined sugar. An anti-inflammatory or elimination diet (page 285) may be helpful in weeding out potential triggers of inflammation.

LIFESTYLE CONSIDERATIONS FOR DIGESTIVE IMBALANCES: Move your body daily: stretch or do yoga, especially yin yoga, aerobic exercise, weight training, and tai chi. Increase your community connection and meditate to calm your mind and spirit. Eat slowly during meals, making sure to chew thoroughly before swallowing.

ADDITIONAL TESTING TO CONSIDER: GI health panel (must include yeast, fungus, and bacteria culture from stool samples); inflammatory markers (must include lysozyme, calprotectin, and alpha 1-antichymotrypsin); digestive enzyme markers (must include chymotrypsin, pancreatic, and elastase); SIBO (including lactulose breath test/hydrogen/methane breath test); secretory immunoglobulin A (IgA); neurotransmitters, food sensitivities.

NAUSEA / VOMITING

Chinese Medicine Interpretation

Energy that runs through the digestive tract is always supposed to move in a downward direction. However, where there is nausea and vomiting, energy is either stuck in the digestive system or moving in the wrong direction (upward). It's a terrible feeling we are all familiar with, and the Chinese medicine approach is to redirect the energy down. Whether due to hormonal changes (as with pregnancy), flu, food poisoning, or having too many cocktails, the patterns can all be fairly similar.

Special Considerations

For pregnancy/morning sickness-related nausea and vomiting, try eating smaller, more frequent meals (or even just a few bites of food). Focus on protein when you do eat. Try bananas, as the high dose of potassium can sometimes squelch the nausea. And find the pattern that most closely fits your symptoms. If you find yourself craving something, try to follow that (within reason), as it is usually your body telling you what it needs.

Some women develop pica (unusual cravings during pregnancy, such as wanting to eat dirt, clay, or rocks), which points to an underlying mineral deficiency. Try taking a multimineral supplement that is safe for pregnancy and see if it curbs your cravings. Otherwise a good prenatal vitamin and a good diet should cover your bases.

Symptoms	Queasiness	
	Persistent nausea	
	Vomiting	
	Dry heaves	
	Loss of appetite	
	Morning sickness during pregnancy	
Chinese Medicine Patterns	Rebellious stomach qi	
	Spleen qi deficiency	
	Liver qi stagnation (can lead to liver invading the spleen)	
Chinese Herbal Formulas	Agastache Powder to Rectify the Chi (*huo xiang zheng qi san*)	
Chinese Herbs	Ginger	Licorice
	Agastache	
Other Herbs	Peppermint	Cardamom
	Chamomile	
Nutritional Supplements	Vitamin B_6	
	Potassium	
Acupressure Points	Pericardium 6	Stomach 36
	Large Intestine 4	

HEARTBURN

Chinese Medicine Interpretation

While this can be another accompanying symptom of pregnancy, many people experience this pattern without such a reward. Similar to the patterns of nausea and vomiting, where all the energies of the digestive system are supposed to be moving downward, in heartburn these energies are moving up and backward. Sometimes there is a physical deficiency, such as when the lower esophageal sphincter doesn't close properly after meals or is weakened in general. This can cause leakage into the esophagus.

I see many clients who experience heartburn and are told by Western doctors that they are producing too much acid; they are put on acid reducers, sometimes for years. First off, it is extremely rare to find someone who is producing too much acid without it being provoked by food allergies or intolerances. Most of the time, after changing the diet, the acidity goes away. Producing too much acid is often the body's way of dealing with having to eat foods that irritate it. Also, antacids have been under much scrutiny in the medical community over the last few years. Taking antacids such as proton pump inhibitors for longer than two weeks has been shown to lead to some pretty serious nutritional deficiencies, putting you at risk for intestinal infections, diarrhea, bone fractures, and low blood magnesium (which can lead to arrhythmias, muscle spasms, and even seizures).[1] Nutritional deficiencies have been linked to all kinds of diseases, including Alzheimer's and dementia. If you find yourself needing to take antacids frequently, go back to the pantry guidelines in Chapter 3, consider doing a cleanse (see Appendix E), and try an elimination diet (see page 285) to find out why this is happening.

HEARTBURN

Symptoms	Burning sensation in the throat and chest Difficulty swallowing Chronic cough Stomach pain or burning in the upper abdomen Persistent sore throat Regurgitation of food or liquid with a taste of acid in the throat Persistent hoarseness or laryngitis	
Chinese Medicine Patterns	Stomach yin deficiency Liver chi stagnation (can lead to liver invading the stomach)	
Chinese Herbal Formulas	Preserve Harmony Pills (*bao he wan*)	
Chinese Herbs	Licorice	
Other Herbs	Slippery elm	Marshmallow root
Nutritional Supplements	Digestive enzymes Probiotics	Collagen L-Glutamine
Acupressure Points	Conception Vessel 12 and 14 Stomach 36	Pericardium 6 Stomach 19

Special Considerations

Lifestyle changes, such as not eating too close to bed or naptime, avoiding hot and spicy foods, avoiding acidic foods (such as tomatoes), lying propped up in bed at night, and taking a short walk after meals will all help to redirect digestive energy downward, while you work on the underlying pattern and make any necessary dietary changes.

IRRITABLE BOWEL SYNDROME

Chinese Medicine Interpretation

For the most part, this is a pattern involving dampness with occasional heat. It is very uncomfortable and can lead to all kinds of nutritional deficiencies, so it must be worked with right away.

IBS		
Symptoms	Abdominal pain, cramping, or bloating that is relieved (or partially relieved) by passing stool Excessive gas Diarrhea or constipation, sometimes alternating Mucus in the stool Nausea	
Chinese Medicine Patterns	Spleen chi deficiency (can lead to dampness and heat in the gallbladder) Damp heat in the large intestine Liver chi stagnation (can lead to liver invading the spleen)	
Chinese Herbal Formulas	Curing Pills (*kang ning wan*)	
Chinese Herbs	Curcumin	
Other Herbs	Slippery elm	Peppermint
Nutritional Supplements	Probiotics Digestive enzymes	L-Glutamine
Acupressure Points	Stomach 36 Spleen 6 Stomach 25 (for constipation)	Spleen 15 (for diarrhea) See guidelines for diarrhea or constipation if present

Special Considerations

Nearly one in five people in the United States are said to experience IBS.[2] What I have found in clinical practice is that this often develops as a result of a weakened microbiome due to chronic exposure to food allergies or intolerances or simply as the result of a poor diet (full of fried foods, iced or frozen foods, sugary or processed foods). Restoring your microbiome would be the best place to start. Referring to the pantry guidelines in Chapter 3 and the elimination diet (page 285) will guide you.

LEAKY GUT SYNDROME
Chinese Medicine Interpretation

Leaky gut syndrome is a modern-day malady. It is not found in the classical Chinese medicine texts, which further confirms that there is something wrong with the way we eat these days. The first culprit for leaky gut is often found in the chronic use of antibiotics (or exposure to antibiotics before age two and a half), NSAIDS, steroids, and/or antacids at some point in a patient's history. All these drug exposures lead to chronic stress on the system, and chronic stress is another cause of leaky gut. From what I have seen, it is this exposure that seems to set the stage for all the secondary symptoms of food allergies/intolerances. From there all kinds of inflammatory symptoms begin to show up. I have seen many cases of supposed rheumatoid arthritis and degenerative disc disease where the symptoms completely resolve after treating the patient for leaky gut syndrome.

SOOTHING BELLY TEA

Make a hot infusion out of equal parts comfrey, plantain, slippery elm, and curcumin. Steep the herbs for 20 to 30 minutes and drink one to three cups a day to support healing from leaky gut.

Special Considerations

Leaky gut is becoming a common presentation in clinical practice. It is a reflection of a sustained poor diet, long-term exposure to food allergies/intolerances, overuse or long-term use of NSAIDS, and/or overuse of antibiotics (or antibiotics used on an already fragile system). This exposure leads to chronic intestinal inflammation that wears on the lining of the intestines. Eventually the lining becomes so thin that you have full-body reactions to meals or what feels like a systemic response to food or drink (*systemic* means all over the body or pain in multiple joints). Not only that, but with the associated inflammation and irritation to the gut, nutritional deficiencies abound and lead to immune system deficiencies. Consider starting with a cleanse (see Appendix E) and return to the pantry guidelines in Chapter 3.

LEAKY GUT SYNDROME

Symptoms	Chronic diarrhea, constipation, gas, or bloating	
	Nutritional deficiencies	
	Multiple food allergies/intolerances	
	Poor immune system	
	Headaches, brain fog, memory loss	
	Excessive fatigue	
	Skin rashes and problems such as acne, eczema, or rosacea	
	Symptoms that are exacerbated after meals	
	Cravings for sugar or carbs	
	Arthritis or joint pain	
	Depression, anxiety, ADD, ADHD	
	Autoimmune diseases such as rheumatoid arthritis, lupus, celiac or Crohn's disease	
Chinese Medicine Patterns	Spleen chi deficiency	
	Spleen yang deficiency	
Chinese Herbal Formulas	Six Gentleman Plus (*xiang sha liu jun zi tang*)	
Other Herbs	Curcumin	Marshmallow root
	Aloe vera	Plantain
	Slippery elm	Comfrey
Nutritional Supplements	Probiotics (bifidobacteria in particular)	Digestive enzymes
	L-Glutamine	Collagen
	EPA/DHA	Quercitin
	Gamma linoleic acid (GLA)	Butyrate
Acupressure Points	Large Intestine 4	Stomach 36
	Liver 3	

YEAST OVERGROWTH / CANDIDA

Chinese Medicine Interpretation

Yeast can grow not only on and inside of our genitals but also in our digestive tract. Have a look at your tongue, as you can often see a fairly heavy white and/or yellow coating with a yeast infection. This is because the digestive tract produces mucus to deal with the overgrowth of yeast, and the overgrowth of yeast can turn that thick white coating into a cottage cheese–like coating (in severe cases, it is called thrush).

Special Considerations

Candida is just one type of yeast, and it is healthy in the gut in small amounts. It's important to remember that this diagnosis all comes back to the gut. If the gut were in good shape and the pH was stable, then the environment of the gut would not provide a home for yeast to grow out of balance. Some yeast is natural and healthy. However, when the gut is in a state of dysbiosis (meaning microbial imbalance; see page 202 on the microbiome), yeast and other bacteria can proliferate. Antibiotics, birth control pills, oral corticosteroids, and the sugar highs and lows of diabetes can all lead to yeast overgrowth. Don't forget about stress as well.

ANTIFUNGAL SUPPLEMENTS

You can find a number of supplements that will supposedly kill yeast, but there is a caveat. Certain types of yeast respond better to certain herbs and supplements. But any type of yeast can become resistant after fourteen days or so. Without doing a yeast sensitivities test, it is difficult to know which herb or supplement will kill the type of yeast you have growing. So try only one or two items from the list of yeast-killing herbs and commit to that for fourteen days. If you are still having symptoms, commit to a different set of herbs. Above all, stop feeding the yeast! Yeast thrives on sugar and things that turn into sugar quickly like breads and other "white foods" (rice, potatoes, and so on). The categories of yeast-killing and gut-supporting herbs need to be taken about two hours apart.

VAGINAL YEAST INFECTION PROTOCOL

Supplies needed: Oregano oil capsules, probiotics, Yin Care, organic cotton tampons with applicators

Oral Supplement Protocol

Begin taking oregano oil capsules with food as directed for fourteen days.

Take probiotic capsules as directed, twice a day with food (even a light snack) for thirty days. Leave a minimum of two hours between probiotics and the oregano oil.

Topical and Vaginal Protocol

Create a 1 to 5 dilution of Yin Care to water. Push about a third of a tampon out of the applicator and dip it in the solution. Insert the tampon at night before bed and take it out in the morning and dispose. Repeat for seven nights in a row.

If you are also having external symptoms (such as redness, irritation, and itching), sprinkle the dilution on a sanitary pad and wear during the day and/or night.

Sleep without underwear to "cool" things down when you are not needing to wear a pad to treat external symptoms. In fact, if you are prone to yeast infections, sleeping without underwear can be a good general rule of thumb to prevent them while you are working on your microbiome.

Avoid sex or contact with anything that could introduce new bacteria.

Dietary Protocol

Avoid sugar, sweet-tasting foods, grains, potatoes, alcohol, and dairy products. Consider cleansing for fifteen to thirty days (see instructions in Appendix E). If you frequently get yeast infections, you may consider the longer cleanse and an overhaul of your diet and lifestyle.

Note: If after fourteen days there has been no change, repeat the protocol, but instead of using oregano oil, switch to *both* grapefruit seed extract and caprylic acid for fourteen days, following the manufacturer's instructions. If after thirty days there is still no change, see your practitioner, consider long-term dietary changes, and take a microbiome stool test. I have seen this situation with patients who have had chronic and/or long-term antibiotic use. In this case, your gut flora may need more specific boosting.

◆

Symptoms	Digestive problems (gas and bloating)
	Cravings for sweets
	Bad breath
	White coating on tongue
	Brain fog
	Exhaustion
	Joint pain
	Loss of sex drive
	Chronic sinus and allergy issues
	Weak immune system
	Chronic urinary tract infections
	Chronic vaginal yeast infections
Chinese Medicine Patterns	Spleen chi deficiency
	Spleen yang deficiency
Chinese Herbs	Atractylodes
	Cardamom
	Orange peel
	Poria
	Mume
Other Herbs (all yeast-killing)	Oregano oil
	Berberine (barberry)
	Grapefruit seed extract
	Garlic
	Coconut oil (also a natural antifungal)
Nutritional Supplements	Probiotics (gut-supporting)
	Prebiotics (gut-supporting)
	Caprylic acid (yeast-killing)
Acupressure Points	Spleen 6
	Stomach 36
	Conception Vessel 12
	Gallbladder 34 and 39

GAS AND BLOATING

Chinese Medicine Interpretation

The spleen needs warmth, energy, and movement to stay healthy, so often when there is gas and bloating, there is a spleen chi deficiency that leads to chi stagnation in the intestines. Gas and bloating are not a normal part of digestion. They are the result of faulty digestion, usually from foods that are foreign to the gut or from a deficiency in the digestive system. Warm and cooked foods, as well as warming herbs, nourish the spleen and, therefore, the entire digestive system. When you notice an imbalance beginning in your digestive tract, consider switching to only warm and cooked foods until your symptoms resolve.

Special Considerations

When there is lots of gas and bloating, there are often food allergies/intolerances as well. The body will produce a lot of extra air when it is confused about how to digest something (which is why taking digestive enzymes helps with gas and bloating). Additionally, yeast overgrowth tends to produce extra gas, and dairy intolerance will produce foul-smelling gas. (If this is happening due to constipation, see page 279). Occasionally this pattern may be due to very little hydrochloric acid in the stomach, which requires a supplement. I recommend getting a hydrogen breath test before beginning supplements.

Adhesions in the digestive system from long-term inflammation can restrict the needed peristalsis in the digestive system, leading to gas and bloating. Bodywork with a visceral therapist is warranted if you have ruled out food allergies/intolerances. Due to the spleen's dependence on movement, making sure to get some sort of exercise after meals could be a way to mitigate some of the distress until you figure out what is causing the gas and bloating.

Symptoms	Pain in the abdomen relieved by passing gas Feeling of unusual fullness after meals Gas Bloating Distended abdomen
Chinese Medicine Patterns	Spleen chi deficiency
Chinese Herbal Formulas	Curing Pills (*kang ning wan*)
Chinese Herbs	Ginger Hawthorn Tangerine peel Poria Licorice
Other Herbs	Peppermint Dandelion root
Nutritional Supplements	Digestive enzymes Probiotics
Acupressure Points	Conception Vessel 6 and 12 Stomach 25 and 36 Spleen 3

DIGESTIVE TEA

Put ½ teaspoon each of fennel seeds, caraway seeds, and anise seeds in a coffee grinder and grind to a fine powder. Pour the mixture into a mug and fill it with boiling water. Steep for ten minutes, strain, and enjoy. The same mixture can be steeped up to three times.

DIARRHEA

Chinese Medicine Interpretation

Acute diarrhea is most often caused by poor diet, food allergies/intolerances, bacterial imbalances, and emotional stress, all of which lead to spleen chi deficiency. Food poisoning is also a common cause of acute diarrhea. Chronic diarrhea is often caused first by spleen chi deficiency which turns into yang deficiency, becoming more cold in nature. A hallmark of yang deficient diarrhea is having diarrhea first thing in the morning (called cock's crow diarrhea).

DIARRHEA		
Symptoms	Loose and/or watery stools Abdominal pain or cramps Urgency and frequent bowel movements (more than 3/day) Increased thirst	
Chinese Medicine Patterns	Spleen chi deficiency Liver attacking the spleen (in cases of emotional stress) Damp heat in the large intestine	**If left unaddressed can lead to:** Spleen yang deficiency Kidney yang deficiency
Chinese Herbal Formulas	Ginseng, Poria, and Atractylodes (*shen ling bai zhu san*)	
Chinese Herbs	Cinnamon Poria Jujube seeds	Licorice Atractylodes
Other Herbs	Aloe vera Chia seeds (soaked, 1 tablespoon 2 times/day) Blackberry	
Nutritional Supplements	Probiotics Digestive enzymes Potassium	Quercitin L-Glutamine
Acupressure Points	Spleen 6 and 15 Conception Vessel 12 Stomach 36	

Special Considerations

In cases of either acute or chronic diarrhea, it's best to simplify your diet until the condition resolves, as diarrhea strips your body of nutrients and fluids, leaving you dehydrated and tired. Drink plenty of water and broth or stock.

CONSTIPATION

Chinese Medicine Interpretation

The ancient Chinese texts say that the healthiest person would pass stool after each meal. Nowadays that has decreased to a healthy person passing stool at least once a day. In Western medicine you aren't considered constipated unless you pass fewer than three stools each week. In my opinion, three stools a week is serious constipation and tells me that your bowels are not functioning well. When you get that constipated, it becomes a vicious cycle because the backup makes it even harder to pass stool! Once a day is my ideal for clients. Sometimes treating constipation is as easy as increasing water intake to a healthy amount (half your body weight in ounces each day. See page 75 for details).

Special Considerations

Food allergies/intolerances can cause constipation as they can create heat and inflammation, thereby drying up all the fluids in the large intestine. Emotions also have a big influence on the large intestine. For children who are constipated (and for whom food allergies/intolerances have been ruled out), inquire about their emotional health. Are they expressing their emotions? If you can catch constipation early, you will save the child a lifetime of always wondering when he or she is "going to go."

If as an adult you have experienced chronic constipation, begin by changing your diet as needed, taking the appropriate supplements and herbs, *and* wake up and sit on the toilet for at least fifteen minutes during large intestine time (between 5 A.M. and 7 A.M. on the Meridian Clock, see page 46), even if nothing is happening. Do that every day and your bowels will start to wake up. Note that strong medications (pain medication, in particular) can cause constipation as a side effect. If this sounds like your situation, you can still address the pattern and add in the appropriate herbs to support you while on the medication. Always consult a practitioner when mixing herbs and prescription medications.

CONSTIPATION

Symptoms	Skipping a day without passing stools
	Having lumpy or hard stools
	Straining to have bowel movements
	Feeling blocked/distended
	Feeling as though bowels are never completely empty
Chinese Medicine Patterns	Heat and dryness in the large intestine
Chinese Herbal Formulas	Hemp Seed Pill (*ma zi ren wan*)
Chinese Herbs	Persica
	Cistanche
Other Herbs	Chia seeds
	Senna
Nutritional Supplements	Magnesium
Acupressure Points	Stomach 25
	Large Intestine 4
	Triple Burner 6

IMMUNE SYSTEM IMBALANCES

Immune system imbalances are often the result of long-term, weakened defenses. In Chinese medicine we call these defenses wei qi, the energy that circulates on the surface of the body, protecting us from the everyday onslaught of pathogens such as bacteria, viruses, and so on. Wei qi is produced and strengthened by the activity of our microbiome and our respiratory system. When our wei qi is deficient, we become more vulnerable to pathogens, and when we have a surplus, we are less vulnerable. When a pattern of imbalance reveals chronic susceptibility to bacteria and pathogens, we call it a wei qi deficiency (see page 227). There are many ways to support wei qi deficiency, but the first is to repair the microbiome. A leading cause of wei qi deficiency is the overuse of antibiotics and the lack of repair after taking them. I recommend giving yourself about one year to repair after a course of antibiotics.

The idea that pathogens and bacteria are everywhere, all the time, goes against the common Western medical model that describes pathogens as something that can appear and suddenly "attack" even a healthy person. In Chinese medicine, we view pathogens as a constant presence, and what determines whether or not we succumb to them is how strong or challenged our wei qi is.

What challenges wei qi? Stress; the consumption of foods that are irritating to the digestive system; and chronic exposure to toxins, mold, and other environmental stressors (creating a high toxic burden) all lead to inflammation. Chronic exposure to inflammation requires attention from the immune system for such a long time that the system begins to do one of two things: it either wears down, creating a state of reduced defenses (leading to more colds, flu, allergies); or it becomes overstimulated and unable to recognize what may be a threat to the system versus the system itself (autoimmune disease).

SUPPORTING IMMUNE SYSTEM IMBALANCES WITH DIET: Eat nourishing, easy-to-digest foods (warm and cooked, nothing raw or cold). Focus on increasing your intake of healthy fats and eliminating inflammatory foods (especially nightshades such as tomatoes, eggplant, potatoes, and peppers); food additives; preservatives; and refined sugar. Simplify your diet and be patient, as these imbalances may take a little while to heal.

LIFESTYLE CONSIDERATIONS FOR IMMUNE SYSTEM IMBALANCES: Gentle daily activity (such as yin yoga, tai chi, walking, hiking, swimming) will maintain good circulation throughout your body without increasing stress. Meditation and the cultivation of mindfulness has a positive effect on the immune system. Grow your community and laugh often.

ADDITIONAL TESTING TO CONSIDER: Food sensitivities; inflammatory markers (must include lysozyme, calprotectin, alpha 1-antichymotrypsin); salivary cortisol; GI health panel

FOOD ALLERGIES AND INTOLERANCES
Chinese Medicine Interpretation
The development of food allergies and intolerances is considered a deficiency pattern. The development of allergies in adults is often due to stress and inflammation. Stress weakens the immune system and creates inflammation in the body. A weak immune system is more vulnerable to even typical foods or pollens. Try doing a cleanse that includes an elimination diet first (page 285) to make sure you aren't continuously exposing yourself to what is irritating you.

Special Considerations
Why are there so many food allergies these days? Many of us have developed irritation toward some of the more common foods that we have eaten all our lives. While there are very few true food allergies, there are significantly many more cases of food intolerances. These intolerances are not life-threatening. They reveal themselves as insidious discomforts that slowly build in intensity and wreak havoc on the body over time. Many of the initial symptoms of food intolerance are headaches, migraines, earaches, skin rashes, emotional swings, immune system imbalances, and (obviously) digestive disturbances.

INCREASING FOOD INTOLERANCES

People are often in denial about food allergies/intolerances and how these conditions are affecting them. This is partly due to rampant food addiction based on using food as emotional comfort. This is understandable given all the opportunities for emotional imbalances in daily life. Denial is also partly due to an addiction to the stimulating effects of eating something to which we are a little bit allergic (an increase in inflammation followed by an increase in cortisol, giving a surge of energy). Food allergies/intolerances are serious because they continue to breach the health of the microbiome, so constant exposure to them takes us into "one step forward, two steps back" terrain—the energy burst makes us feel better but does more and more damage to our system.

The rapid increase in food intolerances is due to (1) stress, inflammation, and medications weakening our microbiomes; (2) depletion of the soil and over-processing of foods, leading to nutritional deficiencies; and (3) the addition of chemicals such as pesticides, preservatives, artificial flavorings, and colorings to our food.

An example of this is what has happened to wheat. In nature, wheat has its own enzymes to help us break it down and with its own fibers to help us push it through our digestive system. Yet we have not only depleted the soil in which wheat grows, but we have added pesticides to it to support its growth by killing insects. We have stripped this plant of its wholeness, turning it into a bright white flour that makes baked goods gluey, and we even have to enrich it to restore the vitamins and minerals that were originally found in the plant. Now when we eat wheat, we are simply getting what's left of the plant after processing. So I am never surprised when someone has a wheat/gluten allergy. There are just too many things wrong with this picture. Is it a true allergy like celiac disease, or is it an intolerance? Are we allergic to the pesticide (glyphosate) commonly used on wheat crops? Or have we taken so many antibiotics that we no longer have the proper enzymes to break it down?

FOOD ALLERGIES AND INTOLERANCES

Symptoms	Unexplained mood swings after meals
	Hives (reddish, swollen, itchy areas on the skin)
	Eczema flare-ups (a persistent dry, itchy rash)
	Redness of the skin, particularly around the mouth or eyes
	Tiredness after meals
	Itchy mouth or ear canal
	Nausea or vomiting
	Diarrhea (or constipation)
	Cramps after eating
	Nasal congestion or a runny nose
	Sneezing
	Slight, dry cough
Chinese Medicine Patterns	Lung chi deficiency
	Liver chi stagnation
	Spleen chi deficiency
	Kidney yin deficiency
Chinese Herbal Formulas	Jade Windscreen Formula (*yu ping feng wan*)
Chinese Herbs	Astragalus
	Codonopsis
	Eleuthero
	White peony
	Bupleurum
Other Herbs	Nettles
	Garlic
	Rose hips
	Bee pollen (local raw honey)
	Curcumin
Nutritional Supplements	Collagen L-Glutamine
	Digestive enzymes Quercitin
	Probiotics
Acupressure Points	Large Intestine 4 and 20
	Stomach 2
	Bladder 2
	Spleen 5

Most patients want to know which foods are triggering their uncomfortable and sometimes debilitating responses without doing extensive food allergy testing. Such testing is still not a perfect science. If you test while you are already inflamed, the results will tell you that you are allergic to loads of foods, some of which you have never even heard of. Due to this inaccuracy, I recommend the time-tested, number-one way to check for food intolerances: elimination and reintroduction. Addressing the most common culprits first will save you time and energy: wheat/gluten, dairy, corn, soy, and eggs. I cannot count how many times I have seen the elimination of these foods lead to the complete elimination of a patient's symptoms!

If you can muster the courage, eliminate all five of the top food culprits at the same time for thirty days to three months (wheat/gluten takes an especially long time to leave the system, hence the "gluey" label). If you can't face this, then choose just one of the five to start with. With a cleanse of all the categories, after you have eliminated them for a minimum of thirty days, reintroduce them one at a time with a meal focused on that specific category. For instance, eat a plate of pasta when you reintroduce wheat/gluten or a few scrambled eggs when you reintroduce eggs. Make sure not to reintroduce more than one at a time so that if you have a reaction, you know exactly which food is causing it. Reactions can take anywhere from five minutes to three days and can look like any of the symptoms listed for allergies and food intolerances.

RECURRENT COLDS, FLU, AND SINUSITIS
Chinese Medicine Interpretation

Chinese medicine isn't too concerned with whether someone has a cold or a flu. The only clinical difference between the two is the typical rapid onset of a flu versus the gradual onset of a cold, and usually with a flu, the symptoms are much more intense than with a cold. Sinusitis is often tangled in with both of them as it can be either a precursor for them or linger after recovery from them. In Chinese medicine, we are only concerned with the pattern, and the pattern tells us one thing primarily: your wei qi is down. When your wei qi is down, you are vulnerable to every bacteria, virus, or ounce of stress you meet. So many recurrent sinus infections are cleared up by removing food allergies/intolerances from the diet. Start there if you haven't done this already.

Special Considerations

Each of us processes stress through our most vulnerable organs and systems. If you are someone who processes stress through your respiratory system, take extra precautions when you find yourself revving up or running down in response to stress. As the front line of defense for your immune system, it's important to keep not just your lungs but also your sinus passages coated in healthy mucus, which provides a good environment for beneficial bacteria. Using a neti pot or something similar, do a nasal rinse a couple of times each week, even when you feel well, just so you can stay ahead of the curve. I personally like to use Alkalol (a mucus solvent) and a little bit of salt in warm distilled water.

NASAL STEAM

If your sinuses are already clogged up, try a nasal steam each day until your symptoms release. Place a pot on the stove with about one to two inches of water in the bottom. Bring it to a boil. Once it is boiling, sit down at your kitchen table with the pot on a heat-friendly surface. Put two to ten drops of one of the following essential oils in the pot: rosemary, thyme, ravensara, spearmint, or eucalyptus. Lean your head over the pot so the steam can get to your face and sinuses, keep your eyes closed, and toss a towel over your entire head so you are sitting in the darkness underneath it. Stay there for ten to fifteen minutes. One of the reasons this works so well is because many of the troublemaking bacteria that can grow in unhealthy sinuses only thrive there because the temperature stays cool (we are always moving air in and out of our sinuses). Doing a Nasal Steam puts moist heat into your sinuses, which kills the naughty bacteria. Expect some nasal drip afterward; try to cough as much of it out as possible rather than swallowing.

RECURRENT COLDS, FLU, AND SINUSITIS

Symptoms	Fever and/or chills
	Body aches and pains
	Fatigue/weakness
	Sinus pressure and/or headache
	Facial tenderness
	Pressure or pain in the sinuses, around the eyes, in the ears and teeth
	Stuffy nose
	Cloudy, discolored nasal or postnasal drip
	Nasal stuffiness
	Sore throat
	Cough
	Facial swelling (occasional)
Chinese Medicine Patterns	Lung chi deficiency
Chinese Herbal Formulas	Jade Windscreen Formula (*yu ping feng wan*)
	Sinus Inflammation Pills (*bi yan pian*)
	Common Cold Remedy (*gan mao ling*; best taken at the start of a cold or preventively)
Chinese Herbs	Ginger
	Mint
	Cinnamon
	Eleuthero
Other Herbs	Garlic
	Echinacea
Nutritional Supplements	Vitamin C
	Probiotics
Acupressure Points	Kidney 3
	Liver 3
	Spleen 6
	Stomach 36
	Large Intestine 4 and 11

A NOTE ON EAR INFECTIONS

When ear infections present in children or adults, they are a beacon to let us know something is out of balance underneath. The trajectory of children who get ear infections is often the same—it usually starts with a few rounds of antibiotics. Then once it becomes clear that the antibiotics are not working, tubes are placed in the child's ears. At that point the child usually develops some wheezing or perhaps even full-blown asthma. After being prescribed steroid inhalers, the child finally exhibits patches of eczema (also known as skin asthma) and is prescribed topical steroid creams. Diet and food allergies/intolerances are typically not explored until the child is much older and, by that time, has developed a weekend immune system from the significant antibiotic and steroid use at such a young age.

Ear infections develop as the result of weakened wei qi due to chronic inflammation. Inflammation most often arises from irritation cause by diet, which then preoccupies the immune system and weakens wei qi. Typical inflammation symptoms begin with digestive problems such as gas, bloating, diarrhea, or constipation, as well as mood swings. If you happen to catch the inflammation response in a child at this stage, it would be a great time to experiment with eliminating potential food triggers before they become intolerances or allergies. By the time the child develops an ear infection, the inflammation is often chronic, and it will take more time to see the relationship between the different foods that trigger the response. Since wei qi is the buffer between the body and harmful bacteria and viruses, when it becomes challenged, we lose our protection and succumb to infection.

Ear infections are nearly always the result of a viral infection rather than bacteria. This helps to explain the high number of ear infections that reoccur despite several rounds of antibiotics.[1] I feel sad that other options (like diet) are not explored first, especially with children, because it leads to unnecessary suffering.

Ear Infection Protocol
Items needed:
Garlic and mullein ear drops (I like the Wise Woman brand)
A wet, warm washcloth
A hot water bottle

Instructions: Lay on your side with the affected ear facing upward. Place three to eight drops of oil in the affected ear (the amount depends on your age and the size of your ear, so follow the manufacturer's instructions). Stay on your side for about ten minutes (if you're dealing with an antsy child, this can be five minutes). Then switch sides, lying with your affected ear facing downward. Drape the wet, warm washcloth over the hot water bottle (warm for children) and lay with your affected ear directly on that; rest there for twenty minutes (less for children who can't wait). Repeat two to four times, depending on the severity of your symptoms. The warmth and moisture help to draw out the inflammation and fluids that are usually backed up in the ear (which causes most of the pain). Repeat on the opposite ear if both sides are affected.

HERPES

There is nothing like a cold sore, shingles rash, or herpes outbreak to stop you dead in your tracks. Herpes is a virus that many people struggle with. The virus lives in the body permanently and makes itself known only when you are under a significant amount of stress: physical, emotional, or environmental (harsh and prolonged sun exposure will do it). This causes an increase in inflammation, a precursor for the expression of the virus. Herpes inflames the nerves of a particular area, producing excruciating pain that can last for days or even weeks.

Whenever I see a cold sore, shingles, or herpes breakout, I immediately think that the person must be under a lot of stress. Consider slowing things down, bringing more yin activities into your life, and consuming more cooling and moistening foods and herbs (see pages 93–95). An important amino acid called lysine is known to prevent outbreaks, reduce their severity, and shorten their duration. Taking 1,000 milligrams a day is an excellent strategy to prevent outbreaks, and the same dose taken three times a day will support the treatment of outbreaks. Lysine is best taken on an empty stomach unless you experience digestive sensitivity. Topical lysine is also available.

Another important amino acid called arginine is known to aggravate the herpes virus. Consider eliminating all foods and herbs high in arginine such as seeds, nuts, chocolate, grains (especially oats and wheat), squash, and spirulina. I also recommend avoiding heating foods and certainly sugar and alcohol.

SKIN CONDITIONS (ECZEMA, DERMATITIS, ACNE, ROSACEA, HERPES)

Chinese Medicine Interpretation

Skin conditions develop, according to Chinese Medicine, when there is a weakness in lung chi and therefore wei qi. In fact, skin conditions such as dermatitis and eczema are often referred to as "skin asthma" (see the next section in this chapter). When this weakness is present, heat and dampness can arise and affect the skin. Most often there is heat somewhere inside the body (lungs, large intestine, or stomach), and if the body can't get rid of the heat through other organs, it will push the heat out via the skin. It's actually quite smart, if a bit unsightly in a culture where aesthetics are everything. Food allergies/intolerances seem to underlie most skin conditions. Frequently I see eczema linked with dairy/lactose intolerance and gluten sensitivity.

Special Considerations

It's important to remember that skin conditions usually come about due to an underlying internal imbalance. (The rare exception is something that is transmitted directly from the outside, although with a strong microbiome and healthy wei qi, the body should still be able to fend off just about anything.) We need to address the aesthetic aspect of the condition as well as the underlying cause, which will be internal. So while you will likely be putting topical creams and salves on your skin, it is a good idea to take herbs and supplements internally to address the root cause of your symptoms. When the skin condition clears, work on building up your wei qi and microbiome to prevent it from returning.

Skin conditions that are red, hot, and damp are mostly acidic in nature. One way to counter the acidity and help restore the pH of your skin biome is to take an alkaline bath. A warm bath with half a cup of baking soda and/or half a cup of raw, unfiltered organic apple cider vinegar can soothe very hot and irritated skin. You could also just make your way to the beach; between the sand, sun, and saltwater, many skin rashes will simply go away! Always be patient with skin conditions. They can take a while to clear because, as already mentioned, they are often the body's last-ditch effort to clear heat from deep inside.

Note: Undiagnosed skin conditions that persist should be brought to the attention of a dermatologist. With the changes in our atmosphere, we are at much higher risk for skin cancers than ever before.

RASH PERSONALITIES

Rashes have something of a personality. Some like to be covered in oil, whereas some like to remain dry. Some like heat, while others prefer cool. The only way to know is to see how the rash reacts after applying a topical medication to it. If your rash looks "angrier" or gets itchier after applying the medication, remove it and try something else.

SKIN CONDITIONS

Symptoms	Raised red or white bumps	Ulcers
	Rash (may be painful or itchy)	Open sores or lesions
	Scaly or rough skin	Dry, cracked skin
	Welts, papules, pustules	Discolored patches of skin
	Peeling skin	
Chinese Medicine Patterns	Lung chi deficiency	
	Liver blood deficiency	
	Liver fire blazing (herpes, all kinds)	
Chinese Herbal Formulas	Clear Wind-Heat Pills (when heat, redness is present) (*sang ju yin wan*)	
	Indigo Combo Pills (*fu fang qing dai wan*)	
	Eliminate Wind Powder (*xiao feng san*)	
Chinese Herbs	Seeds of Job's tears	
	Siler root (for itchy skin)	
	Angelica	
Other Herbs	Aloe	
Nutritional Supplements	Vitamin A (best from food, supplement under supervision)	
	Vitamin C	
	Zinc	
Topical Formulas	Yin Care	Comfrey salve
	Vitamin E	Calendula
	Aloe vera	St. John's wort
	Lavender essential oil	Neem oil
Acupressure Points	Large Intestine 11	Bladder 40
	Lung 5 and 7	Spleen 10

ASTHMA

Chinese Medicine Interpretation

In Chinese medicine, phlegm is considered to be the main culprit behind all asthma. But the question becomes, is the phlegm present because of a weakness in the lungs, spleen, or kidneys, or vice versa? Lung and spleen involvement mostly present acute cases of asthma, whereas more chronic asthma patterns are linked with the kidneys and chronic exposure to stress.

Special Considerations

As mentioned previously, asthma is often accompanied by skin conditions and digestive disturbances, mostly due to food allergies/intolerances. Remember to support the underlying cause of the asthma; in particular, look for the relationship between foods and presentation of asthma symptoms. Consider doing a cleanse (see Appendix E) and returning to the pantry guidelines in Chapter 3 to fully address this.

ASTHMA	
Symptoms	Shortness of breath Coughing Chest tightness or pain Trouble sleeping or lying horizontal Whistling or wheezing sound when exhaling Coughing or wheezing attacks that are worsened by a respiratory virus, such as a cold or the flu Feelings of not being able to exhale fully
Chinese Medicine Patterns	Lung chi deficiency Spleen chi deficiency Kidney yin or yang deficiency
Chinese Herbal Formulas	Jade Windscreen Formula (*yu ping feng wan*) Sinus Inflammation Pills (*bi yan pian*) Common Cold Remedy (*gan mao ling*; best taken at the start of a cold or preventively)
Chinese Herbs	Cordyceps Pinellia Cinnamon Lobelia
Other Herbs	Mullein $\rightarrow$

ASTHMA		
Nutritional Supplements	Quercetin Vitamin C	N-Acetylcysteine
Acupressure Points	Lung 1 and 5 Ding Chuan	Ren 17

AUTOIMMUNE DISEASE

Autoimmune disease has many variations. Among them are psoriasis, rheumatoid arthritis, lupus, Hashimoto's disease, Graves' disease, Crohn's disease, ulcerative colitis, multiple sclerosis, and Sjogren's syndrome.

Chinese Medicine Interpretation

You don't just wake up with an autoimmune condition. Usually you will have a lung or stomach chi deficiency or chronic exposure to stress that prevents your immune system from maturing from a young age. This, combined with the daily onslaught of toxins and inflammation from the environment and food allergies/intolerances you face, further weakens your organs and wei qi. Underneath almost all presentations of autoimmune conditions lie internal heat and inflammation that has been present for a very long time and has had nowhere to go. This latent heat begins to attack a certain organ or tissue. Stress, overwork, depression, and frustration are key players in any autoimmune condition.

Special Considerations

In Western medicine, autoimmune conditions are often treated with corticosteroids and/or immune-suppressing drugs. As an acute response to help you get comfortable, this makes sense because autoimmune flare-ups can be excruciating. If you choose to go this route in the long term, however, it is important to track any side effects you may have and know that while you are taking these drugs, your immune system is at risk. Building up your wei qi is of utmost importance and should be a constant focus.

Consider assessing your food allergies/intolerances (especially for celiac disease) and check your microbiome for hidden infections such as yeasts, bacteria, Lyme disease, and viruses. Also get tested for heavy metal toxicity. And above all, go back to the pantry guidelines in Chapter 3.

Symptoms	Unexplained and prolonged fatigue
	Joint pain and swelling, usually in multiple joints
	Skin conditions
	Abdominal pain or digestive issues
	Recurring fever
	Swollen glands
Chinese Medicine Patterns	Kidney yin deficiency
	Kidney yang deficiency
Chinese Medicine Patterns Most Common to Western Diagnoses	Damp heat in the large intestine (Crohn's disease or ulcerative colitis)
	Stomach and spleen deficiency, kidney and liver deficiency (multiple sclerosis)
	Stomach and liver blood deficiency (Sjogren's syndrome)
	Spleen chi deficiency and kidney yang deficiency (Hashimoto's disease or Graves' disease)
	Spleen chi and liver blood deficiency leading to damp heat in joints (rheumatoid arthritis)
	Heat in, deficiency of, or stasis of the blood (psoriasis)
	Kidney yin deficiency (lupus)
Chinese Herbal Formulas	Work closely with an herbalist to create a formula for your unique presentation of autoimmune symptoms and Chinese medicine patterns.
Chinese Herbs	Reishi
	Boswellia
Other Herbs	Curcumin

Nutritional Supplements	EPA/DHA	Probiotics
	Vitamin C	Quercitin
	Vitamin D	

Acupressure Points	Liver 3	Stomach 36
	Large Intestine 4	Gallbladder 41
	Spleen 4	Governing Vessel 20

CANCER

Chinese Medicine Interpretation

The basic presentation of cancer is the loss of wei qi and the consequential accumulation of toxins, including heat. This burdens the body, and its ability to create a smooth flow of chi is hindered, hence the growth of cancer cells and the formation of masses or tumors. In my experience, there is always an emotional component, usually of repressed emotions, that begins with a liver chi stagnation pattern and moves on from there. The best overall approach to cancer is to remember to address it holistically, using the pantry guidelines in Chapter 3 and the underlying pattern. In addition to this, make sure to support the organs most affected by the masses or tumors and the meridians that pass through those masses or tumors.

Special Considerations

It's not likely, but the American Cancer Society says some patients *could* have no symptoms whatsoever. However, I have found that no matter what stage cancer patients are in, they always say they had some unusual symptoms preceding the diagnosis. One patient who had breast cancer developed unexplained headaches, which she managed with over-the-counter NSAIDS, for about a year. Then after six months, she developed her first (of about five in one year) urinary tract infection, for which she was prescribed antibiotics each time. It was after all that, that tests found the malignant lump in her breast. Another patient who had lower back pain and urgent urination for about two years, was practically living on over-the-counter pain medications, and drank minimal water discovered he had developed prostate cancer. These are two examples of why it is important not to mask symptoms, but to explore them further in order to find the root cause of what is happening.

In cases of cancer, blood tests can be very helpful for early detection because the blood will have too many or too few of certain kinds of blood markers, and this can be an early indicator of your body responding to the cancer.

A hot infusion tea of elecampane flowers is excellent for chemotherapy-related nausea. Use 2 to 4 grams of dried flowers per 8-ounce cup of boiling water. Let steep for ten to fifteen minutes, then strain and enjoy.

CANCER

Symptoms	Immune system vulnerability Painless lumps that grow Digestive changes (usually more diarrhea) Low-grade fever Persistent lumps or swollen glands Bloody discharge from any orifice Unexplained anemia Unexplained weight loss Night sweats Abnormally slow or nonhealing sores	
Chinese Medicine Patterns	Liver chi stagnation Spleen chi deficiency (with dampness and/or phlegm accumulation)	**If left unaddressed can turn into:** Liver chi stagnation and blood stasis Kidney yin deficiency (with heat or Fire accumulating in response to chemotherapy and radiation) Kidney yang deficiency (late-stage cancer)
Chinese Herbs	Wormwood Skullcap Solomon's seal Astragalus	Coriolus (turkey tail mushrooms, shown by Johns Hopkins to reduce tumors) Licorice Poria
Other Herbs	Red clover Curcumin	Garlic Green tea
Nutritional Supplements	Vitamin C (preferably intravenously) Selenium	Melatonin
Acupressure Points	Heart 7 Pericardium 6 Large Intestine 4	Spleen 8 and 9 Governing Vessel 20

— 9 —

PAIN AND INFLAMMATION IMBALANCES

Pain and inflammation can sap your will to make it through the day. I hear this from new clients in my office all the time: "A life of chronic pain is hardly worth living." That's because pain is debilitating and distracting. It's difficult to enjoy anything when you are in pain. So the sooner you can address it the better. When imbalances that bring pain and inflammation arise, it's important to see them as warning signs from your body. Though it can be tempting to go for a "quick-fix," try to avoid using substances that mask the symptoms right away; working to unearth the root cause will serve you in the long term. Of course, sometimes you just need to get through the day. Pain and inflammation over a long period of time actually degrades your tissues the same way that chronic exposure to cortisol (the stress hormone) does.

Acute pain and inflammation are a part of life. A twisted ankle or a crick in your neck are fairly typical and shouldn't require much troubleshooting. A little Epsom salts in your bath or arnica salve on the injury, and you may be good to go. However, the chronic pain and inflammation that sometimes comes your way requires your full attention, investigation, and treatment strategies. Western medicine's pain management protocols aren't amazing. Over-the-counter NSAIDS eat away at your stomach lining, and acetaminophen is hard on your liver. Anything stronger than that, and you compromise your clear-headedness for slight sedation. It's important to find something that works but still leaves you with energy to investigate the root cause.

Many of my pain clients also have unresolved emotional imbalances along with digestive imbalances. The most supportive strategy in such cases is to address the underlying imbalances at the same time that we are managing the pain and inflammation.

SUPPORTING PAIN AND INFLAMMATION IMBALANCES WITH DIET: Eat nourishing, easy-to-digest foods (warm and cooked, nothing raw or cold). Focus on increasing your intake of healthy fats and anti-inflammatory foods. Avoid nightshades (such as tomatoes, eggplant, potatoes, and peppers), and eliminate food additives, preservatives, and refined sugar. Investigate your possible food allergies/intolerances.

LIFESTYLE CONSIDERATIONS FOR PAIN AND INFLAMMATION IMBALANCES: Continue to move painful joints or affected areas as this will bring new blood flow to the area. Avoid sitting for long periods of time. Address past trauma, increase stress management strategies, heal your digestive system, and continue to broaden your support network and community. Try meditation techniques that focus on pain management. Epsom salt baths with at least four cups of salt also help to increase circulation.

ADDITIONAL TESTING TO CONSIDER: Food sensitivities, neurotransmitters, salivary cortisol, GI health panel, inflammatory markers (must include lysozyme, calprotectin, and alpha 1-antichymotrypsin)

ACUTE PAIN AND INFLAMMATION
Chinese Medicine Interpretation

An ancient Chinese medicine axiom says, "If there is free flow of chi, there is no pain; If there is no free flow of chi, there is pain." The sooner you can treat pain and/or inflammation, the quicker it will resolve, and you will avoid developing any chronic patterns.

ACUTE PAIN		
Symptoms	Sharp or dull pain from a recent injury or trauma	
Chinese Medicine Patterns	Chi stagnation Blood stagnation Liver chi stagnation	
Chinese Herbs	Corydalis Cyperus Tangerine peel Persica	Myrrh Boswellia Curcumin
Other Herbs	Willow bark	Kava kava
Nutritional Supplements	Quercitin B-complex	Vitamin B_6
Topical Formulas	Arnica oil, cream, or salve Tiger balm	St. John's wort oil (for nerve pain and inflammation)
Acupressure Points	Bladder 60 (the "Aspirin Point") Large Intestine 4	Liver 3

Special Considerations

The medical community is only just learning how destructive the chronic use of NSAIDS is on the system. These over-the-counter drugs—like ibuprofen, naproxen, and aspirin—can burn a hole in your stomach or cause stomach bleeding in only a few uses. Over-the-counter pain medication that is not an NSAID, such as acetaminophen, also comes with a price because it can cause toxicity of the liver. So it's important to have a few things on hand that will assist you with immediate relief and not be detrimental to your long-term health.

HEADACHES AND MIGRAINES

Chinese Medicine Interpretation

The difference between headaches and migraines in Chinese medicine is that they exist on a spectrum where migraines are at the more painful, longer-lasting end. Location is key with headaches in Chinese medicine. Headaches that are one-sided are often due to stress that has irritated the Liver and Gallbladder meridians that run along the side of the head. Headaches at the back of the head are often related to stress and tension as well. Headaches around the eyes are often related to dehydration, as the Bladder meridian ends at the corner of the eye. Headaches at the top of the head are often related to the kidneys and liver. Headaches in the forehead are often related to the stomach and challenges with digestion (food allergies/intolerances).

Special Considerations

In addition to these patterns, I tend to see headaches and migraines that are responses to structural imbalances (which of course can come from imbalances in the meridians as well). Often these stem from a stress pattern involving the shoulders, and specifically the trapezius muscle (which the Gallbladder meridian runs through) and the sternocleidomastoid (SCM) muscle. In cases like this, there are also trigger points (places in the body that are super-sensitive, and when you massage them, you can feel the sensation refer to another area). Trigger points, if you can locate them, are often the golden ticket for getting pain relief. Deep massage of the trigger point, muscle, and meridian; gua sha; cupping; reducing stress; and developing better ergonomics—all of these can make a considerable impact on chronic headaches and migraines.

Another imbalance to consider when it comes to headaches and migraines is magnesium deficiency. The body depends on magnesium for a number of processes, including muscle relaxation (giving it the nickname "nature's muscle relaxer"). Magnesium ensures the proper expansion and release of muscles after contractions. When there is a magnesium deficiency, you have lots of tension in your muscles, which can restrict blood flow and cause aches and pains. Rest seems to be key with *all* headaches as they tend to get worse with exertion.

Food allergies/intolerances are also at the root of many headaches and migraines. Trying an elimination diet (page 285) may be the way to go to rule out this potential imbalance. When all else fails, Chinese medicine has a folk remedy for headaches and migraines: put your bare feet under rushing water (a bathtub faucet at full blast), switching back and forth each minute from hot (not burning) to cold for about ten or fifteen minutes total, or until the headache/migraine is gone. This revitalizes your chi and blood and removes stagnation from the meridians.

HEADACHES AND MIGRAINES

Symptoms	Headache:	Migraine:
	Feelings of a band of pressure wrapped around the head Onset without warning signs Dull pain of mild to moderate nature Duration from 30 minutes to several days (several hours is more typical)	Moderate to severe throbbing pain at the front or sides of the head Duration from several hours to several days Resulting developing auras (visual, auditory, psychological, or physiological) Onset with warning signs Double vision Loss of balance
Chinese Medicine Patterns	Invasion of pathogenic wind (in the meridian most affected) Liver chi stagnation (can lead to liver fire blazing; there will be heat signs) Chi deficiency (most often of the kidney) Liver blood deficiency	
Chinese Herbal Formulas	Pain and inflammation supports listed in the "Acute Pain" section Clear the Liver Wind (*tian ma gou teng yin*) Decoction to Drain Liver Fire (*long dan xie gan tang*) $\rightarrow$	

HEADACHES AND MIGRAINES	
Other Herbs	Feverfew
Nutritional Supplements	Magnesium Caffeine B-complex
Topical Formula	Peppermint essential oil Lavender essential oil
Acupressure Points	Liver 3 Large Intestine 4 Gallbladder 41 Stomach 8 Yin Tang Tai Yang Bladder 2 and 10 Gallbladder 1, 20, and 21

ARTHRITIS

Chinese Medicine Interpretation

Arthritis is considered to be an obstruction to the free flow of chi due to either chi stagnation, blood stagnation, or both. Arthritis tends to appear after chronic overuse of a joint or as a response to chronic inflammation, usually related to the diet.

Special Considerations

Since arthritis is yet another disease of inflammation, much of this can be addressed through your diet. Head back over to the pantry guidelines in Chapter 3 and see how much impact a good diet can make on your inflamed joints. I have often seen weekly acupuncture sessions combined with a good anti-inflammatory diet completely resolve arthritis. Also, soaking in Epsom salt baths can relieve pain and swelling. Use a minimum of four cups of salt for your whole body, or one cup for a hand or foot.

ARTHRITIS		
Symptoms	Pain Stiffness Swelling	Redness Decreased range of motion
Chinese Medicine Patterns	Chi and blood stagnation	
Chinese Herbal Formulas	Du Huo and Loranthus (*du huo ji sheng tang*)	
Chinese Herbs	Cinnamon Ginger	Boswellia
Other Herbs	Aloe vera Eucalyptus	Willow bark
Nutritional Supplements	EPA/DHA Vitamin C Magnesium	Methylsulfonylmethane (MSM) Glucosamine sulfate Collagen
Topical Formulas	Thunder God Vine	
Acupressure Points	Governing Vessel 12 Gallbladder 34	Liver 3 Large Intestine 4 and 11

FIBROMYALGIA AND CHRONIC PAIN

Chinese Medicine Interpretation

Fibromyalgia and chronic pain comprise a slow progression of pain (physical and/or emotional) that has gone unresolved. Often stemming from liver chi stagnation, this progression leads to more chronic patterns.

Special Considerations

This has become a much more common diagnosis over the last several years and seems to perplex many Western doctors, which explains the influx of people with this diagnosis to Chinese medicine. The ancient system has shown considerable support in studies of people with this diagnosis. Relief comes not just from the acupuncture and herbs, but largely from the overall decrease in inflammation thanks to these treatments *plus* a healthier diet. Returning to the pantry guidelines in Chapter 3 and making sure to protect yourself from any unnecessary stress while you are focused on healing.

FIBROMYALGIA AND CHRONIC PAIN

Symptoms	**Symptoms will linger for weeks, months, and even years after an injury, illness, or trauma:** Pain that is dull, achy, throbbing, burning, shooting, squeezing, or stinging Pain, soreness, or stiffness in various regions of the body, including the joints Tender points that are abnormally sensitive to touch, with certain areas being supersensitive Stiffness or spasms in the muscles Fatigue Poor sleep (waking up not refreshed) Cognitive disorders (problems with memory and concentration, slowed or confused speech) Emotional symptoms (anxiety, depression)	
Chinese Medicine Patterns	**Acute patterns:** Chi stagnation Blood stagnation Liver chi stagnation	**If left unaddressed can turn into:** Liver-spleen disharmony Kidney deficiency (chi, yin, or yang)
Chinese Herbs	Supports listed in the "Acute Pain" section Bupleurum Angelica Astragalus Eleuthero	
Other Herbs	Valerian St. John's wort	Willow bark
Nutritional Supplements	Magnesium Vitamin C	Vitamin D Melatonin
Acupressure Points	Gallbladder 20 Bladder 10 Liver 3, 8, 9, and 10 Spleen 5 and 10 Stomach 36	

NATURE'S OPIOIDS

The body has built-in mechanisms for helping you manage pain. These are neuro-transmitters called endorphins, serotonin, and gamma-aminobutyric acid (GABA). You build neurotransmitters from amino acids naturally found in high-protein foods. The body takes protein, breaks it down into amino acids, and then turns the acids into important neurotransmitters that help you naturally mitigate your pain receptors. This is nature's opioid system. When someone is experiencing pain, I recommend anywhere from 90 to 100 milligrams of protein each day and a complete elimination of inflammatory foods like sugars or things that turn to sugar quickly. Here are some foods that have at least 50 percent protein content:

- Poultry
- Seafood
- Beef
- Pork
- Lamb
- Eggs
- Cottage cheese

And here are some foods that have between 20 and 30 percent protein content:

- Green vegetables
- Beans
- Nuts

In addition to eating these foods, consider taking the following supplements:

- Essential amino acids
- D-Phenylalanine (DPA)
- 5-HTP (or L-tryptophan)
- GABA
- L-Glutamine

ENERGY-ZAPPING IMBALANCES

As you read in the beginning of this book, sometimes being exhausted is simply a matter of spending more energy than you have available (yin and yang balance). If you have a mostly yin nature and your career requires mostly yang energy, you *will* get exhausted. It sounds like common sense—match your life to your nature—but is often overlooked and could be contributing to your lowered energy levels. If the preceding example sounds like you, finding ways to bring more yin energy to your job may be helpful. For example, if you are a yin-natured person working at a retail store, perhaps cashiering part-time and stocking the rest of the time to cut down on stress from working with customers might work. Or if you are cubicle-bound in a busy office, how about making sure you get a cubicle on the edge and not in the middle? Little changes like this might make all the difference to your energy at the end of the day.

Sometimes we spent more energy than we had *in the past* and have never recouped our loss. A stressful childhood could require a lifetime of repair. Going through difficult times such as experiencing a death in the family, an illness, an accident—and even beautiful things like planning a wedding or having a baby—all require energy. If we aren't equipped with energy-restoring practices and are living at the mercy of impossible twenty-first-century standards, we may have a one-way ticket to exhaustion.

Many of us are wildly overstimulated and overwhelmed. We have more on our plates than we will ever get through, try as we might. This situation takes some serious brainstorming to resolve. Do you carve out and enjoy quality downtime? I'm not talking about watching TV; I mean taking baths, getting acupuncture and massages, reading books, and doing other yin activities. The point is you've got to make more energy than you're spending, and you will notice that all of the dietary and lifestyle suggestions are all about this. Occasionally I have patients who simply don't produce energy well. This often happens because their body is preoccupied by something, or because they aren't getting the nutrients they need to support themselves.

SUPPORTING ENERGY-ZAPPING IMBALANCES WITH DIET: Eat nourishing, seasonal, easy-to-digest foods (warm and cooked, nothing raw or cold). Focus on increasing your intake of healthy fats and anti-inflammatory foods; eliminate food additives, preservatives, and refined sugar. Drink lots of bone stocks that are rich in collagen.

LIFESTYLE CONSIDERATIONS FOR ENERGY-ZAPPING IMBALANCES: Slow down. Build yin activities into your schedule every day. Gentle exercise such as walking, yin yoga, tai chi, stretching, and slow dancing are helpful. Assess your yin-yang balance. Grow your community around a hobby rather than career.

ADDITIONAL TESTING TO CONSIDER: Salivary cortisol, salivary hormone, neurotransmitters, food sensitivities, GI health panel, nutritional deficiencies

HPA AXIS DYSFUNCTION (ADRENAL FATIGUE)

Chinese Medicine Interpretation

As with most patterns of imbalance, stress is a huge culprit here. We begin to spend more chi than we have to give. This leads to liver chi stagnation and spleen chi deficiency and then the presenting patterns of adrenal fatigue begin.

Special Considerations

HPA axis dysfunction exists on a spectrum and may also be called adrenal exhaustion and adrenal dysfunction. There are typically four phases involved in HPA axis dysfunction with an increase in symptoms as the imbalance progresses. No matter the stage, an overhaul is in order, starting with reducing stress and increasing rest. Repairing from HPA axis dysfunction takes patience (a six-month minimum if you are in phase 1 or 2, eighteen months for phase 3 or 4).

PHASE 1: Symptoms are mild (2 through 4 in the table on page 307). There is intermittent tiredness and difficulty sleeping. Cortisol, adrenaline, dihydroepiandrosterone (DHEA), and insulin levels usually elevated.

PHASE 2: Symptoms progress (4 through 8 in the table). Wired-but-tired feeling during the day ends with crashing hard at night. All hormones maybe low except for cortisol.

PHASE 3: Symptoms get more intense (8 through 12 in the table). Exhaustion is prevalent, as are low libido and lowered immunity. Hormones (possibly including cortisol) drop significantly.

PHASE 4: Symptoms are across the board (1 through 15 in the table). You feel burned out and extremely tired and find it difficult to function. All hormones, including cortisol, are low.

HPA AXIS DYSFUNCTION

Symptoms	Anxiety	Depression
	Asthma, allergies, or respiratory complaints	Extreme tiredness (especially in the morning and after exercise)
	Weakened immune system	Insomnia (sometimes feeling wired at night)
	Dark circles under the eyes	
	Salt cravings	Back and joint pain
	Dizziness	Low blood pressure
	Low tolerance for stress	Low blood sugar
	Cravings for caffeine and sugar	Low libido
Chinese Medicine Patterns	Kidney yin deficiency	
	Kidney yang deficiency	
Chinese Herbs	Ashwaganda	Rhodiola
	Licorice	Ginkgo
	Eleuthero	
Other Herbs	Chamomile	Maca
	Lavender	
Nutritional Supplements	Probiotics	
	B-complex	
	Vitamin E	
	Vitamin C	
	Magnesium	
	EPA/DHA	
	Coenzyme Q_{10} (CoQ_{10})	
	Tyrosine	
	Bovine adrenal glandulars (for Phase 3 and 4)	
Acupressure Points	Kidney 3, 7, and 16	
	Liver 3	
	Large Intestine 4	
	Conception Vessel 4 and 6	

CHRONIC FATIGUE SYNDROME (CFS)

Chinese Medicine Interpretation

In most cases of CFS, more than one pattern is present so take a quick look at each pattern listed in the table below, even after finding one that fits your current experience.

Special Considerations

I see this pattern present after long-standing overwork and stress due to lifestyle, trauma, or repeated insults to the system such as overuse of antibiotics. All of this wear and tear creates a vulnerable system. Then the fatigue sets in and leads to many more imbalances such as poor diet (it takes energy to think, plan, and prepare meals), a lack of exercise, a lack of socialization, and isolation. These things in turn lead to a further weakening of the body, mind, and spirit. It's a vicious cycle, one that requires support from many angles and patience at all times. Go back to the pantry guidelines in Chapter 3 to stock up on foods that will support your pattern; consider restoring your microbiome and boosting your wei qi.

CHRONIC FATIGUE SYNDROME		
Symptoms	Debilitating fatigue lasting six months or more (not arising from exertion, and not relieved by rest) Sore throat Persistent low-grade fever Swollen lymph nodes Weak and aching muscles Headache	Joint pain Confusion Depression Agitation Impaired memory or concentration Appetite loss or gain Need for excessive sleep
Chinese Medicine Patterns	Kidney yin deficiency Kidney yang deficiency Lung yin deficiency	Spleen chi deficiency Liver chi stagnation
Chinese Herbs	Rhodiola Ashwagandha Radix ginseng Eleuthero	Schisandra Astragalus Skullcap (if heat is present)
Other Herbs	Evening primrose oil Lemon balm	St. John's wort

$\rightarrow$

Nutritional Supplements	B-complex		CoQ$_{10}$
	Vitamin C		Magnesium
	Tyrosine		N-Acetylcysteine
Acupressure Points	Stomach 36		Kidney 3
	Governing Vessel 4 and 20		Spleen 6
	Conception Vessel 6 and 12		

SLEEP IMBALANCES

Chinese Medicine Interpretation

Sleep has a lot to do with the shen, or spirit. When your spirit is relaxed and at home inside your heart, Chinese medicine says that sleep will come easily and you will wake feeling fully rested. However if your shen is disturbed, sleep is difficult and then so is everything else. If you are trying to go to bed after 11 P.M., forget about it. In Chinese medicine that time is reserved for the liver, which has lots of creative energy that is meant for detoxing and dreaming. I know it's tempting to stay up because you can get that second wind later, but trust me, your liver needs that time to rejuvenate. Make sure to get to bed before your 11 P.M. curfew.

DREAMS

Chinese medicine considers dreams a vital marker for health, especially that of the digestive system. The content isn't as important as the fact that they are happening—so long as they aren't nightmares. The ability to dream and remember your dreams, even if only briefly upon waking, tells a practitioner that your digestive system is working well and your body is not so preoccupied by toxins that it's not allowing you to dream.

Not only that, but spirits are associated with each organ. The liver is home to a spirit referred to as the *hun*, and the heart is home to the shen. We each have our own unique hun and shen, and the quality of our dreams reveals the health of these spirits. If we are healthy and our bodies are peaceful when we are resting, the shen will stay rooted in the heart while the hun takes off and finishes our business for us. The classical texts tell us that what we remember of our dreams is actually what the hun experiences while we are sleeping.

Special Considerations

We need uninterrupted hours of sleep each night to reset our bodies and brains. When falling asleep is easy and we can reach deep sleep, it is such a gift. Six to eight hours of sleep is generally considered maintenance level, whereas eight to ten hours is considered restorative. With our lives as busy and full as they are, sleep is crucial.

It's important to note that there are different types of "sleep personalities." In Chinese medicine it is considered typical to fall asleep between 10 and 11 P.M. and to stay asleep for seven to eight hours. It's not that anything outside of that is considered an imbalance, but if you are having symptoms in addition to unusual sleep patterns, then it is a pattern of imbalance to address.

Sleep apnea is more complicated. It can be due to issues with the chi of the lungs, spleen, or kidneys; phlegm; blood stasis; or liver excess. These patterns may arise from food allergies/intolerances that create heat and phlegm deep in the body. Or there could be a physical obstruction in the sinuses, nose, or jaw. It's best to see a practitioner for a full diagnosis.

SLEEP IMBALANCES

Symptoms	Difficulty falling asleep
	Difficulty staying asleep
	Insomnia (can't fall asleep or stay asleep)
	Insomnia due to vivid dreams
	Insomnia due to disturbing dreams
	Insomnia due to restless leg syndrome
	Insomnia due to indigestion
	Insomnia due to sleep apnea
Chinese Medicine Patterns	Liver chi stagnation (leading to shen disturbance)
	Liver blood deficiency
	Spleen chi deficiency
	Kidney yin deficiency
Chinese Herbal Formulas	Emperor's Heart Yin (*tian wang bu xing dan*)
	Restore the Spleen Decoction (*gui pi tang*)
	Jujube Seed Decoction (*suan zao ren tang*)
	Preserve Harmony (*bao he wan*)
Chinese Herbs	Schisandra
	Skullcap →

Other Herbs	Valerian	Chamomile
	Passionflower	Hops
	Kava kava	
Nutritional Supplements	Melatonin	GABA
	Magnesium	L-Theanine
Acupressure Points	Anmian	Kidney 6
	Heart 7	Bladder 62

WAKING PATTERNS

Are you waking up at a certain time each night? If so, check the Meridian Clock on page 46 for insights into which organ might need some extra attention.

THYROID DISEASES
Chinese Medicine Interpretation
Hyper- and hypothyroidism are the ultimate expression of an imbalance between yin and yang. Symptoms of hyperthyroidism, for instance, lead to excessive yang energy, whereas symptoms of hypothyroidism lead to excessive yin energy. Both patterns, however, signal a deficiency. Technically thyroid diseases, when left unaddressed, can develop into autoimmune disease.

Special Considerations
Aside from hormonal changes in pregnancy (which can radically change thyroid function), most thyroid imbalances can be address through the diet. Return to the pantry guidelines in Chapter 3; consider doing a cleanse (see Appendix E); and then address the underlying pattern with foods, herbs, supplements, and practices.

Symptoms	Hypothyroidism:	Hyperthyroidism:
	Fatigue	Irritability
	Increased sensitivity to cold	Increased sweating
	Constipation	Heat intolerance
	Dry skin	Heart palpitations
	Weight gain	Unexpected weight loss
	Puffy face	Changes in appetite (both increased and decreased)
	Hoarseness	Insomnia
	Muscle weakness	Fatigue
	Elevated blood cholesterol	Diarrhea
	Muscle aches, tenderness, and stiffness	Hair loss
	Joint pain, stiffness, or swelling	Muscle weakness/tremors
	Thinning hair	Bulging eyes
	Slowed heart rate	Nervousness
	Depression	Mood swings
	Impaired memory	Panic attacks
	Heavier than normal or irregular menstrual periods	
Chinese Medicine Patterns	Kidney yang deficiency (hypothyroidism) Kidney yin deficiency (hyperthyroidism)	
Chinese Herbal Formulas	Hypothyroidism: Kidney Qi Pills from the Golden Cabinet (for kidney yang deficiency) Restore the Right Kidney (for kidney yang deficiency)	Hyperthyroidism: Gardenia Decoction to Clear the Liver (*zhi zi qing gan tang*) Emperor's Heart Yin (*tian wang bu xin dan*) Six Ingredient Pill with Rehmannia (for kidney yin deficiency) (*liu wei di huang wan*)
Chinese Herbs	Hypothyroidism: Ashwagandha Cinnamon Licorice Rhodiola Schisandra Radix ginseng Eleuthero Astragalus	Hyperthyroidism: Rehmannia Chinese yam

Other Herbs	Hypothyroidism: Tulsi Raspberry leaf	Hyperthyroidism: Curcumin Lemon balm
Nutritional Supplements	Hypothyroidism: B-complex Tyrosine Iron (if deficient) Selenium	Hyperthyroidism: B-complex L-Carnitine
Acupressure Points	For all thyroid imbalances: Kidney 3, 6, 7, and 27 Stomach 8 Large Intestine 4 and 18	

— 11 —

WOMEN'S HEALTH IMBALANCES

Women's health imbalances are becoming more and more common. There are several reasons for this, including the ongoing struggle for equality; the stress endured by millions of women who are responsible for raising families, maintaining sanity in their households, and holding down careers; and last but not least, every-day exposure to toxins like bisphenol A (BPA) in plastics and phytoestrogens in food, which wreak havoc on our hormones. All of these factors seem to contribute to many of the most common women's health issues.

A PERSONAL MESSAGE

To the women reading this book, I would like to say, "You are enough." If you are running yourself ragged and compromising your health because of underlying feelings of inadequacy, I have so much love and empathy for you; you are not alone. I cannot emphasize this enough. Work on those feelings just as you would if you were diagnosed with cancer. Give it all you've got to transform them into core messages of love, value, and healing. You *are* enough!

Back to the yin-yang balance. Especially for women who are menstruating, our lives depend on us being able to cycle through yin and yang energies each month. If we push through this by drinking insane amounts of coffee and not stopping until we crash at night, we will burn out. Birth control pills, implants, rings, and intrauterine devices may very well be the death of us because they toy with our cycles and, therefore, our natural yin-yang balance. I would rather teach women about their cycles, to know when they are fertile, and to feel empowered about the choices they make to be intimate during these times. Birth control *always* comes at a price. And if you have taken birth control at all, but especially for more than two years of your life, it's important to have your hormones and nutritional levels checked.[1]

The emotional component of women's health imbalances is often a feeling of being backed up emotionally, and in particular, with anger. Not surprisingly, women are still encouraged to withhold feelings of anger or strong opinions for fear of coming across as you-know-whats. This gets so exaggerated that even women who speak their minds the way many men do on a daily basis are criticized and not taken seriously. Many of these women may also develop cysts and fibroids, the body's signal that it too is backed up.

SUPPORTING WOMEN'S HEALTH IMBALANCES WITH DIET: Eat nourishing, easy-to-digest foods (warm and cooked, nothing raw or cold). Focus on increasing your intake of healthy fats and anti-inflammatory foods; eliminate food additives, preservatives, and refined sugar. Eat more frequently to maintain a balanced blood sugar level. An anti-inflammatory or elimination diet (page 285) may be helpful to weed out potential triggers of inflammation.

LIFESTYLE CONSIDERATIONS FOR WOMEN'S HEALTH IMBALANCES: Reread "Menses and the Moon" on page 42 if you are still menstruating. Address unresolved emotional wounds, especially trauma. Exercise daily, especially during the more yang phase of your cycle or the moon's cycle. Listen to your body.

ADDITIONAL TESTING TO CONSIDER: Salivary hormones, neurotransmitters, salivary cortisol, nutritional deficiencies

PROGESTERONE: A LIFESAVER

Many of the women's health imbalances presented in this book can be linked to progesterone insufficiency. As mentioned previously, we are overexposed to estrogens in our world and underexposed to progesterone (and all the other hormones we need to keep estrogens in check). I recommend working with a skilled practitioner to get tested if you experience any of the following imbalances.

PREMENSTRUAL SYNDROME

Chinese Medicine Interpretation

The three organs primarily responsible for an easy and regular menstrual cycle are the liver, spleen, and kidneys. Emotional stress, overwork, and feeling overwhelmed tax the liver like nothing else, so the smooth flow of blood and chi gets interrupted and begins to stagnate. The most common pattern that underlies all PMS symptoms is liver chi stagnation. The quality, quantity, and viscosity of our blood is something we can witness each month and gives us insight into our organs and systems. Blood that is thick and clotting is a sign that we need to support the liver. A period that comes too soon (spotting) or lasts too long (bleeding for more than five days) is a sign that we need to support the spleen. If our cycle comes with changes in sleep habits (most notably insomnia), changes in body temperature (like hot flashes), and cramps that radiate into the lower back, then we know that we need to support the kidneys.

Let's talk about a typical menstrual cycle for a moment. Society has normalized PMS symptoms—the whole "that time of the month" mindset—but PMS is not normal; it's only common. When all of our energy is flowing properly, our cycles flow without drama, without pain, and sometimes even without noticing the physical changes (except when we are bleeding, of course). In a normal healthy cycle, we will still feel that tug of yin energies around our bleeding time and yang energies around ovulation, but aside from that, our cycles should feel easy and be consistent. Blood should be red in color and without clots.

Special Considerations

Often I find that PMS reflects a deeper yin-yang imbalance than the standard patterns are able to describe. Our cycles give us both a yin and a yang aspect to each month. When we are bleeding, we are having yin time in our bodies, and when we are ovulating (about two weeks after the start of our cycle), we are having yang time in our bodies. During bleeding, it is normal and natural to want more alone time, to need more space, and to feel more internal. Our drop in hormones (which is what signals the cycle to begin) is also a drop in the extremely yang hormone progesterone, leaving us with our highly yin hormone, estrogen. Slowly over the next two weeks, progesterone starts to creep back up, giving us more energy for ovulation, which tends to feel more yang. It is normal and natural to want to be more social, more sexual, more creative, and more energetic at this time because it is when we are more fertile.

This world is not a soft place for women to land during their yin time. We still have to show up and do everything we normally do without faltering, despite this radical change in hormones. And with our society being so yang and rewarding those who are more yang as well, women who are bleeding can try to keep up, but it is very unnatural. I so often feel that it is because of this conundrum each month that we begin to build up and stagnate our blood and chi. What would happen if we could create a world where we could actually listen to the wisdom of our bodies and participate in more yin work during this time?

If you lose a lot of blood during menstruation, it's important to replenish your stores right away. Liquid, plant-based iron and blood-building foods, along with Chinese medicine herbs are great and easily assimilated (see page 96 for blood-building foods). Otherwise red meat is a wonderful alternative, and in severe cases of anemia, taking iron supplements may be the best medicine. Adding raw, unfiltered organic apple cider vinegar to your greens will help you absorb more iron.[2] In cases of amenorrhea, you might do well to eat red meat daily until you bleed.

BREAST TENDERNESS AND SWELLING DURING PMS

Working on the pattern that underlies this imbalance will help with all the symptoms you experience during PMS. However, one way to work with the liver chi stagnation aspect in the breast tissue is to massage and skin brush your breasts. It's best to do this midcycle, when your breasts are not so tender. Using your hands, massage in lotion or oil from the center of each breast out toward the base. Don't be afraid to massage deeply, especially if you wear underwire bras, as they tend to stop the lymph from flowing around your breasts. Alternate between massaging and skin brushing, always in the same direction. Do this for five minutes each day to move chi and lymph fluid out of your breasts. Cutting out caffeine and wearing more supportive bras (no underwire) can also reduce the amount of stagnation in your breasts.

NOTE: Cases of a much more severe form of PMS, called premenstrual dysphoric disorder (PMDD), have been steadily increasing over the years. This is basically severe PMS with the addition of extreme mental health imbalances, mostly depression and anxiety. Western medicine views the development of PMDD as a reaction to the change in hormones, but doctors haven't found much to do for it except to prescribe antidepressants (which only work for an extremely small part of the population) and recommend pain medications. On the other hand, Chinese medicine practitioners are well equipped to treat PMDD. In fact, this is where Chinese medicine really shines. Finding the underlying pattern of imbalance, along with following the dietary, lifestyle, and herbal recommendations can completely reverse PMDD in as little as three months.

PREMENSTRUAL SYNDROME

Symptoms	Swollen or tender breasts
	Constipation or diarrhea
	Fatigue
	Sleep problems (sleeping too much or too little)
	Bloating or gas
	Cramping
	Headache or backache
	Irritability or hostile behavior
	Appetite changes or food cravings
	Trouble with concentration or memory
	Tension or anxiety
	Depression, feelings of sadness, or crying spells
	Mood swings
	Low libido
Chinese Medicine Patterns	Liver chi stagnation
	Kidney yin deficiency
	Liver blood deficiency
Chinese Herbal Formulas	Free and Easy Wanderer
	Free and Easy Wanderer Plus (when heat signs are present)
	Four Ingredient Pills with Safflower and Peach Pit (tao hong si wu tang)
	Eight Treasure Combination
Chinese Herbs	Ginkgo
	White peony (for hot flashes, cramps, and muscle pain)
	Motherwort
	Fenugreek

$\rightarrow$

Other Herbs	Raspberry leaf	Evening primrose oil
	Chaste tree berry	Cramp bark
	St. John's wort	
Nutritional Supplements	B-complex	GLA
	Magnesium (especially when headaches or migraines precede start of cycle)	Calcium
		Zinc
	EPA/DHA, all essential fatty acids	
Acupressure Points	Liver 3	Spleen 6
	Large Intestine 4	Bladder 30, 31, and 32
	Conception Vessel 5	

FIBROIDS

Chinese Medicine Interpretation

While most women will develop fibroids at some point in their lives, many will have no idea they have them because the growths can be so small that they don't cause any symptoms and simply go away on their own. However, for some women, the development of fibroids can be a sign that something has gone out of balance underneath. In Chinese medicine, once the correct pattern has been diagnosed, it takes about three months of regular acupuncture treatments and herbs to clear the fibroids and rebalance the system.

Special Considerations

One of the biggest factors that makes women prone to developing fibroids is their exposure to plastics (plastic water bottles, Tupperware, and so on) and phytoestrogens (such as consuming large amounts of soy). Cleaning up your environment and your life so that you are reducing your toxic burden is a crucial step to getting rid of fibroids. Avoiding plant-based estrogen products is also important to allow for the healthy restoration of your hormones and uterus. Increase your intake of flaxseeds and discuss with your practitioner the possibility of bringing on board lipotropic supports such as inositol and choline. Daily castor oil packs applied directly on the abdomen (over the uterus) have been shown to support the reduction and elimination of fibroids.

FIBROIDS		
Symptoms	Heavy menstrual bleeding Menstrual periods lasting more than a week Pelvic pressure or pain Frequent urination Difficulty emptying the bladder Constipation Backache or leg pains	
Chinese Medicine Patterns	Liver blood deficiency Spleen chi deficiency Kidney yang deficiency Blood stasis	
Chinese Herbal Formulas	Cinnamon Twig and Poria (*gui zhi fu ling wan*)	
Chinese Herbs	Hawthorn Curcumin	
Other Herbs	Chaste tree berry Milk thistle	Maca
Nutritional Supplements	B-complex EPA/DHA	Vitamin C Iron (after menstruation)
Acupressure Points	Stomach 25 Conception Vessel 5 and 7	Zigong Spleen 6

LOW LIBIDO

Chinese Medicine Interpretation

To be intimate with another person requires a balancing of yin and yang energy, both the energy to initiate intimacy as well as the energy to receive intimacy from your partner. Sex itself is a perfect blend of yin-yang energy. Yang energy is very active and engaging, whereas yin energy allows for the production of sexual fluids (including those that make us fertile) and for deeper connection. When this desire is lost, either individually or for both partners, it's important to look at the underlying patterns because being intimate can be so healing when it's healthy and desired.

Special Considerations

A common block to libido is stress. When you are stressed, your body is not going to be focused on producing and secreting sexual fluids and connecting deeply with your partner. It will be focused on surviving the next meeting or the next day. Stress is a huge factor in libido. If you can work on your body's ability to manage stress (while lowering the amount of it in your life), not only will you experience drastic health benefits, but your libido is also likely to increase. Other common blocks to libido for women are grief, changes in hormones, and PTSD (especially after a sexually based trauma).

LOW LIBIDO		
Symptoms	Lack of interest in sex and/or intimacy Lack of sexual fluids Difficulty orgasming Pain or discomfort during intercourse	
Chinese Medicine Patterns	Liver blood deficiency Kidney yin deficiency Liver chi stagnation	
Chinese Herbs	Horny goat weed Schisandra Radix ginseng	
Other Herbs	Damiana Passionflower Saw palmetto Maca Tribulus Fenugreek	
Nutritional Supplements	Dihydroepiandrosterone (DHEA) Vitamin C Iron	
Acupressure Points	Governing Vessel 20 Conception Vessel 6 Kidney 1	Spleen 4 Liver 3 Pericardium 8

INFERTILITY

Chinese Medicine Interpretation

Chinese medicine has become very popular in the successful treatment of women and men who have been deemed infertile by Western medicine. Why? Perhaps because a successful pregnancy is so much more than a healthy sperm meeting a healthy egg. It's also implantation (providing a cozy home for the fetus); it's proper hormones that keep the pregnancy viable and prevent miscarriages; it's good, nourishing blood that goes to support the growing fetus; and much more. Infertility has become a growing field within Chinese medicine because we address all of these things while at the same time reducing stress and anxiety (which I believe is a large culprit in causing infertility).

To get the clearest information regarding your cycle and where there might be a hiccup, track your cycle so you can look at the particular phases and ask, "Is it the follicular phase where I'm having trouble? The ovulation phase? Or the luteal phase?" Then support can be tailored to be much more specific. (See page 368 for resources on learning to track your cycle.)

Electrical stimulation on the acupuncture point Zigong has been well researched as an effective tool for opening up all the circulation to the uterus and assisting with implantation and gestation.[3]

Special Considerations

While 25 percent of pregnancies are lost naturally within the first twelve weeks, it still comes as a shock and causes significant grief when it happens. Of course, if you are one of the women to whom this happens again and again, it can also be very frustrating. To promote a successful pregnancy, one of the first things I look at is the stress level of both parents, followed by the quality of their blood and whether or not they have potential hormonal challenges. Chinese medicine focuses on addressing these three things in order to help a couple have a successful pregnancy.

When you begin working on infertility, give yourself three months to find the underlying pattern and address that before trying to conceive again. This will give your body the greatest chance of success. I know it's hard not to try for three months, but just think of how healthy you and your baby will be if you take your challenges with pregnancy as a sign that something underneath is out of balance and choose to rebalance it before bringing a baby in.

NOTE: If you and your partner consider yourselves fairly healthy and you have still had multiple miscarriages, I recommend getting genetic testing for methylenetetrahydrofolate reductase (MTHFR). While much of the research on MTHFR is focused on its role in mental health, there are significant links between MTHFR and frequent miscarriages (For more information, see the "Resources for Delving Deeper" section at the end of this book.)

Also, if you have used hormonal birth control, I recommend taking two years off from this method before trying to conceive. Take this time to replenish your lost nutrients (especially folic acid).

INFERTILITY		

Symptoms	Frequent miscarriages
	Six months without pregnancy,
	    despite regular unprotected sex
	Fibroids
	PCOS
		Hormonal imbalances
		Endometriosis
		Premenstrual dysphoric disorder
		    (PMDD)

Chinese Medicine Patterns	Liver chi stagnation Spleen chi deficiency Kidney yin or yang deficiency Liver blood deficiency	
Chinese Herbal Formulas	Dang Quai and Peony (*dang quai xiao yao san*) Ba Zhen Tang (for chi and blood deficiency)	
Chinese Herbs	Cinnamon Angelica	White peony Eleuthero
Other Herbs	Red clover Raspberry leaf	Chaste tree berry Maca
Nutritional Supplements	Prenatal vitamins Vitamin C Folic acid Inositol	N-Acetylcysteine Progesterone cream (during second half of cycle)
Acupressure Points	Conception Vessel 3, 4, and 6 Stomach 30 Kidney 9 and 16	Yin Tang Zigong

POLYCYSTIC OVARIAN SYNDROME

Chinese Medicine Interpretation

Chinese medicine's treatment for PCOS can include all five patterns from the table below but mainly begins with nourishing the kidneys, regardless of the pattern of imbalance. Nourishing the kidneys will relieve some of the emotional symptoms that accompany PCOS, lowering cortisol and other androgens and assisting in rebuilding your energy. You will also need to work to strengthen your spleen so you can dry up the dampness and phlegm (cysts). Making sure that you tend to your emotions will relieve the liver stagnation and help to free up blood stasis.

POLYCYSTIC OVARIAN SYNDROME		
Symptoms	Irregular or missed periods Anovulatory cycles Cysts on ovaries Weight gain Fatigue Unwanted hair growth Thinning hair on head	Infertility Acne Mood changes Pelvic pain Headaches Sleep problems
Chinese Medicine Patterns	Spleen chi deficiency Kidney yang deficiency Liver chi stagnation	Liver blood deficiency Blood stasis
Chinese Herbal Formulas	Bupleurum Soothe the Liver Formula Drive Out Blood Stasis Below the Diaphragm	
Chinese Herbs	Angelica Cinnamon Eleuthero	Licorice Poria
Other Herbs	Milk thistle Dandelion root	Saw palmetto Chaste tree berry
Nutritional Supplements	B-complex Multimineral vitamin EPA/DHA	Inositol (for egg quality) N-Acetylcysteine (for egg quality and blood sugar regulation)
Acupressure Points	Conception Vessel 5 and 12 Large Intestine 11 Liver 3 and 14	Spleen 6, 8, and 9 (massaging the whole lower Spleen meridian)

Special Considerations

There is often a strong relationship between hormones and metabolism when you have PCOS. Typically some insulin resistance develops, which will be largely curbed by eliminating sugar from the diet and returning to the basics introduced in Part Two. Additionally, androgens (our more masculine hormones) can start to creep up with PCOS, so I will recommend doing a hormone panel (preferably salivary) to see what all three estrogens as well as DHEA, testosterone, and cortisol are doing so we can support the patient even more. While acupuncture and dietary and herbal changes can sometimes be enough, adding hormonal support can often expedite healing, especially if pregnancy is a goal.

ENDOMETRIOSIS

Chinese Medicine Interpretation

In Chinese medicine the uterus and the liver are closely related, so we often find liver patterns at the heart of uterine and/or menstrual imbalances (in case you haven't noticed). When the liver is taxed, as with significant emotional stress, it can't support the flow of chi and blood, and blood stasis occurs. Occasionally there is also a coldness in the pattern as well as in one or more of the meridians that run through the uterus: Liver, Kidney, and Spleen. Endometriosis seems to be exacerbated by internal and external coldness. Plan on anywhere from three to six months of supporting yourself through this diagnosis.

Special Considerations

Warm castor oil packs assist in moving blood stasis, warming the cold uterus, and relieving pain. I've met many women with this diagnosis over the years and some who have had complete hysterectomies (even before age twenty-five) due to the severity of the pain associated with this condition. I have also seen countless women completely reverse debilitating endometriosis in six months through acupuncture, diet, and herbs. It takes patience and dedication, but it does happen! It's important to remember that endometriosis is just a symptom of something being out of balance underneath. Remembering to treat the whole person as well as the symptoms can create lifelong, sustainable change.

Symptoms	Painful periods
	Pain during intercourse
	Painful bowel movements and/or urination
	Excessive bleeding during menstrual cycles
	Infertility
	Nausea
	Fatigue
	Bloating
	Diarrhea or constipation
Chinese Medicine Patterns	Liver chi stagnation
	Blood stasis
Chinese Herbs	Bupleurum
	Red peony
	White peony
	Cyperus
	Angelica
	Salvia
	Rehmannia
	(Also see herbs for acute pain on page 298)
Other Herbs	Pine bark (pycnogenol)
	Cramp bark
	Chaste tree berry
Nutritional Supplements	Magnesium
	B-complex
	N-Acetylcysteine
	Melatonin
	EPA/DHA
	Progesterone cream
Acupressure Points	Spleen 6
	Zigong
	Stomach 36
	Liver 3
	Kidney 3
	Conception Vessel 4 and 6

MENOPAUSE

Chinese Medicine Interpretation

For most women, perimenopause and menopause begins in the late forties. As discussed earlier in this book, we have both yin and yang aspects to our lives, and menopause moves us into a more yin phase. With the decline of our yang hormones (progesterone, cortisol, DHEA, testosterone, and so on), we naturally begin to feel more internal, with less drive to engage in the world like we did in our twenties and thirties (of course, this is not true for everyone).

Special Considerations

We all tend to assume that menopause is the same the world over and that it's difficult for all women, but that isn't true. Having traveled around the world more than a few times and worked in urban and rural communities, I have seen plenty of women begin this chapter of their lives with few to no symptoms—in fact, they meet it with something more like welcome relief.

One of the complications of menopause in the developed countries is that we have burned our candle at both ends. We are not only trying to raise families or take care of our elders; we are also trying to have careers, contribute to our society, and hopefully one day make a difference. With all of this extra expenditure of energy throughout our lives, we tax our adrenal glands (the ones responsible for our energy and stress response). By the time we enter menopause, we should theoretically be using our adrenal glands to get that extra estrogen output for the remaining years of our lives. However, when that time comes, we realize we've spent it all already and don't have the extra hormones to use. This is what makes our transition from menstruation to menopause more like a steep decline rather than a gradual shift.

A diet rich in phytoestrogens may be one of the factors that separates those who experience severe menopause symptoms from those who don't. These are estrogen-like compounds found in fruits, legumes, and vegetables. Soy is one of the most phytoestrogen-rich foods on the planet. Because the current data on plant estrogens is controversial, I recommend doing a hormone test before increasing their presence in your diet.

Symptoms	Perimenopause:	Menopause (in addition to perimenopause symptoms):
	Less frequent menstruation	One year or more without a cycle (or pregnancy or illness)
	Heavier or lighter periods than normal	Insomnia
	Hot flashes	Vaginal dryness
	Night sweats	Unexplained weight gain
	Flushing	Depression
		Anxiety
		Difficulty concentrating, memory problems
		Reduced libido or sex drive
		Dry skin, mouth, and eyes
		Increased urination
		Sore or tender breasts
		Headaches
		Racing heart
		Reduced muscle mass
		Painful or stiff joints
		Reduced bone mass
		Less full breasts
		Hair thinning or loss
Chinese Medicine Patterns	Kidney yin deficiency	
	Kidney yang deficiency	
	(or a combination of the two)	
Chinese Herbal Formulas	Eight Flavor Rehmannia	
	Two Immortals Decoction	
	Women's Precious Formula	
Chinese Herbs	Radix ginseng	Fenugreek
	Eleuthero	Motherwort
	Angelica	Siler
Other Herbs	Black cohosh	Passionflower
	Red clover	St. John's wort
	Chaste tree berry	Valerian
Nutritional Supplements	Multimineral vitamin	Probiotics
	Vitamin D	Calcium
	Vitamin A	Magnesium

MENOPAUSE		
Acupressure Points	Kidney 1 and 3 Yin Tang Conception Vessel 3 and 4	Governing Vessel 4 and 20 Triple Burner 5 Spleen 6

SOY: TO EAT OR NOT TO EAT

To supplement with it or not to supplement with it. The reality is that we are likely already consuming soy products every day. It's downright scary how many ways soy is snuck into our foods. This, in conjunction with the fact that most soy is now genetically modified, has contributed to our current Western epidemic of soy allergies. Almost all soy in the United States is genetically modified. If you are going to eat soy, source it organically (most likely outside the States) and eat it fermented so you can get all the rich probiotics out of it along with the phytoestrogens. Tempeh, miso, and natto are all varieties of soy products you can try. After all, Japan is one of the healthiest places on earth, and unmodified and fermented soy is a staple in the national diet.

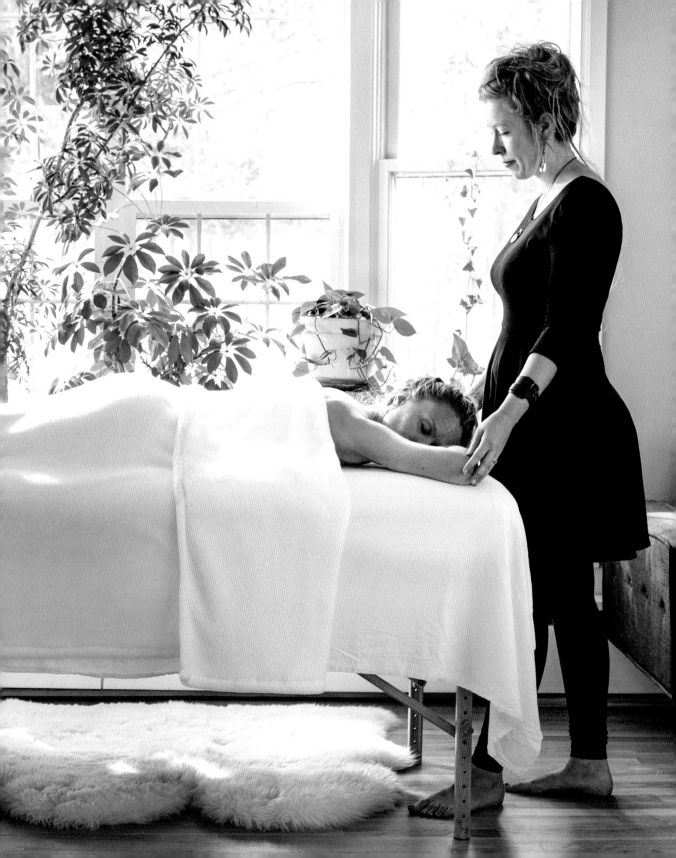

CONCLUSION

— ◆ —

As you can see, this book is about bringing us home into the very heart of ourselves, to make sense of some of our life experiences, and to do what we came here to do with as much energy and spirit as possible. We all want to live in a world with less suffering, more love, and greater connection. As you open and close the many chapters of your life, may this book serve as your compass to finding your way home again and again. I hope you have found the tools needed to understand your personal as well as our collective suffering so you can now become a catalyst for your own healing and, in turn, the much-needed healing of our world.

If you still crave more from this ancient system of medicine, or from me, head over to my website (www.mindikcounts.com) to find resources and other ways to continue working with me, including workshops, retreats, and blogs. And be on the lookout for a second book where I dive deeper into the Five Elements as pathways to authenticity, purpose, and soul-centered living!

Be patient with yourself and your healing, for you are already on the path.

Much love and many blessings,
Mindi

APPENDICES

— ♦ —

APPENDIX A. ACUPRESSURE POINTS AND MERIDIANS

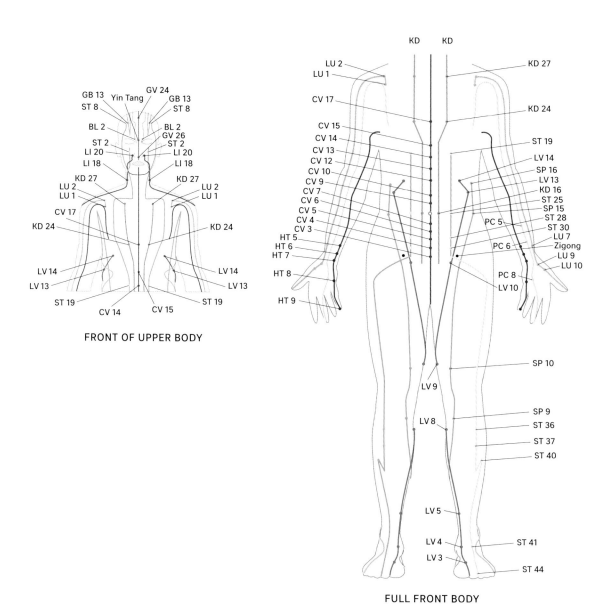

FRONT OF UPPER BODY

FULL FRONT BODY

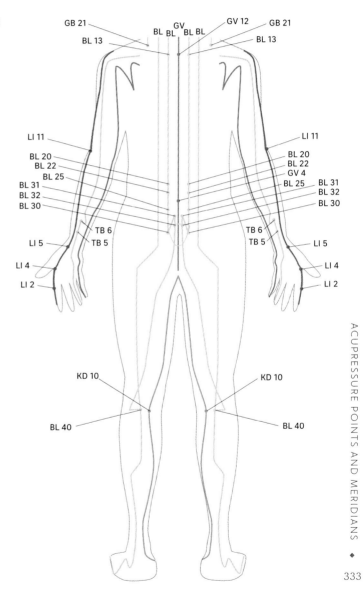

BACK OF UPPER BODY

GV 20
GV 19
BL 10
GB 20
Ding Chuan
GB 21
BL 13

BL 10
GB 20
Ding Chuan
GB 21
BL 13

GV 12

BL 20
BL 20

GB 21
BL 13

GV
BL BL BL BL

GV 12
GB 21
BL 13

LI 11
BL 20
BL 22
BL 25
BL 31
BL 32
BL 30

LI 11
BL 20
BL 22
GV 4
BL 25
BL 31
BL 32
BL 30

TB 6
TB 5
LI 5
LI 4
LI 2

TB 6
TB 5
LI 5
LI 4
LI 2

KD 10
BL 40

KD 10
BL 40

FULL BACK BODY

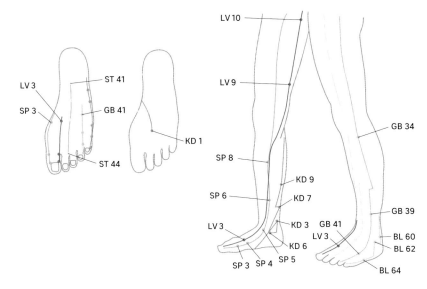

FEET AND LEGS

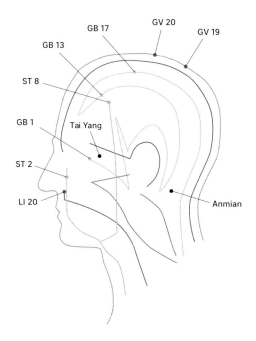

LATERAL SIDE OF HEAD

Acupressure Points

Point Number	Point Name	Point Action
Anmian	Peaceful Spirit	Relieves anxiety and insomnia (empirical point for these conditions)
Bladder (BL) 2	Gathering Bamboo	Relieves headaches and dizziness, clears the sinuses and sinus pressure, calms anxiety and manic behavior
BL 10	Heavenly Pillar	Relieves headaches, dizziness, congestion, sinus pain and pressure, and sore or swollen throat and tonsils
BL 13	Lung Association	Balances all lung imbalances
BL 20	Spleen Association	Balances all spleen-related imbalances
BL 22	Triple Burner Association	Balances all triple burner imbalances
BL 25	Large Intestine Association	Balances all large intestine imbalances
BL 30	White Ring Association	Regulates menstruation, balances lower back issues, reduces hemorrhoid pain
BL 31	Upper Sacral Bone	Regulates the lower burner, facilitates urination and defecation, regulates menstruation
BL 32	Second Sacral Bone	Regulates menstruation, relieves diarrhea, promotes urination
BL 40	Equilibrium Middle	Cools the blood, stops nausea and vomiting, relieves diarrhea, benefits the back and knees
BL 60	Kunlun Mountain	Clears heat in the body, relieves pain (sometimes called the "Aspirin Point")
BL 62	Extended Meridian	Calms the spirit, eliminates internal wind, alleviates pain, benefits the head and eyes
BL 64	Capital Bone	Calms the spirit, relaxes the body, alleviates pain, clears the head and eyes, eliminates wind
Conception Vessel (CV) 3	Utmost Middle	Provides sense of balance and calm, relieves urinary disorders caused by excess heat, stagnation, and dampness
CV 4	First Gate	Stimulates energy; treats yin, yang, chi, and blood deficiencies; relieves exhaustion, weakness, and chronic fatigue
CV 5	Stone Gate	Provides a sense of movement when feeling stuck; relieves urinary tract imbalances, diarrhea, undigested food in stools, and poor appetite

CV 6	Sea of Chi	Stimulates energy; relieves hernia pain, uterine bleeding, irregular menstruation, dysmenorrhea, impotence, and fatigue
CV 7	Yin Crossing	Relieves abdominal pain, bloating, edema, hernia pain, genital pain, irregular menstruation, uterine bleeding, and leukorrhea
CV 9	Water Division	Relieves water stagnation, edema, urinary issues, poor digestion, gas, bloating, gastroesophageal reflux disease (GERD), and vomiting after eating
CV 10	Lower Duct	Treats issues with the lower intestines such as stagnation, bloating, diarrhea, and undigested food in the stool
CV 12	Middle Duct	Treats middle burner issues such as pain, bloating, acid reflux, vomiting, diarrhea, and jaundice
CV 13	Upper Duct	Treats upper burner issues such as vomiting, hiatal hernia pain, hiccups, and epigastric pain
CV 14	Great Deficiency	Relieves heart/shen-related issues arising from an excess or a deficiency, nausea, acid reflux, vomiting, and abdominal pain
CV 15	Dove Tail	Relieves all heart/shen-related psychological issues, epilepsy, heart palpitations, mania, and upper digestive issues
CV 17	Within the Breast	Promotes feelings of safety, security, and calm; tonifies the upper burner; relieves chronic lung, breast, and chest/throat issues
Ding Chuan	Asthma Point	Relieves cough, neck rigidity, and pain in the shoulder and back (empirical point for asthma)
Gallbladder (GB) 1	Orbit Bone	Benefits the eyes and promotes clear sight in body, mind, and spirit; relieves headache, eye problems, and any conditions with rising heat in the head
GB 13	Root of the Spirit	Regulates the liver and gallbladder; eliminates wind; calms the mind; relieves stiff neck, headache, and epilepsy
GB 17	Upright Living	Clears heat, regulates the gallbladder, relieves headache and dizziness
GB 20	Wind Pond	Eliminates exterior and interior wind; relieves fever/chills, stiff neck, twitching, tremors, numbness, dizziness, headaches, and all head issues
GB 21	Shoulder Well	Relaxes the whole body; induces labor; relieves occipital headaches, tight trapezius muscles, neck and shoulder pain, phlegm-related issues, and pain in the head, neck, breast, and chest
GB 34	Yang Mound Spring	Relieves cramping, pain, spasms, weakness, and numbness anywhere in the body (empirical point for all ligament and tendon issues)

GB 39	Hanging Cup	Lowers rising liver and gallbladder heat; relieves dizziness, tinnitus, neck issues, stiffness, arthritis, strains, sprains, whiplash, and headache
GB 41	Foot above Tears	Moves stuck liver chi, relieves depression, menstrual disorders, breast pain, lateral headaches, migraines, and lateral foot issues
Governing Vessel (GV) 4	Gate of Destiny	Reunites you with your sense of purpose, will, and strength; clears heat from the whole body; tonifies kidney chi; relieves menstrual disorders and lower back pain
GV 12	Body Pillar	Relieves all psychological imbalances; clears heat in the lungs and chest; relieves asthma, chest pain, whooping cough, and chronic conditions affecting the lungs
GV 19	Posterior Summit	Relieves headache, vertigo, dizziness, neck pain, wind, insomnia, psychological issues with manic symptoms, and epilepsy
GV 20	Meeting of 100 Ancestors	Relieves headache, dizziness, eye pain and redness, irritability, hypertension, and excess yang in the upper body (an empirical point)
GV 24	Spirit Courtyard	Relieves anxiety and restlessness (empirical point for frontal headache, chronic sinusitis, nosebleed, and nasal discharge)
GV 26	Middle of Man/ Woman	Restores consciousness from fainting, combats shock, treats acute lower back sprain, helps relieve pain, moves stagnation
Heart (HT) 5	Penetrating the Inside	Calms the spirit, regulates heart rhythm, benefits the tongue, activates the meridian, alleviates pain
HT 6	Yin Mound	Regulates heart and blood, calms the spirit, moderates acute conditions, clears fire deficiency
HT 7	Spirit Gate	Calms the spirit, regulates and tonifies the heart, relieves insomnia and muddled thinking, clears heart and phlegm fire
HT 8	Lesser Palace	Clears heat from the heart and small intestine, calms the spirit, regulates chi, alleviates pain
HT 9	Little Rushing In	Revives the heart; benefits the tongue, eyes, and throat; regulates heart chi and emergency heart attack point
Kidney (KD) 1	Bubbling Spring	Reduces excess energy from the head, calms the spirit, restores consciousness, rescues yang, tonifies kidney and heart yin
KD 3	Greater Mountain Stream	Nourishes kidney yin, clears heat deficiency, tonifies kidney yang, anchors chi, strengthens the lumbar spine
KD 6	Illuminated Sea	Provides a sense of ease and calm, benefits the throat, nourishes the kidneys, clears heat deficiency, regulates the lower burner

KD 7	Returning Current	Benefits the kidneys, regulates the water passages, relieves edema, regulates sweating, clears damp heat
KD 9	Building for a Guest	Increases fertility, clears heat and dissipates phlegm, regulates chi, alleviates pain in the lower burner
KD 10	Yin Valley	Clears damp heat from the lower burner, benefits the kidneys, activates the meridian, and alleviates pain
KD 16	Vitals Correspondence	Regulates chi, alleviates pain, regulates and warms the intestines, relieves constipation and abdominal pain
KD 24	Spirit Burial Ground	Provides a sense of hope and feelings of recovery after trauma and PTSD, unbinds the chest, lowers rebellious lung and stomach chi, benefits the breasts, relieves heart palpitations and abdominal bloating
KD 27	Storehouse	Unbinds the chest, dissipates phlegm, alleviates cough and wheezing, harmonizes the stomach, reduces rebellious chi
Large Intestine (LI) 2	Second Interval	Eliminates wind, clears heat, reduces swelling, alleviates pain all over the body
LI 4	Joining of the Valleys	Regulates wei qi; reduces sweating; eliminates wind; regulates the face, eyes, nose, mouth, and ears; restores yang balance
LI 5	Yang Stream	Clears heat, calms the spirit, benefits the wrist
LI 11	Crooked Pond	Clears heat, cools the blood, eliminates wind, dries dampness, alleviates itching, regulates chi and blood, relieves skin conditions
LI 18	Support and Rush Out	Reminds you of your connection to the spirit; benefits the throat and voice; alleviates cough, wheezing, asthma, sore throat, and sudden loss of voice; shrinks goiter
LI 20	Welcome Fragrance	Opens nasal passages; eliminates wind; clears heat; relieves frontal headaches, itching, and swelling of the face
Liver (LV) 3	Supreme Rushing	Spreads liver chi; clears the head, eyes, and sinuses; regulates menstruation; nourishes liver blood and liver yin
LV 4	Middle Seal	Spreads liver chi, regulates the lower burner, clears the Liver meridian of stagnant heat, promotes urination, relieves hernia pain
LV 5	Insect Ditch	Relieves skin conditions, calms feelings of irritation, clears heat in the liver and gallbladder
LV 8	Crooked Spring	Invigorates the blood, benefits the uterus and genitals, nourishes blood and yin, relieves lower abdominal pain

LV 9	Yin Wrapping	Regulates menstruation and the lower burner, relieves lumbosacral and lower abdominal pain
LV 10	Five Miles	Clears damp heat, benefits the lower burner, relieves lower abdominal pain and distention, promotes urination
LV 13	Chapter Gate	Harmonizes the liver and spleen; regulates the middle and lower burners; relieves vomiting, diarrhea, and indigestion
LV 14	Gate of Hope	Provides a sense of relief and hope; relieves depression; spreads stuck liver chi; harmonizes the liver and stomach; alleviates abdominal pain and distention, hiccups, and acid reflux
Lung (LU) 1	Middle Palace	Restores your connection to the heavens; relieves coughing, wheezing, and asthma
LU 2	Cloud Gate	Eliminates congestion in the lungs and phlegm, relieves coughing and wheezing, clears the mind and heart
LU 7	Narrow Defile	Relieves coughing and sore throat, restores wei qi
LU 9	Very Great Abyss	Relaxes the lungs, reduces coughing, relieves chronic sense of grief
LU 10	Fish Region	Clears heat from the throat, lungs, and Lung meridian; reconnects you to your heart
Pericardium (PC) 5	The Intermediary	Unbinds the chest, regulates chi, harmonizes the stomach, alleviates nausea and vomiting, clears heat
PC 6	Inner Frontier Gate	Reduces anxiety, induces feelings of calm and security, regulates the heart, harmonizes the stomach, alleviates nausea and vomiting, relieves cardiac pain and heart palpitations
PC 8	Palace of Weariness	Reduces anxiety and feelings of weariness, clears heat, restores consciousness, cools the blood
Spleen (SP) 3	Supreme White	Tonifies the spleen; strengthens the spirit; clears dampness and damp heat; relieves gastric pain, constipation, vomiting, and dysentery and diarrhea
SP 4	Grandmother-Granddaughter/ Grandfather-Grandson	Regulates chi, clears dampness, fortifies the spleen, harmonizes the middle burner, benefits the heart and chest, reminds you of your purpose
SP 5	Merchant Mound	Fortifies the spleen, renews feelings of self-worth, clears dampness, benefits the sinews and bones, alleviates pain in the foot and ankle, relieves hemorrhoid pain

SP 6	Three Yin Crossing	Relieves anxiety, exhaustion, and adrenal fatigue; clears dampness; tonifies the spleen and stomach; regulates menstruation and urination; benefits the genitals; induces labor
SP 8	Earth Motivator	Resolves eating disorders
SP 9	Yin Mound Spring	Regulates the spleen, clears dampness, opens the waterways (i.e. kidneys and bladder) and moves water, relieves pain in the external genitals and dysmenorrhea
SP 10	Sea of Blood	Invigorates the blood and dispels stasis, cools the blood, regulates menstruation, relieves skin conditions
SP 15	Great Horizontal	Promotes body-mind balance; moves chi; regulates the intestines; relieves abdominal pain and distention, diarrhea and dysentery, and constipation
SP 16	Abdomen Sorrow	Regulates the intestines, relieves sadness, eating disorders, abdominal pain, indigestion, constipation, and dysentery
Stomach (ST) 2	Four Whites	Eliminates wind; clears heat; benefits the eyes and sinuses; relieves eye redness, pain, and itching; eases facial paralysis and pain
ST 8	Head Tied	Reduces anxiety and worry, eliminates wind, alleviates pain, benefits the eyes, relieves headaches and blurred vision
ST 19	Not at Ease	Brings a feeling of relaxation and ease; reduces chi; alleviates nausea, cough, and wheezing; harmonizes the middle burner; reduces rebelliousness
ST 25	Heavenly Pivot	Balances the body-mind connection, relieves constipation, clears dampness and damp heat, regulates chi and blood, eliminates stagnation
ST 28	Water Passage	Regulates the lower burner and dispels stagnation, benefits the bladder and uterus, relieves lower abdominal pain and distension
ST 30	Rushing Chi	Regulates chi in the lower burner; relieves abdominal pain, gas, bloating, hernia pain, and impotence
ST 36	Leg Three Miles	Reduces anxiety, stress, and fatigue; stimulates energy (empirical point for any digestive issues)
ST 37	Upper Great Void	Regulates the intestines, eliminates stagnation, clears damp heat, alleviates diarrhea and dysentery
ST 40	Abundant Splendor	Clears phlegm and dampness; relieves cough, asthma, excessive mucus, and swelling or paralysis in the lower extremities

ST 41	Released Stream	Clears heat from the stomach and its meridian; relieves headache, dizziness/vertigo, abdominal distension, and constipation; reconnects you with your heart/shen
ST 44	Inner Courtyard	Harmonizes the mind and intestines; clears damp heat; relieves toothache, sore throat, gastric pain, and acid reflux
Tai Yang	Great Sun	Relieves temporal, one-sided, and migraine headaches; eye issues; toothache; and facial paralysis and pain
Triple Burner (TB) 5	Outer Frontier Gate	Supports the immune system; relieves fever, headache, and pain in the upper limbs; promotes sense of security in self
TB 6	Branch Ditch	Relieves constipation caused by stagnation and heat in the body, treats chest issues, supports detoxification
Yin Tang	Hall of Seal	Calms the spirit; relieves insomnia, anxiety, stress, frontal headache, and sinus issues
Zigong	Ovarian Association Point	Regulates the lower burner, treats infertility, regulates menstruation and the reproductive organs

APPENDIX B. CHINESE HERBS (SINGLE)

Chinese Herbs (Single)			
English Name	Pinyin Name	Flavors, Temperatures, and Actions	Daily Dosage in Grams, for Decoction
Agastache	Huo Xiang	Pungent, slightly warm. Enters the Lung, Spleen, and Stomach meridians, drains dampness and reduces rebellious chi. Used in formulas for summer colds and flu with symptoms of low fever, stomachache, diarrhea with sensation of having to defecate after finishing, nausea, vomiting, bloating, headache, scanty and dark urine, and sensation of heaviness in arms and legs. See page 214.	5–10 grams
Angelica	Dang Gui	Sweet, pungent, bitter, and warm. Enters the Heart, Liver, and Spleen meridians. Useful for dysmenorrhea, amenorrhea, female infertility, anemia, tinnitus, hair loss, blurred vision, mental fogginess, and heart palpitations. See page 185.	4.5–15 grams
Ashwagandha	Nan Fei Zui Jia	Sweet, bitter, pungent, and warm. Enters the Lung, Spleen, and Heart meridians. Powerful adaptogen. Reduces anxiety and stress, helps counter depression, boosts fertility and testosterone in men, and may even boost brain function.	6–12 grams
Astragalus	Huang Qi	Sweet, slightly warm. Enters the Lung and Spleen meridians. Boosts the body's immune system, tonifies chi and blood, and is useful in wei qi deficiency. Has also been used with conditions including heart disease. Contraindicated for use with immunosuppressive drugs. See page 128.	9–15 grams
Atractylodes	Bai Zhu	Bitter, sweet, slightly pungent, and warm. Enters the Spleen and Stomach meridians. Useful with spleen, stomach, and kidney chi deficiencies. Useful in cases of diarrhea, edema, fatigue, vomiting, and a generally weakened immune system. See page 214.	5–15 grams
Boswellia (Frankincense)	Ru Xiang	Bitter, pungent, and warm. Enters the Heart, Liver, and Spleen meridians. Major anti-inflammatory, promotes tissue regeneration by increasing chi circulation and blood. Relieves pain and swelling. Contraindicated in pregnancy.	3–9 grams
Bupleurum	Chai Hu	Bitter, pungent, and cool. Enters the Gallbladder, Liver, Pericardium, and Triple Burner meridians. Reduces fevers and spreads liver chi (good for vertigo, emotional instability, and menstrual problems). Raises yang chi in spleen/stomach deficiencies. See page 158.	3–12 grams

Chinese Yam	Shan Yao	Sweet and neutral. Enters the Kidney, Lung, and Spleen meridians. Tonifies the spleen and stomach chi. Useful for diarrhea, fatigue, spontaneous sweating, lack of appetite, chronic cough/wheezing, spermatorrhea, vaginal discharge, and frequent urination. Strengthens the uterus and reproductive organs.	15–30 grams
Chrysanthemum	Ju Hua	Bitter, sweet, slightly pungent, and cold. Enters the Lung and Liver meridians. Cools liver fire and tonifies a deficient liver. Useful for the common cold, acute bronchitis, headache, fatigue, red eyes, and prostate issues. See page 155.	5–15 grams
Cinnamon	Rou Gui	Pungent, sweet, and hot. Enters the Heart, Kidney, Liver, and Spleen meridians. Reinforces fire and strengthens yang, dispels cold and stops pain, warms meridians. See page 128.	1–6 grams
Cistanche	Rou Cong Rong	Sweet, salty, and warm. Enters the Large Intestine and Kidney meridians. Often used for constipation and traditionally used as a tonic to reverse symptoms of wasting diseases. Considered an aphrodisiac for men and used to cure impotence; useful for menstrual difficulties, gonorrhea, and problems related to the female reproductive organs.	10–20 grams, up to 30 grams for severe symptoms
Codonopsis	Dang Shen	Sweet and neutral. Enters the Lung and Spleen meridians. Invigorates lung and spleen chi by nourishing the blood and promoting the generation of body fluid.	3–10 grams
Coptis	Huang Lian	Bitter and cold. Enters the Heart, Large Intestine, Liver, and Stomach meridians. Drains fire and relieves toxic heat. Calms insomnia due to heart fire and drains dampness. Useful for all heat conditions, but use caution with long-term consumption or in cases of yin, blood, or spleen chi deficiency. Contraindicated during the last four weeks of pregnancy and in children under age two.	1.5–9 grams
Cordyceps	Dong Chong Xia Cao	Sweet and warm. Enters the Lung and Kidney meridians. Useful for wei qi deficiency, coughs, chronic bronchitis, all respiratory disorders, kidney disorders, nighttime urination, male sexual problems, anemia, irregular heartbeat, high cholesterol, liver disorders, dizziness, weakness, ringing in the ears, and unwanted weight loss. Contraindicated for use with immunosuppressive drugs. (It is endangered, so source it well.) See page 237.	3–6 grams
Coriolus	Yun Zhi	Sweet and slightly cold. Enters the Spleen, Lung, and Liver meridians. Used widely for cancerous tumors. Replenishes essence and chi, and provides general enhancement of energy and immunity.	6–9 grams

Corydalis	Yan Hu Suo	Pungent, bitter, and warm. Enters the Heart, Liver, and Lung meridians. Considered to be nature's NSAID. Used as a mild sedative and tranquilizer, to lower blood pressure, and to relax spasms in the small intestine. Good for mild depression, mild mental disorders, emotional disturbances, and severe nerve damage. Contraindicated in pregnancy.	3–10 grams
Curcumin (Turmeric)	Jiang Huang	Pungent, bitter, and warm. Enters the Spleen, Stomach, and Liver meridians. Breaks up blood stasis, moves chi, unblocks the meridians, and stops pain and inflammation. Contraindicated in pregnancy.	3–9 grams
Cyperus	Xiang Fu	Pungent, slightly warm, and slightly sweet. Enters the Liver, Triple Burner, and Spleen meridians. Soothes the liver, regulates the flow of chi, regulates menses, and relieves pain. See page 159.	6–12 grams
Elecampane	Xuan Fu Hua	Pungent, bitter, and warm. Enters the Lung, Spleen, Stomach, Large Intestine, and Liver meridians. Aids lung chi deficiency, blood stagnation, and liver chi stagnation. Useful for relief of wheezing, nausea, vomiting, diarrhea, hypochondriac pain, abdominal distention, chest pain, and fetal irritability. See page 238.	3–9 grams
Eleuthero (Siberian Ginseng)	Wu Jia Shen	Pungent, slightly bitter, and warm. Enters the Spleen, Kidney, and Heart meridians. Potent adaptogen, can also build blood, tonify chi and calm the shen. An effective antifatigue herb and immune system tonic. See page 130.	9–30 grams
Fenugreek	Hu Lu Ba	Bitter and warm. Enters the Kidney and Liver meridians. Primary herb for kidney yang deficiency with accumulation of cold.	3–10 grams
Ginger	Sheng Jiang	Pungent and warm. Enters the Lung, Spleen, and Stomach meridians. Improves circulation, regulates digestion, and reduces nausea and pain from menses by warming and therefore strengthening the triple burner. Also warms the lungs and reduces coughing. See page 238.	3–9 grams
Ginkgo	Bai Guo	Sweet, bitter, astringent, and neutral. Enters the Lung meridian primarily. Clears dampness and calms asthma, wheezing, and chronic cough (especially wet cough). Can be toxic at higher doses or if used long term.	1.5–9 grams
Ginseng (Notoginseng)	San Qi	Sweet, slightly bitter, and warm. Enters the Liver, Stomach, and Large Intestine meridians. Stops bleeding and transforms blood stasis, reduces swelling, and alleviates pain. Excellent herb for acute physical trauma.	6–9 grams

Ginseng (Radix)	Ren Shen	Sweet, slightly bitter, and slightly warm. Most potent of all the ginsengs in its ability to tonify chi, especially lung and spleen chi. Increases energy.	3–9 grams
Goji Berry	Gou Qi Zi	Sweet and neutral. Enters the Liver, Lung, and Kidney meridians. Tonifies chi and blood, promotes good eyesight, and slows down aging.	5–18 grams
Green Tea	Lu Cha	Sweet, bitter, cooling, and astringent. Enters the Spleen, Stomach, Large Intestine, Kidneys, Heart, and Liver meridians. Supports a calm, stable mind and the immune system. Considered to be protective to the heart.	3–12 grams (served in 3–10 cups/day)
Hawthorn	Shan Zha	Sour, sweet, and slightly warm. Enters the Liver, Spleen, and Stomach meridians. Enhances digestion, relieves food retention, promotes qi circulation, and removes blood stasis. Powerful herb for all heart- and blood-related conditions.	9–12 grams
Horny Goat Weed	Yin Yang Huo	Pungent, sweet, and warm. Enters the Kidney and Liver meridians. Increases energy and stamina, tonifies yang. Used for weak back and knees, joint pain, osteoarthritis, mental and physical fatigue, and memory loss. Use caution in cases of headaches and high blood pressure.	3–9 grams
Jujube Seed	Suan Zao Ren	Sweet, sour, and neutral. Enters the Gallbladder, Heart, Liver, and Spleen meridians. Nourishes the heart and calms the spirit. Supportive in clearing dampness, losing weight, and prolonging life. Major herb used for insomnia.	6–15 grams
Licorice	Gan Cao	Sweet and neutral. Enters all meridians but especially the Lung, Heart, Spleen, and Stomach. A powerful digestive aid and nervous system tonic, can be used as a general vitality-promoting herb. Use caution in cases of high blood pressure.	1.5–9 grams
Lobelia	Ban Bias Lian	Sweet and neutral. Enters the Heart, Lung, and Small Intestine meridians. An excellent herb to clear the lungs, reduce wheezing/asthma symptoms, and curb nicotine cravings.	3–15 grams
Mint (Chinese)	Bo He	Pungent, astringent, and cooling. Enters the Lungs, Spleen, and Stomach meridians. Vents hot and/or damp skin rashes. Wakes up a sluggish digestive system. Supportive in cases of the common cold with heat symptoms.	1.5–6 grams (add to decoction last 5 minutes)
Motherwort	Yi Mu Cao	Pungent, bitter, and slightly cold. Enters the Heart, Liver, Bladder, and Pericardium meridians. Promotes blood circulation, dispels blood stasis, regulates menses, reduces masses, promotes urination, and relieves swelling and edema. Contraindicated in pregnancy.	9–15 grams, maximum dose of 30 grams

Mugwort	Ai Ye	Bitter, pungent, and warm. Enters the Spleen, Liver, and Kidney meridians. Stops bleeding, resolves phlegm, relieves asthma, and eliminates cough. Often used in combination with other herbs to calm the fetus and prevent miscarriage. Please work with a practitioner if pregnant.	3–9 grams
Mume	Wu Mei	Sour, warm, and astringent. Enters the Liver, Large Intestine, Lung, and Spleen meridians. Resolves dampness associated with yeast/Candida; eliminates coughing, thirst, and chronic diarrhea.	3–9 grams
Myrrh	Mo Yao	Bitter and neutral. Enters the Heart, Liver, and Spleen meridians. Invigorates the blood, prevents gum disease, alleviates pain, moves stagnant blood (including tumors) from the uterus. Promotes skin healing. Contraindicated in pregnancy.	3–10 grams
Peony (Red)	Chi Shao	Sour, bitter, and slightly cold. Enters the Liver and Spleen meridians. Removes heat from the blood (as in nosebleeds; blood in stool; sore, red, swollen eyes; swelling and joint pain; abscesses and boils) and invigorates blood to remove blood stasis. Useful with amenorrhea, dysmenorrhea, and irregular vaginal discharge. Contraindicated in pregnancy.	4.5–9 grams
Peony (White)	Bai Shao	Bitter, sour, and cool. Enters the Liver and Spleen meridians. Best used as a tonic for the blood and as a heat-reducing herb for the liver. More astringent than red peony (chi shao). Relieves abdominal pain, muscle spasms, and irregular menses.	5–10 grams
Persica	Tao Ren	Bitter, sweet, and neutral. Enters the Heart, Liver, Large Intestine, and Stomach meridians. Invigorates the blood, removes stagnation, and moistens and unblocks the intestines. Contraindicated in pregnancy.	4.5–9 grams
Pinellia	Ban Xia	Pungent and warm. Enters the Lung, Spleen, and Stomach meridians. Transforms phlegm and coldness, stops vomiting, relieves stuffiness, and dissipates nodules. Resolves swelling and alleviates pain; useful with cough that comes with thick mucus.	5–10 grams; toxic at higher doses
Polygonum (Fo Ti)	He Shou Wu	Bitter, sweet, slightly warm, astringent, blood-building, and tonifying. Enters the Liver and Kidney meridians. Supports the immune and respiratory systems. Useful in immune system imbalances, anemia, high cholesterol, allergies, infertility, and erectile dysfunction. See page 130.	4–8 grams (processed)
Poria	Fu Ling	Sweet, bland, and neutral. Enters the Heart, Spleen, and Lung meridians. Regulates water in the body, drains dampness and edema, and relieves diarrhea and other gastrointestinal and urinary problems. Calms the shen.	10–15 grams

Rehmannia	Shu Di Huang	Sweet, slightly warm, blood-building, moistening, and tonifying. Enters the Liver, Kidney, and Heart meridians. Supports the respiratory system. Strong blood tonifier and builder. Useful with PMS, heart palpitations, anxiety, allergies, and chronic lung imbalances. See page 131.	9–15 grams; up to 30 grams, depending on treatment
Reishi	Ling Zhi	Sweet and neutral. Enters the Heart, Liver, and Lung meridians. Nourishes the heart and calms the spirit. Reverses wei qi deficiency. Useful for migraines, headaches, gout, osteoarthritis, and rheumatism. Contraindicated for use with immunosuppressive drugs. See page 187.	3–15 grams
Rhodiola	Hong Jing Tian	Sweet, bitter, calming, and tonifying. Enters the Lung and Heart meridians. Powerful adaptogen. Useful in recovery from chronic illness, respiratory illness with coughing, restlessness, agitation, and fatigue (both acute and chronic).	3–9 grams
Rose	Mei Gui Hua	Bitter, sweet, sour, and warm. Enters the Heart, Liver, Spleen, and Stomach meridians. Useful with heart chi deficiency and liver chi stagnation. Relieves symptoms of PMS, anxiety, depressive symptoms, headache, nausea, and pain.	1.5–6 grams
Royal Jelly	Feng Wang	Bitter and neutral. Enters the Kidney and Triple Burner meridians. Tonifies kidney yin and yang and reverses blood deficiency. Excellent for exhaustion, sore throat, weak muscles, chronic and recurrent colds and flu, as well as digestive disturbances.	6–10 grams
Rhubarb	Da Huang	Bitter and cold. Enters the Heart, Large Intestine, Liver, and Stomach meridians. Drains and purges heat from the body. As a strong laxative, evacuates the bowels, improves digestion; useful in cases of jaundice, endometriosis, burns, and skin ulcers (when used topically). Contraindicated in pregnancy.	3–12 grams
Salvia	Dan Shen	Bitter and slightly cold. Enters the Heart, Pericardium, and Liver meridians. Invigorates and moves the blood and clears stagnation. Useful in cases of heart palpitations and insomnia due to heat in the heart and heart blood deficiency.	3–15 grams
Schisandra	Wu Wei Zi	Sour and warm (though known as containing all five flavors). Enters the Heart, Kidney, and Lung meridians. Powerful adaptogen. Supports vitality, tonifies the lungs, dries dampness, and clears skin.	1.5–6 grams

Seeds of Job's Tears	Yi Yi Ren	Sweet and slightly cold. Enters the Spleen, Lung, and Kidney meridians. Most often used in cases of dampness, especially dampness expressing through the skin such as with acne or cases of diarrhea, arthritis, and muscle spasms. Acts as a mild diuretic and can be used to support spleen chi deficiency.	9–30 grams
Siler	Fang Feng	Pungent, sweet, and slightly warm. Enters and strengthens the Bladder, Liver, and Spleen meridians. Useful for the common cold, headaches, body aches, and all windy conditions including itchy skin.	3–9 grams
Skullcap (Baikal)	Huang Qin	Bitter and cold. Enters the Gallbladder, Large Intestine, Lung, and Stomach meridians. Clears heat and dries dampness. Used for insomnia, anxiety, and yellow phlegm in the lungs.	6–15 grams
Solomon's Seal	Yu Zhu	Sweet and slightly cold. Enters the Lung and Stomach meridians. Tonifies yin, supports all lung disorders, and is used as an astringent and anti-inflammatory herb.	6–15 grams
Tangerine Peel	Chen Pi	Pungent, bitter, and warm. Enters the Lung, Spleen, and Stomach meridians. Regulates chi and strengthens the spleen and stomach. Removes dampness, reduces phlegm, and stops cough.	3–9 grams
Tiger Balm	Wan Jin You	Cooling topical liniment. Relieves minor muscle or joint pain. Also used as a chest rub to soothe congestion and relieve cough caused by the flu or common cold.	Rub a pea-size amount into the affected area, repeat as needed.
Tribulus	Bai Ji Li	Pungent, bitter, and warm. Enters the Liver and Lung meridians. An important herb for resolving headaches, dizziness, vertigo, blurry vision, high blood pressure, PMS, allergic skin conditions, and other windy and hot conditions.	6–10 grams
Turmeric		*See* Curcumin.	
Wormwood	Qing Hao	Bitter and cold. Enters the Kidney, Liver and Gallbladder meridians. Clears heat and transforms dampness. Relieves fever, headaches, vomiting, bloating, cramping, fatigue, and anemia. Can also be used as an appetite stimulant. When used fresh, combats malaria.	3–10 grams

APPENDIX C. OTHER HERBAL MEDICINES

Other Herbal Medicines		
Herb	**Action**	**Daily Dosage**
Alfalfa	Bitter, sweet, and cooling. Considered highly nutritive, blood-building, and tonifying. Useful for recovery from illness or as a daily tonic to support energy, balance, and immunity	15–30 grams
Aloe Vera	Useful for abdominal pain, especially with heat and inflammation (burning pain, ulcers, GERD, etc.); pelvic congestion; kidney inflammation; constipation; and weight loss. Used topically for acne and sunburn relief	2–6 tablespoons
Arnica	Useful for pain, bruising, and inflammation in the muscles and joints; applied topically	Apply topically as needed for pain and inflammation
Bacopa	Adaptogenic; improves memory and concentration; useful for anxiety and ADHD; reduces stress response	5–10 grams
Barberry (Berberine)	Useful for bacterial and fungal infections in the digestive and urinary tracts; helps lower cholesterol; supports reversal of fatty liver (Berberine, the active constituent, is easy to find in capsules.)	Capsules: 1,500 mg taken in three doses of 500 mg each
Bee Pollen	Increases energy and stamina; helps relieve respiratory problems; soothes digestion; balances hormones	5–20 grams | Eat pollen grains or granules plain or mixed with food
Blackberry	Soothes sore throats, wounds, and skin irritation; dries up diarrhea; regulates menstrual flow	3–10 grams
Black Cohosh	Useful for symptoms of menopause, PMS, headaches, hot flashes, mood changes, sleep problems, heart palpitations, and joint inflammation; known as a powerful phytoestrogen and often prescribed in cases of low estrogen	3–6 grams
Burdock Root	Supports liver detoxification; useful for a variety of skin problems; aids in digestion	6–9 grams
Calendula	Soothes irritated gut lining; promotes metabolism of proteins and collagen; useful for itchy skin (topically)	6–9 grams, hot infusion For topical use, follow directions on product
Cardamom	Used as an appetite stimulant; useful for abdominal discomfort and pain, nausea, diarrhea, and other digestive troubles (Grind and brew with coffee to offset negative effects of caffeine.)	3–10 grams
Catnip	Gentle, calming herb for occasional sleeplessness, fevers, cough, cold, and stomachaches; gentle enough for children and infants	2–4 grams, hot infusion

Chamomile	Nourishes the heart; calms the spirit; supports liver detoxification; useful for colds; clears up skin irritations such as eczema, acne, and hives; soothes the stomach	9–15 grams, hot infusion
Chaste Tree Berry	Increases the production of progesterone, which helps regulate the menstrual cycle, combating PMS symptoms	3–6 grams
Chia Seeds	Supports the digestive system in collecting debris inside the intestines and moving stool; assists in weight loss and reducing glucose levels, which can benefit diabetics and those with high blood pressure	5–20 grams
Chickweed	Salty herb useful for relieving constipation, asthma, inflammatory skin conditions, and moving stubborn weight	1–5 grams, hot infusion
Chicory Root	Supports the liver; acts as a detoxifier; cools heat in the body, including inflammatory conditions; useful for high blood pressure, high cholesterol, kidney disease, indigestion, anemia, abdominal disease, acid reflux, angina, jaundice, liver disease, asthma, and acne	3–5 grams
Coconut Oil	Naturally antifungal; excellent source of medium-chain triglycerides (MCTs); useful for colds, flu, herpes outbreaks, respiratory infections, and UTIs; boosts energy, endurance, and the immune system	1–3 tablespoons in divided doses
Comfrey	Heals external wounds, sprains, strains, and broken bones (not approved by the Food and Drug Administration for internal use)	For topical use, follow instructions on product
Cramp Bark	Soothes muscle cramps (especially PMS); reduces swollen glands and fluid retention; useful for eye disorders	2–4 grams
Damiana	Stimulates sexual fluids; useful for sexual health, managing stress, supporting the digestive system, and maintaining energy levels	2–4 grams
Dandelion Root	Supports the liver in detoxification; useful for problems relating to the liver, gallbladder, kidneys, skin, and joints; relieves constipation, indigestion, and heartburn; acts as a diuretic	3–5 grams
Echinacea	Supports healthy immune system; useful for infections like colds and flu, bites, stings, and toothaches	5–9 grams
Elderberry/ Elderflower	Immune system tonic herb; boosts wei qi; supports healing of respiratory illnesses, colds, flu, and other conditions that bring fever	10–15 grams | Elderberry best made in decoction; elderflower best made in hot infusion
Eucalyptus	Immune system tonic herb; boosts wei qi; supports healing of respiratory tract infections, bronchitis, sinusitis, colds, flu, and wheezing from asthma; clears fevers; can be used as an expectorant	4–6 grams, hot infusion Can inhale essential oil several times a day to open sinuses and congested lungs

Evening Primrose Oil	Soothes skin disorders such as eczema, psoriasis, and acne; reduces symptoms of PMS, endometriosis, and menopause	4–12 capsules, at a dose of 500 mg per capsule
Feverfew	Useful for migraines, headaches, fever, common cold, arthritis, and caffeine withdrawal	3–9 grams, hot infusion
Fumitory	Soothes intestinal spasms; quiets IBS; useful for skin conditions, eye irritation, fluid retention, and constipation; cleanses the liver and kidneys	2–4 grams, hot infusion
Garlic	Stimulates digestive and immune systems; removes stagnation and blockages of chi; detoxifies; stops diarrhea; useful for bacterial infection in the digestive system	2–5 grams fresh raw garlic; 0.5–1.5 grams dried garlic powder
Grapefruit Seed Extract	Useful for bacterial or fungal infection in the digestive system and high cholesterol; known to restore venous sufficiency	50–300 mg in capsules
Hibiscus	Useful for lung chi deficiency leading to coughing, hypertension, hypercholesterolemia, heart disease, arteriosclerosis, diabetes, burning sensations during urination, menstrual disorders, and fever	3–6 grams, hot infusion
Hops	Useful for anxiety, insomnia and other sleep disorders, restlessness, tension, excitability, ADHD, nervousness, and irritability	1–3 grams
Kava Kava	Useful for anxiety, nervousness, heart palpitations, chest pains, headaches, dizziness, and stomach upset; should be used with caution in cases of preexisting liver conditions	Follow instructions on product, can also put herb into bath water for relaxation
Lavender	Nourishes the heart; calms the mind and spirit; useful for anxiety; can be used topically as an essential oil to reduce acne and other skin irritations	1–3 grams, hot infusion 1–4 drops essential oil in 8 oz. water, sipped throughout the day
Lemon Balm	Useful for anxiety, heart palpitations, insomnia, cold sores, high cholesterol, genital herpes, indigestion, and heartburn	3–6 grams | Consult with practitioner before use if you have thyroid imbalances
Maca	Enhances energy and stamina; supports reproductive organs; useful for anemia, chronic fatigue syndrome, and memory loss	2–6 grams | Consult with practitioner if you are also on birth control, pregnant, or breast-feeding
Marshmallow Root	Useful for digestive issues that are hot and/or dry in nature, such as constipation, acid reflux, and GERD; useful for cough and bronchitis as it is highly mucilaginous	6–9 grams
Milk Thistle	Supports liver detoxification; lowers cholesterol; useful for natural treatment of liver problems, including cirrhosis, jaundice, hepatitis, and gallbladder disorders.	250- to 500-mg capsules, 1–2 times/day

Mullein	Used internally for skin and lung diseases, but added to a smoking blend in some cultures; useful for all inflammatory diseases, especially in the respiratory and urinary tracts	3–4 grams
Neem	Useful for treatment of eczema, dermatitis, acne, rosacea, and herpes	Use topically as needed
Nettles	Salty, adaptogenic, and blood-building herb; useful for painful muscles and joints, eczema, arthritis, gout, anemia, and UTIs	6–9 grams, hot infusion left overnight
Oatstraw (Wild Oat)	Adaptogenic. Reduces cortisol and soothes stress response. Useful for high blood pressure; high cholesterol; diabetes; and digestion problems such as IBS, diarrhea, and constipation	3–6 grams
Oregano Oil	Useful for bacterial or fungal infection in the digestive system; calms allergies and inflammation	2 capsules, 2–4 times/day Do not use essential oil internally. Use as directed by health care practitioner
Passionflower	Useful for anxiety; an herbal sleep aid; helps lower blood pressure	1–5 grams, hot infusion
Peppermint	Useful for inflammation and pain, and to reduce heat and inflammation in the digestive system	5 drops essential oil in 10 ml water, 3 times/day
Pine Bark	Reduces symptoms of PMS; boosts antioxidant levels; combats erectile dysfunction; reduces inflammation; fights off the common cold; balances blood sugar; active compound in Pycnogenol	100- to 300-mg in capsules
Plaintain	Supports healing of a weakened intestinal lining (from leaky gut, ulcers, gastritis) and urinary tract	4–8 grams, hot infusion
Raspberry Leaf	Soothes the uterus and thyroid; supports the body in building a healthy uterine lining; useful for PMS, irregular cycles, diarrhea, and colds	4–8 grams
Red Clover	Reduces chi stagnation, cysts, nodules, and tumors; useful for symptoms of menopause such as hot flashes and breast pain or tenderness, PMS, skin sores, burns, and more chronic skin diseases	4–8 grams
Rose Hips	Strengthens the immune system (loaded with vitamin C); helps maintain healthy digestion and circulation; eases stress, headaches, and dizziness; heals tissues; has been used as an antidepressant	3–6 grams
Saw Palmetto	Used to enhance energy by increasing circulating testosterone; decreases symptoms of an enlarged prostate (benign prostatic hypertrophy)	1–2 grams

Senna	Best known as a colon-cleansing agent and assists with detoxing; useful for a variety of conditions like constipation, IBS, bloating, and hemorrhoids; can cause cramping	1–3 grams, hot infusion 30 minutes before bed
Slippery Elm	Highly mucilaginous; soothes coughs, sore throat, colic, diarrhea, constipation, hemorrhoids, IBS, bladder and urinary tract infections, syphilis, and herpes; useful for expelling tapeworms	1.5–3 grams
Spearmint	Useful for diarrhea and painful menstruation; promotes perspiration and dissipates body heat; helps in the treatment of ADD/ADHD with its calming effects on the nervous system	2–5 grams
St. John's Wort (internal and external)	Useful for anxiety and depression, having had better research results than most prescription antidepressants (without all the side effects); also used topically for nerve-pain relief	Standard dosage for adults with depression and other mood disorders = 300 mg 3 times/day in capsules.
Tulsi (Holy Basil)	Adaptogenic; reduces cortisol levels; useful for managing symptoms of stress, anxiety, and depression	6–9 grams
Valerian	Useful for insomnia and anxiety; known to increase the brain level of GABA, a natural muscle relaxer	2–3 grams, hot infusion 30 minutes before bed
Vervain	Antibacterial and analgesic; useful for headaches and gallstones; tonifies the liver and heart	2–4 grams
Willow Bark	Famously known as "nature's aspirin"; reduces pain and inflammation	2–5 grams

APPENDIX D. NUTRITIONAL SUPPLEMENTS

Nutritional Supplements			
Name	**Actions**	**Dosage**	**Precautions**
5-Hydroxy-tryptophan (5-HTP)	Natural antidepressant; increases serotonin; helps with smoking cessation, mental health disorders, athletic performance; emotional symptoms in women with PMS and PMDD; supports healthy sleep patterns	200–300 mg/day given in 3–4 divided doses to prevent possible nausea	If you are on a selective serotonin uptake inhibitor (SSRI) or have high blood pressure or diabetes, talk to your doctor first
B-Complex	Contains all the important building blocks of the body; helps maintain good health, energy, and stable mood	1–2 capsules/day	Caution is advised if you have diabetes, alcohol dependence, liver disease, or phenylketonuria
Bovine Adrenal Glandulars	Used for low adrenal function, fatigue, stress, lowered resistance to illness, severe allergies, asthma, certain skin conditions	450–1,000 mg/day (typical dosage)	Contraindicated for pregnant and breast-feeding women
Butyrate	Short-chain fatty acid used in healing of leaky gut syndrome, autoimmune disease, IBS, and colon cancer	200–400 mg, 3 times/day	
Caffeine	Stimulant, promotes alertness and feeling more awake/ less tired; treats or manages drowsiness, headaches, and migraines	5–400 mg/day	Not recommended for children under 12 years, older or pregnant/nursing women, those with heart conditions or type 2 diabetes
Calcium	Prevents weak teeth and bones and issues with muscle contractions; supports metabolism of magnesium and healthy heart tissue	1,000–1,500 mg/day	Tell your doctor or pharmacist if you have any allergies; kidney, heart, lung, or pancreas disease; kidney stones; or stomach acid issues
Caprylic Acid	Antibacterial, antiviral, and antifungal properties; supports relief from yeast infections, Candida, thrush, and fungal infections	1,000–2,000 mg, 2–3 times/day, 30 minutes before every meal	Not recommended for women who are pregnant or breast-feeding
Chromium	Effective at improving the body's response to insulin or lowering blood sugar in those with diabetes; reduces cravings; supports hypoglycemic response	1,000 mcg/day in divided doses	Psychiatric or behavioral disorders possible from high doses

Coconut Oil	Increases good HDL cholesterol and may help turn bad LDL cholesterol into a less harmful form; contains caprylic acid to fight fungal, yeast, candida infections internal and externally	2–6 table-spoons/day	
Collagen	Improves skin health, relieves joint pain, prevents bone loss, boosts muscle mass, promotes heart health and weight loss, soothes irritated intestinal lining	Up to 30 grams/day	
Coenzyme Q_{10} (CoQ_{10})	Antioxidant that protects cells from damage and helps metabolism, slows down effects of aging, increases energy and stamina, supports the heart, maintains healthy blood sugar levels	30–100 mg/day	May not be safe for women who are pregnant or breast-feeding
Complete Amino Acid Blend	Building blocks of muscle, bone, neurotransmitters, and hormones; assists with pain management	12 mg/kilo of bodyweight	Some blends sourced from whey (if allergic to dairy products, find different source)
Digestive Enzymes	Supports the breakdown and digestion of food and absorption of nutrients	1 capsule/meal, or as directed by a practitioner	
Dihydroepi-androsterone (DHEA)	Increases energy; helps with depression; precursor for testosterone and progester-one; useful for adrenal insufficiency, mood disorders, and erectile dysfunction	25–200 mg/day	Appropriate testing advised before taking hormones
D-Phenylala-nine (DPA)	Useful for vitiligo (skin disease), depression, ADHD, grief, weight loss, and alcohol withdrawal symptoms	150–5,000 mg/day	Contraindicated with levodopa; exercise caution if pregnant or breast-feeding
Eicosapen-taenoic acid (EPA)/doco-sahexaenoic acid (DHA) (Fish Oil)	Essential nutrients for preventing and managing heart disease	2,400–8,400 mg/day total (720–2,200 mg of EPA and 480–1,500 mg of DHA daily)	Should be high-quality fish oil, made from small fish rather than large fish, and tested for mercury levels
Folic Acid	Helps produce and maintain new cells; useful for preventing changes to DNA that may lead to cancer; a must after getting off birth control	400–600 mcg/day	
Gamma-aminobutyric acid (GABA)	Works to regulate muscle tone, works as a calming agent in the brain	300–1,500 mg/day in divided doses	Not recommended for women who are pregnant or breast-feeding; can cause sleepiness in high doses

Gamma linoleic acid (GLA)	Plant-derived omega-6 fatty acid; vital for healing chronic inflammation, skin conditions, heart disease, and PMS; borage oil and evening primrose oil are excellent sources	500–1,000 mg taken 2 times/ day (evening primrose oil) 350–500 mg taken 3 times/day (borage oil)	Ideally taken with food for maximum absorption
Glucosamine Sulfate	Maintains healthy joint function, promotes cartilage strength, lubricates joints by supporting building of cartilage and mucopolysaccharide (thick fluid that surrounds joints)	1,000–1,500 mg/day in divided doses	Exercise caution if pregnant or breast-feeding
Glutathione	Amino acid considered the "master antioxidant" because it can regenerate itself in the liver; powerful aid against free radicals; helps to prevent cancer, heart disease, dementia, and other chronic imbalances; used intravenously in post-chemo treatment and recovery from alcoholism	200–500 mg/ day in divided doses	Consult health care practitioner before use if pregnant
Inositol	Supports egg quality for fertility; useful for PCOS, menopause, diabetes, and other metabolic imbalances	1,000–1,200 mg/day in divided doses	Monitor blood sugar carefully in cases of diabetes
Iron	Helps metabolize proteins; plays a role in the production of hemoglobin and red blood cells	20–60 mg/ day in divided doses (with food if iron deficiency is present)	Note: start with a liquid, plant-based iron supplement; if no noticeable changes, switch to capsule. Always take with vitamin C for absorption
L-Carnitine	Helps the body produce energy; important for heart and brain function, muscle movement, and mood stabilization	500–1,000 mg/day in divided doses	Caution advised for those with hypothyroidism, seizures, peripheral vascular disease (PVD), hypertension, diabetes, and for pregnant/breast-feeding women
L-Glutamine	Promotes healthy gastrointestinal function, aids in tissue growth, supports the growth of muscle mass and healthy sugar metabolism	2,000–5,000 mg/day in divided doses	Not for use by women who are pregnant or breast-feeding
L-Theanine	Supports stress resistance, promotes relaxation and focus, helps maintain a sense of well-being	100–200 mg/day, can repeat dosage	Not for use by women who are pregnant or breast-feeding

Lysine (and Lysine Salve)	Supports the immune system and healthy tissue in gums, lips, and mucus membranes; antiviral used to treat herpes outbreaks and cold sores	500–4,500 mg/day	Topical creams can be used for cold sores and herpes and shingle outbreaks to manage pain and reduce duration of outbreak
Magnesium	Helps keep blood pressure normal, bones strong, and heart rhythm steady; "nature's muscle relaxer," maintains emotional wellness during PMS and PMDD	300–800 mg/day	*Likely safe* for women who are pregnant or breast-feeding when taken in doses less than 350 mg daily
Melatonin	Assists with insomnia	3–10 mg/day	
Methylsulfonylmethane (MSM)	Helps support joint health, promotes flexibility, preserves collagen, supports the immune system	2,000–6,000 mg/day in divided doses	
Multimineral	Potentially beneficial in preventing/treating chronic medical conditions and inadequacies in micronutrient intake	Brands vary, follow instructions on bottle	
N-Acetylcysteine (NAC)	Promotes normal mucus levels in healthy sinus and respiratory systems, provides immune system support, maintains healthy liver function	1,200–1,800 mg/day in divided doses, with food	May be toxic in doses higher than 7,000 mg
Potassium	Helps maintain consistent blood pressure the balance of muscle relaxation and contraction, useful for morning sickness	3,000–5,000 mg/day in divided doses	
Prebiotics	Acts as a fertilizer for the good bacteria in the gut, enhances and strengthens the immune system, supports calcium and magnesium absorption	25–40 grams/day	
Prenatal Vitamins	Helps cover any nutritional gaps in mother's diet; ensures sufficient intake of vitamins and minerals; reduces risks for pregnancy complications	Brands vary, follow instructions on bottle	
Probiotics	Used for immune system deficiencies, digestive problems, eczema, vaginal yeast infections, lactose intolerance, and UTIs	4 billion cfu minimum a day	The more diverse the species, the better
Progesterone Cream	Balances hormones and mood, protects the uterine lining	50–200 mg/day	Appropriate testing advised before taking hormones
Quercetin	Supports normal sinus and respiratory function, lowers inflammation and histamine response in allergies	800–1,200 mg/day in divided doses	Not for use by women who are pregnant or breast-feeding

Selenium	Increases immunity, assists in antioxidant activity that defends against free radical damage and inflammation, supports thyroid function, is a potent antioxidant	50–100 mcg/day	Can be toxic in larger doses
Tryptophan	Natural antidepressant; increases serotonin; useful for smoking cessation, mental health disorders, athletic performance, emotional symptoms in women with PMS and PMDD; supports healthy sleep patterns	250–500 mg/day in divided doses	If you are already on an SSRI or have high blood pressure or diabetes, talk to your doctor first
Tyrosine	Supports healthy adrenal glands, promotes healthy thyroid functioning, supports a healthy immune system, useful when withdrawing from caffeine	200–800 mg/day in divided doses	Use with caution if migraine headaches, anxiety, hyperthyroidism, or Graves' disease is present
Vitamin A	Supports healthy vision and immune system function, maintains healthy skin and mucus membranes	4,000–10,000 IU/day	Can be toxic in high doses (fat-soluble)
Vitamin B$_6$	Supports healthier skin, detoxifies the liver, enhances the health of blood vessels, improves cognitive function, helps with protein breakdown and metabolism	1.5–2.5 mg/day	High doses (100 mg) may be unsafe and cause problems with the brain and nervous system in long-term
Vitamin B$_{12}$	Promotes healthy nerve and blood cells, provides energy, helps make DNA, prevents certain types of anemia	2–3 mcg/day	Consider a blood test for B$_{12}$
Vitamin C	Heals wounds; supports healthy formation of scar tissue; assists in the growth of healthy skin, tendons, and ligaments; increases immune system function	400–1,000 mg/day in divided doses, with food	Can cause loose stools in high doses, lower dosage if this happens
Vitamin D	Builds and maintains healthy bones, stabilizes mood, supports healthy colon, aids calcium absorption	600–2,000 IU/day, take as recommended by practitioner	Blood test to check optimal levels
Vitamin E	Antioxidant that prevents damage to cells and their DNA by neutralizing harmful free radicals; promotes healthy blood vessels	60–75 IU/day	Check with health care provider before use if pregnant
Zinc	Supports the immune system, stabilizes mood	10–30 mg/day, with food	Simple liquid zinc test to test for optimal levels; use with caution if kidney function is impaired

APPENDIX E: YIN AND YANG CLEANSING
The Four Phases
— ◆ —

I'm excited to share with you how eating healthy can be easy *and* delicious and come with the added benefits of cleaning you up and clearing you out. Cleansing is like pushing the reset button on your body, mind, and spirit. While I am not interested in deprivation-style cleansing, I do think there are times we could all use a break from our usual eating habits. You may want to cleanse for only a few days or for an entire month. My goal is to help you feel empowered and excited to try something new and *not* to create an opportunity for shame to creep in.

Before you begin cleansing, decide what length of time feels right for you and works with the current demands of your energy. Above all else, listen to your body. Spring and autumn are my favorite times to cleanse because the weather is typically less demanding on the body and the energy of nature is either winding up (spring) or winding down (autumn), and we can mimic this energetically.

Consider cleansing only after you have mastered the practices of living according to the seasons and your constitution, as presented in this book. If after following the seasonal guidelines in each chapter, which naturally support your detoxification pathways, you are still experiencing unpleasant symptoms, consider the following four phases: eliminate, replace, reduce, and target.

Phase 1: Eliminate

Here you temporarily say good-bye to the foods that notoriously hijack your system whether by causing inflammation, forming mucus, knocking your blood sugar out of balance, requiring more energy to process than the energy that is returned, and eating foods that are questionably supportive to your overall health goal. You could easily spend a week just getting through this part. This phase will give your body access to food that comes directly from the earth, hasn't been treated or modified in any way, and requires little cooking or processing to break down. Make a list of foods to eliminate and stick to it for the whole month. A week should be enough time to target these foods and remove them from your kitchen for the time being. Here is a suggested list of foods to eliminate:

Grains (especially corn and wheat)
Legumes (especially soy)
Dairy
Prepackaged salad dressings (often toxic vegetable oils, even the organic ones)
Food coloring
Artificial flavoring (or flavoring of any kind)
Preservatives
Nightshades (such as tomatoes, eggplant, potatoes, peppers)
Tap water
High-fat foods
Fried foods
Nonorganic fruits and vegetables (often sprayed with pesticides)
Roasted nuts and seeds or nut butters
Refined sugar
Alcohol
Caffeine

Phase 2: Replace

Here you can bring in the most nutrient-dense foods on the planet to make sure you are getting access to all the good stuff in your meals. While you are busy thinking of all the foods and beverages you love that you won't be able to have during this phase, spend some time looking at the following list of everything you can add in to nourish yourself:

Bone stock
Vegetable broth
Cultured dairy (if you have no reactions to it, try kefir, especially goat)
Fermented vegetables (and their juice)
Coconut oil and coconut kefir (if you can't do cow or goat dairy)
Avocados

Egg yolks (omit if you're concerned about food allergies/intolerances)

Ghee/butter (omit if you're concerned about food allergies/intolerances)

Lemons/limes in anything

All organic vegetables (except for nightshades such as tomatoes, eggplant, potatoes, peppers)

Dandelion greens

Grass-fed lean beef

Bison

Chicken

Wild-caught salmon

Steamed fruit (low-sugar fruits like apples, pears, berries)

Raw local honey

Garlic

Turmeric

After you have targeted all the foods to remove, spend about a week integrating these nutrient-dense foods into your daily meals. You may find that going through only the first two phases of cleansing can be enough to reset your system and support you in finding balance. If this doesn't do the trick and you would like more targeted cleansing, consider moving on to phase 3.

Phase 3: Reduce

While I am not interested in depriving you of nutrition as a way to cleanse, I do want to talk about quantity. I believe that most of us overeat. Not at just one meal a day, but at two out of three. Many of us are liable to skip breakfast, then have a decent lunch, and make a big deal about dinner, only to go to bed a couple of hours later without burning any of those calories. We are usually better off eating smaller meals more often, as this stabilizes the blood sugar longer. Since our days are chock-full of activities, and our presence is required for all of them, we do need to eat substantial meals. That being said, it's important that we match our food intake with our lifestyles.

For this phase, make up your plate with exactly as much food as you are used to, and then take a third or half of it off and tuck it away for later.

If you are interested in experiencing a total liver and kidney flush, you can do what's called intermittent fasting. This is where you select one day of the week when you don't consume any food—only water or lemon water (and about a gallon of it). This enables your body to spend all its energy on cleansing rather than on breaking down food. In fact, modern research has concluded that in order for us to be the healthiest versions of ourselves, every week of our lives should include one day of intermittent fasting or, at the very least, one day per week when we consume less than 500 calories.

If we watch animals in the wild (how different *are* we?), they will fast when they are not feeling well. What a lesson for us humans! Another way to practice intermittent fasting without completely cutting out food for a day is to eat all your meals within a six-hour period and fast for the remaining eighteen hours. This is also an excellent way to change how your body uses food as fuel and to give your digestive system a mini-vacation.

A word of caution: if you tend toward hypoglycemia, intermittent fasting might not be of service to your system. Lightheadedness, dizziness, difficulty concentrating, fatigue, and irritability are some signs of hypoglycemia. If any of these symptoms describe you, eating smaller and more frequent meals is more likely to help stabilize your blood sugar and prevent you from having energy crashes.

Phase 4: Target

The last phase is to target the specific organs and patterns that are presenting the most challenges. If you are feeling a resolution of symptoms and increase in energy after phases 1 through 3, you may not need to target specific organs in phase 4. Phase 4 should not last longer than a week.

Answering the following questions will guide you toward a Yin Cleanse or a Yang Cleanse:

YIN CLEANSE QUESTIONS

Is it cold to cool outside?

Are you feeling cold most of the time?

Do you have cold hands and feet?

Are you tired? Or tired and wired?

Are you feeling easily overwhelmed?

Is your tongue swollen and pale? Or with several deep cracks?

Are you experiencing anxiety, irritability, or mood swings?

Are you easily startled?

Do you feel sluggish in energy and/or digestion?

Do you feel weak, especially in your lower back and/or knees?

Is your digestion off? Do you have loose stools?

If you answered yes to these questions, consider doing a Yin Cleanse to reset your system and get your energy back. In addition to performing phases 1 through 3, try the following:

Wake up with one cup of Warm Ginger Lemon Tea with Mint (page 156).

Drink three cups of Nourishing Bone Stock (page 122), Medicinal Vegetable Broth (page 120), or Immunity Stock (page 232) throughout the day.

Take a Nourishing Bath (page 107) each night for thirty minutes.

Dry brush your skin each day either before a shower or after a bath.

Try to get eight to ten hours of sleep each night.

Add in one Nourishing Practice for Winter (page 133) each day, even if it's not wintertime.

Drink rose hip tea each day (it's slightly sour but loaded with Vitamin C).

Simplify your days; reduce activity and your work hours if possible.

YANG CLEANSE QUESTIONS

Is it warm to hot outside?

Are you feeling hot most of the time?

Do you feel wired?

Does your body feel strong and capable?

Are your hands and feet hot and/or sweaty?

Has your digestion been good? Or are you a little constipated?

Is your tongue pink or red with a coating?

Are you experiencing restlessness? Insomnia?

Do you feel like you have too much energy and find it hard to relax?

Do you find yourself drawn to or addicted to substances?

If you answered yes to these questions, consider doing a Yang Cleanse to reset your system and give your nervous system a break. In addition to performing phases 1 through 3, try the following:

Wake up with one cup of Warm Ginger Lemon Tea with Mint (page 156).

Drink one cup of Detox Smoothie (page 154) three to five times per day, depending on your metabolism. (If your body is sensitive to eating lightly and you become light-headed, consider adding raw nut butters like almond or cashew and/or protein powder to the smoothie.)

Drink one cup of Detox Tea (page 155) twice a day.

Take a Detox Bath (page 85) each evening.

Dry brush your skin after your bath every night.

Take 1,000 milligrams of vitamin C with each meal.

Take milk thistle every night before bed.

Incorporate one of these items into every meal during your cleanse: grapefruit, pickles, fermented veggies with live cultures, raw, unfiltered organic apple cider vinegar, cultured products such as kefir and yogurt (cow, goat, or coconut).

NOTE: If you are feeling cold, be sure to make the smoothie with room-temperature ingredients, and consider alternating between the Detox Smoothie (page 154) and Nourishing Bone Stock (page 122) during your cleanse.

NOTES

— ◆ —

CHAPTER 3: PANTRY GUIDELINES

1. U.S. Environmental Protection Agency, *Hydraulic Fracturing for Oil and Gas: Impacts from the Hydraulic Fracturing Water Cycle on Drinking Water Resources in the United States*, final report (Washington, DC: U.S. EPA, EPA/600/R-16/236F, 2016).

2. Irwin H. Putzkoff, Cho Byung-Ho, and Oh Jin-Hwan, "Animal Stress Results in Meat Causing Disease," Internet Archive Wayback Machine, accessed February 23, 2019, https://web.archive.org/web/20161027224500/http://www.scn.org/~bk269/fear.html.

3. "3 Surprising Myths about Cholesterol," Cleveland HeartLab, February 19, 2015, http://www.clevelandheartlab.com/blog/horizons-3-surprising-myths-about-cholesterol.

4. Doug Gurian-Sherman, Michael Hansen, Marcia Ishii-Eiteman, David Schubert, and Ray Seidler, "Are GMOs Safe? No Consensus in the Science, Scientists Say in Peer-Reviewed Statement," Center for Food Safety, February 19, 2015, https://www.centerforfoodsafety.org/press-releases/3766/are-gmos-safe-no-consensus-in-the-science-scientists-say-in-peer-reviewed-statement.

CHAPTER 4: CHINESE HERBAL MEDICINE AND NUTRITIONAL PRINCIPLES

1. Roddy Scheer and Doug Moss, "Dirt Poor: Have Fruits and Vegetables Become Less Nutritious?" *Scientific American*, July 10, 2015, https://www.scientificamerican.com/article/soil-depletion-and-nutrition-loss.

CHAPTER 5: SEASONAL PRACTICES

1. Heidi Godman, "Are Sprouted Grains More Nutritious than Regular Whole Grains?" Harvard Health Publishing, November 2017, https://www.health.harvard.edu/blog/sprouted-grains-nutritious-regular-whole-grains-2017110612692.

2. "Science of the Heart: Vol 1 (1993–2001) Exploring the Role of the Heart in Human Performance," HeartMath Institute, https://www.heartmath.org/resources/downloads/science-of-the-heart.

3. "What Your Gut Bacteria Says about You," WebMD, May 2018, https://www.webmd.com/digestive-disorders/what-your-gut-bacteria-say-your-health#1.

4. Maggie Fox, "Amazon Tsimane People Have the Healthiest Hearts," NBC News, March 17, 2017, https://www.nbcnews.com/health/heart-health/amazon-tsimane-people-have-healthiest-hearts-n734976.

5. Michaeleen Doucleff, "Is the Secret to a Healthier Microbiome Hidden in the Hadza Diet"?

Goats and Soda, August 24, 2017, https://www.npr.org/sections/goatsandsoda/2017/08/24/545631521/is-the-secret-to-a-healthier-microbiome-hidden-in-the-hadza-diet.

6. Christina M. Puchalski, MD, MS, 2001, "The Role of Spirituality in Health Care," https://www.ncbi.nlm.nih.gov/pmc/articles/PMC1305900/.

CHAPTER 6: SUPPORTING EMOTIONAL IMBALANCES

1. National Alliance on Mental Illness, "Mental Health by the Numbers," NAMI, accessed February 23, 2019, https://www.nami.org/learn-more/mental-health-by-the-numbers.

2. Leslie Gutman, Heather Joshi, Michael Parsonage, and Ingrid Schoon, *Children of the New Century: Mental Health Findings from the Millennium Cohort Study* (London: Centre for Mental Health, 2015).

3. Razali Salleh Mohd, "Life Event, Stress and Illness," *The Malaysian Journal of Medical Sciences*, PubMed Central, October 2008, https://www.ncbi.nlm.nih.gov/pmc/articles/PMC3341916/.

4. "Addiction Passed Down through Generations," CRC Health, accessed February 23, 2019, https://www.crchealth.com/drug-addiction-rehab/hereditary-addiction.

CHAPTER 7: SUPPORTING DIGESTIVE IMBALANCES

1. Roni Caryn Rabin, "Ask Well: Taking Heartburn Drugs Long-Term," *The New York Times*, October 15, 2015, https://well.blogs.nytimes.com/2015/10/15/ask-well-taking-heartburn-drugs-long-term.

2. "Irritable Bowel Syndrome," *U.S. News & World Report*, developed with Johns Hopkins Medicine, July 28, 2009, https://health.usnews.com/health-conditions/digestive-disorders/irritable-bowel-syndrome/overview.

CHAPTER 8: SUPPORTING IMMUNE SYSTEM IMBALANCES

1. Infectious Diseases Society of America, "Most Ear Infections Host Both Bacteria and Viruses, Study Shows," *ScienceDaily*, November 7, 2006, https://www.sciencedaily.com/releases/2006/11/061106164651.htm.

CHAPTER 11: SUPPORTING WOMEN'S HEALTH IMBALANCES

1. Monica Reinagel, "How Birth Control Pills Affect Your Nutritional Needs," *Scientific American*, September 23, 2015, https://www.scientificamerican.com/article/how-birth-control-pills-affect-your-nutritional-needs.

2. David Jockers, "13 Ways to Heal Anemia Naturally," DrJockers, September 2017, https://drjockers.com/13-ways-heal-anemia-naturally.

3. "Acupuncture Provides Effective Fertility Treatments," HealthCMi, November 18, 2013, http://www.nccaom.org/wp-content/uploads/pdf/Effect%20on%20Fertility%20Treatments.pdf.

RESOURCES FOR DELVING DEEPER
— ◆ —

CHINESE MEDICINE PRACTITIONERS

Almost all states require national licensure in acupuncture. If you visit the National Certification Commission for Acupuncture and Oriental Medicine website (www.nccaom.org), you can search for practitioners by name, city, and proximity to your zip code. It's an excellent resource for finding a qualified practitioner.

To find Chinese medicine practitioners who offer rates on a sliding scale, consider seeking treatment from students in master's programs through a student clinic. They are always overseen by a senior practitioner, so it can be the best of both worlds.

Community clinics are another great way to receive the care you need at a discounted rate. They can be found in every major city.

It is *always* worth asking your practitioner if he or she has a sliding scale. If not, some will accept insurance. Others may be interested in trading for services (I traded administrative work for many treatments while I was a student).

There are different kinds of Chinese medicine practitioners, so how do you decide what kind to see? There are traditional Chinese medicine (TCM) acupuncturists, classical Chinese medicine (CCM) acupuncturists, Five Element acupuncturists, and more (I call myself a Five Element integrative acupuncturist to reflect how I integrate classical, traditional, and Five Element in my practice). These titles all refer to the training practitioners have received, and while each training program is valuable, there are some significant differences between them.

Traditional Chinese medicine is a blend of old and new practices. Spawned by the Cultural Revolution in China in the 1950s, it integrates the ancient system of medicine that began around 2600 B.C.E. with more modern, Westernized ideas of medicine with a focus on diagnosing and treating the patterns of imbalance as they arise in their clients. Because the Chinese government removed any parts of Chinese medicine that didn't align with the modern understanding of medicine, all things related to spirit, nature, the seasons, and so on are missing from this version.

There is also Five Element acupuncture, which is the interpretation of the classical system of Chinese medicine by Professor J. R. Worsley. He brought this interpretation to the West and has become known for what is now called Worsley Five Element acupuncture. This practice tends to focus on treating the spirit of the person.

CCM and integrative practitioners tend to focus on the patterns of imbalance presenting in their clients as well as supporting the spirit of the person and their constitution.

Above all else, rapport is key when it comes to finding a practitioner. With so many specialized acupuncturists integrating their practices into Western medical settings, it is getting easier to find the right person for you.

HERBS AND SUPPLEMENTS

Wellevate (https://wellevate.me/mindi-counts/#/): Chinese and other herbs and nutritional supplements from Innate Response, Vital Nutrients, Mega Spore Biotics, Klaire Labs, Quicksilver Scientific, Designs for Health, and other personal favorites can be found in my online herbal pharmacy. They are discounted between 15 and 35 percent to support you in achieving your health goals.

CHINESE HERBS

Urban Herbs (www.urbanherbsco.com): Custom herbal formulas in raw, granular, and encapsulated forms. Sliding scale options available.

Golden Flower Chinese Herbs (www.gfcherbs.com): Single and formula herbs in pressed tablet form.

OTHER HERBS

Mountain Rose Herbs (www.mountainroseherbs.com)

Wise Woman Herbals (https://wisewomanherbals.com)

EQUIPMENT

Lhasa Oms (lhasaoms.com): This is a great resource for many of the practice tools mentioned in this book, such as jade rollers, gua sha tools, tiger warmers, moxa sticks, and beyond. Also, some practitioners might carry these items for sale in their office.

BOOKS

Chinese Medicine

Beinfield, Harriet, and Efrem Korngold. *Between Heaven and Earth: A Guide to Chinese Medicine.* New York: Random House, 1991.

Brooks, Marlow. *Singing Our Heart's Song: A Guide to the Five Elements and Plant Spirit Healing.* Self-published, 2017.

Cowan, Stephen. *Fire Child, Water Child: Understanding How the Five Types of ADHD Can Help You Improve Your Child's Self-Esteem and Attention.* Oakland, CA: New Harbinger Publications, 2012.

Kaptchuk, Ted. *The Web That Has No Weaver: Understanding Chinese Medicine*. New York: McGraw-Hill, 2000.

Nutrition

Axe, Josh. *Eat Dirt: Why Leaky Gut May Be the Root Cause of Your Health Problems and 5 Surprising Steps to Cure It*. New York: HarperCollins, 2016.

Mayer, Emeran. *The Mind-Gut Connection: How the Hidden Conversation within Our Bodies Impacts Our Mood, Our Choices, and Our Overall Health*. New York: HarperCollins, 2017.

Pitchford, Paul. *Healing with Whole Foods: Asian Traditions and Modern Nutrition*. Berkeley, CA: North Atlantic Books, 2003.

Ross, Julia. *The Diet Cure: The 8-Step Program to Rebalance Your Body Chemistry and End Food Cravings, Weight Gain, and Mood Swings—Naturally*. New York: Penguin Books, 2012.

Mental Health

Brogan, Kelly Brogan. *A Mind of Your Own: The Truth about Depression and How Women Can Heal Their Bodies to Reclaim Their Lives*. London: Thorsons, 2016.

Hari, Johann. *Lost Connections: Uncovering the Real Causes of Depression—and the Unexpected Solutions*. New York: Bloomsbury USA, 2018.

Larson, Joan Mathews. *Depression-Free, Naturally: 7 Weeks to Eliminating Anxiety, Despair, Fatigue, and Anger from Your Life*. New York: Random House, 1999.

Louv, Richard. *Last Child in the Woods: Saving Our Children from Nature-Deficit Disorder*. Chapel Hill, NC: Algonquin Books, 2008.

Ross, Julia. *The Mood Cure: The 4-Step Program to Take Charge of Your Emotions—Today*. New York: Penguin Books, 2002.

Walsh, William J. *Nutrient Power: Heal Your Biochemistry and Heal Your Brain*. New York: Skyhorse Publishing, 2014.

Hormonal Health

Briden, Lara. *Period Repair Manual: Natural Treatments for Better Hormones and Better Periods*. Greenpeak Publishing, 2018.

Lewis, Randine. *The Infertility Cure: The Ancient Chinese Wellness Program for Getting Pregnant and Having Healthy Babies*. Boston: Little, Brown, 2004.

Vitti, Alisa. *WomanCode: Perfect Your Cycle, Amplify Your Fertility, Supercharge Your Sex Drive, and Become a Power Source.* New York: HarperCollins, 2014.

Weschler, Toni. *Taking Charge of Your Fertility: The Definitive Guide to Natural Birth Control, Pregnancy Achievement, and Reproductive Health.* New York: HarperCollins, 2015.

Addiction

Larson, Joan Mathews. *Seven Weeks to Sobriety: The Proven Program to Fight Alcoholism through Nutrition.* New York: Random House, 1997.

Milkman, Harvey, Stanley Sunderwirth, and Katherine Hill. *Craving for Ecstasy and Natural Highs: A Positive Approach to Mood Alteration.* 2nd ed. San Diego, CA: Cognella Academic Publishing, 2018.

Ross, Julia. *The Mood Cure: The 4-Step Program to Take Charge of Your Emotions—Today.* New York: Penguin Books, 2002.

Cancer

Christofferson, Travis. *Tripping Over the Truth: How the Metabolic Theory of Cancer Is Overturning One of Medicine's Most Entrenched Paradigms.* White River Junction, VT: Chelsea Green Publishing, 2017.

Winters, Nasha, and Jess Higgins Kelley. *The Metabolic Approach to Cancer: Integrating Deep Nutrition, the Ketogenic Diet, and Nontoxic Bio-Individualized Therapies.* White River Junction, VT: Chelsea Green Publishing, 2017.

MICROBIOME RESOURCES

Doctor's Data Lab (www.doctorsdata.com): Microbiome testing

Cultures for Health (www.culturesforhealth.com): Information and products for sprouting and fermenting at home

TOXIC BURDEN RESOURCE

Doctor's Data Lab (www.doctorsdata.com): Multiple tests that assess toxic load through hair, urine, and stool samples. Find a practitioner who can order these tests for you and help you reduce your toxic burden if needed.

MENTAL HEALTH RESOURCES

Labrix (www.labrix.com): Neurotransmitter testing. Testing for methylenetetrahydrofolate reductase (MTHFR), a genetic condition that leads to all kinds of mental health imbalances and frequent miscarriage. If you and other members of your family have struggled all your lives with mental health imbalances, MTHFR is worth looking into. Also testing for catechol-O-methyltransferase (COMT) and single nucleotide polymorphisms (SNPs).

DHA Laboratory (www.dhalab.com): Testing for pyroluria, a likely genetic condition that leads to mental health imbalances, specifically high anxiety and fearfulness.

The Breathe Network (www.thebreathenetwork.org): A wonderful resource for those who have experienced sexual abuse and trauma. This nonprofit is a resource listing practitioners who have had trauma-informed training, many of whom offer sliding-scale services.

HORMONAL HEALTH RESOURCE

Labrix (www.labrix.com): Salivary hormone and cortisol testing.

ADDICTION RECOVERY RESOURCES

Any and all of the testing services listed in other sections will support addiction recovery, as these tests will give you insight into any biochemical imbalances that may be fueling your unique addiction. It is important to address those while simultaneously addressing the emotional and spiritual components of addiction.

National Acupuncture Detoxification Association (https://acudetox.com): NADA is a leading organization devoted to researching and furthering the use of acupuncture treatment for addiction. NADA clinics can be found in every major city.

Refuge Recovery Treatment Center (https://refugerecoverycenters.com): Located in Los Angeles, California, this in-patient treatment center focuses on recovery from addiction. Its philosophy aligns with ancient Taoist and Buddhist concepts, mimicking some of the Eight Branches of Chinese medicine. People of all religious backgrounds have benefitted tremendously from their programs.

CANCER RESOURCE

Euromed Foundation (https://euromedfoundation.com/en): Located in Arizona, this is an alternative medical facility using the best of holistic systems of medicine alongside Western medical approaches to cancer on an inpatient and outpatient basis.

INDEX

— ◆ —

herbal formulas and, 99
quiz to assess, 51–54, 252
soups or stews for, 208
syncing with seasons, 71
temperatures and, 179
See also under individual
element
cooling foods and herbs, 60, 61,
64, 67, 68, 69, 93–94, 289
avoiding, 63, 66, 68, 155
Cooling Watermelon Milk, 182
in summer, 179, 180, 185
topical use, 243
cordyceps, 237, 292
coriolus (turkey tail mushrooms),
47, 296
corn, 80, 89, 93, 118, 180, 204, 285
cortisol, 250–51, 253
adrenal fatigue and, 306, 307
in animal products, 77–78
chronic exposure to, 297
fear and, 109
food intolerance and, 283
at menopause, 327
in winter, 133, 134
corydalis, 298
coughs
asthma and, 292
chronic, 238, 239, 269
dampness and, 56
herbs for, 159, 161, 162, 215,
216, 217, 237, 238, 239–40
immune system imbalances
and, 284, 287
internal wind pathology and,
146
cramp bark, 319, 326
cravings, 74, 170, 171, 197, 256,
267, 272, 274, 307
Crohn's disease, 237, 272, 293–94
cucumbers, 89, 91, 94, 96, 230, 233
cupping, 26, 35, 299
curcumin, 270, 271, 272, 284, 294,
296, 298, 313, 320
cyperus, 159, 298, 326
cysts, 28, 66, 88, 197, 315, 324

D
dairy, 64, 89, 92, 93, 94, 95, 96
avoiding, 118, 148, 204, 274
intolerance, 276, 285
seasonal, 149, 180, 230
skin conditions and, 290

yeast overgrowth and, 274
damiana, 321
damp heat, 58, 69, 159, 217, 270,
278, 294
dampness and phlegm, 56, 58,
217, 324
dandelion, 47, 88, 159–61, 180,
181–82
dandelion root, 88, 95, 96, 180
Digestive Bitters, 181–82
for digestive imbalances, 277
for emotional imbalances, 256,
260, 265
for polycystic ovarian syndrome,
324
roasted, 76
in teas, 155, 237
dates, 89, 93, 95, 96, 125, 204, 210,
211
dementia, 110, 269
depression, 15, 61, 63, 65, 259–60
acupuncture for, 23
adrenal fatigue and, 307
anxiety and, 257
autoimmune disease and, 293
chronic fatigue syndrome
and, 308
fibromyalgia and, 303
Fire and, 170, 171
herbs for, 162, 217
leaky gut syndrome and, 272
menopause and, 328
premenstrual syndrome
and, 318
as shen disturbance sign, 173
stagnation and, 56
thyroid diseases and, 312
Wood imbalance and, 142
yin and yang in, 41
dermatitis, 290–91
detoxification, 75, 91
cholesterol and, 78
cupping for, 35
Detox Smoothie, 154
Detox Tea, 155
herbs for, 130, 188
liver's role in, 143
nutritional supplements and,
99–100
skin's role in, 228
See also cleansing
diabetes, 161, 273. *See also*
blood sugar

diaphoretics, 90
diarrhea, 66, 69, 238, 278–79
cancer and, 296
dampness and, 56
digestive imbalances and, 270,
272
Earth imbalance and, 197, 253
herbs for, 128, 189, 214, 215, 217,
239–40
immune system imbalances
and, 284
inflammation and, 288
thyroid diseases and, 312
tui na for, 34
Water imbalance and, 127
women's health imbalances and,
318, 326
diet, 247
during diarrhea, 279
for digestive imbalances, 266–67
elimination, 285
for emotional imbalances, 250
for energy-zapping imbalances,
306
for immune system imbalances,
282
inflammation and, 288, 301, 303
for pain and inflammation
support, 297
poor, results of, 65, 271–72,
278, 308
thyroid imbalance and, 311
for women's health imbalances,
315, 317, 325
digestion, 56, 90, 91–92
autoimmune disease and, 294
Basic Soup and Stew, 206–8
Chaga Chai, 235–37
Congee, 126–27
Digestive Bitters, 181–82
dreams and, 309
Earth and, 197, 198
eating habits and, 219, 267, 270
emotional imbalance and, 249–50
headaches and, 299, 300
herbs for, 128–30, 159, 189,
214–17, 238
imbalances in, 266–67
microbiome and, 202
pain and, 297, 298
spleen's role in, 201
stress and, 197, 219, 250, 253,
266, 273, 278

integrative medicine, 23, 99, 246
intentions, 102, 164, 219, 241–42, 244
intestine, large, 47, 226, 228
   cleansing action of, 83
   damp heat in, 69, 159, 217, 270, 278, 294
   heat and dryness in, 69, 159, 215, 217, 280
   herbs for, 159, 162, 215, 217
   pungent and, 90
   seasonal cycles and, 44–45
   stress and, 253
   time of, 46, 241, 279
intestine, small, 46, 47, 88, 144, 172, 174, 177, 267
intimacy, 170, 171, 175, 320–21
iron, 143, 149, 209, 313, 317, 320, 321
irritable bowel syndrome (IBS), 61, 66, 69, 181, 197, 270–71

J
jade facial roller, 25
jasmine, 76, 180
jaundice, 142, 145, 161, 162
jing qi (ancestral chi), 36, 112
joint pain, 272, 275, 294, 307, 308, 312, 328
jojoba oil, 26, 31, 243
joy, 47, 170, 171, 189
jujube seeds, 187, 258, 265, 278, 310

K
kale, 94, 120–21, 124, 148, 183
kava kava, 256, 258, 262, 265, 298, 311
kidney chi deficiency, 60, 62, 303
kidney yang deficiency, 60
   addiction and, 255
   adrenal fatigue and, 307
   asthma and, 292
   autoimmune disease and, 294
   cancer and, 296
   chronic fatigue syndrome and, 308
   depression and, 260
   diarrhea and, 278
   fibromyalgia and, 303
   herbs for, 128–30, 131, 237, 238, 239

hypothyroidism and, 312
women's health imbalances and, 320, 323, 324, 328
kidney yin deficiency, 60, 68
   addiction and, 255
   adrenal fatigue and, 307
   asthma and, 292
   autoimmune disease and, 294
   cancer and, 296
   chronic fatigue syndrome and, 308
   fibromyalgia and, 303
   food allergies/intolerances and, 284
   herbs for, 131, 240
   hyperthyroidism and, 312
   infertility and, 323
   low libido and, 321
   menopause and, 328
   premenstrual syndrome and, 318
   sleep imbalances and, 310
kidneys, 47, 60
   asthma and, 292
   cleansing action of, 83
   headaches and, 299
   heart and, 173
   herbs for, 128–30, 131, 161, 215, 217, 237–40, 256
   and liver, relationship between, 144, 145
   menstruation and, 316
   polycystic ovarian syndrome and, 324
   salty and, 90–91
   stones, 110
   stress and, 252, 253
   time of, 46
   Water and, 109, 110, 111, 112–13, 114
   water consumption and, 75
   in winter, 119
kimchi, 90, 91, 151–52, 232
kitchen cleaning, 218
kombu, 91, 94, 96, 120–21

L
lamb, 89, 93, 118, 122–23, 204, 206–8, 304
late summer, 193
   body in, 198–202
   herbs and spices for, 214–17

nourishing practices for, 217–19
nutritional principles in, 203–4
lavender, 90, 96, 180, 184, 307
lavender essential oil, 85, 107, 291, 301
leaky gut syndrome, 23, 66, 271–72
leeks, 90, 92, 93, 118, 120–21, 229, 230, 232
legumes, 80
   blood-building, 96
   calming, 96
   five flavors in, 89, 91, 92
   seasonal, 118, 148, 180, 230
   soaking and sprouting, 81
   three temperatures of, 93, 95
   tonifying, 95
lemon, juice of, 83, 124, 125, 148, 153, 154, 155, 156, 209
lemon balm, 91, 96, 184, 253, 256, 258, 262, 308, 313
lemon essential oil, 85
lemons, 89, 91, 92, 94, 95, 230, 234–35
lentils, 81, 82, 93, 96, 118, 180, 204, 209
Li Shizhen, 17
libido, 60, 61, 320–21
   adrenal fatigue and, 306, 307
   digestive imbalances and, 275
   herbs for, 239–40
   menopause and, 328
   premenstrual syndrome and, 318
   Water imbalance and, 110
   with yang chi deficiency, 56
licorice, 89, 93, 94, 95, 215, 217, 253
   for adrenal fatigue, 307
   for cancer, 296
   for digestive imbalance, 268, 269, 277, 278
   for emotional imbalances, 256, 258
   for hypothyroidism, 312
   for polycystic ovarian syndrome, 324
life force. *See* chi
life-work balance, 141, 197, 218–19, 252
ligaments, 47, 144–45, 252
limbic system, 228

food intolerances and, 283
skin conditions and, 290
wei qi and, 281
microbiome cloud, 227
migraines, 61, 65, 282, 299–301, 319
milk thistle, 78, 83, 91, 256, 260, 265, 320, 324
millet, 80, 81, 89, 91, 94, 95, 126–27, 149–50
mind, 89, 91, 177, 184, 196, 244, 250, 267
mint, 156, 180, 182. *See also* peppermint
mint (Chinese), 216
miso, 91, 125, 230, 329
moistening action, 94–95, 118, 149, 180, 231, 289. *See also* nutrition, five actions/ properties
molasses, 77, 89, 95, 96
moods, 61
blood sugar and, 119
coffee and, 76
digestive imbalances and, 284, 288
grains and, 80
herbs for, 162, 216
meditation for, 18
thyroid diseases and, 312
women's health imbalances and, 318, 324
morning sickness, 214, 238, 267, 268
motherwort, 187, 318, 328
mouth, 47, 55, 201
moxibustion, 24–25, 26–28
mugwort, 24–25, 90
mullein, 288–89, 292
multiple sclerosis, 293–94
mume, 275
mung beans, 82, 94, 95, 96, 148, 180, 204
soaking and sprouting, 81, 149–50
Sprouted Savory Mung Bean Pancakes, 151–52
muscles, 47, 55
chronic fatigue syndrome and, 308
Earth and, 201, 253
menopause and, 328

relaxing, 300
spasms in, 62, 217, 269
thyroid diseases and, 312
mushrooms
Basic Soup and Stew, 206–8
chaga, 235–37
Lentil Pâté, 209
shiitake, 89, 93, 120–21, 209, 232
turkey tail, 47, 296
See also reishi
myrrh, 298

N

Nasal Steam, 286
nausea, 67, 142, 267–68
anxiety and, 258
digestive imbalances and, 270
endometriosis and, 326
herbs for, 158, 188, 189, 214, 215, 217, 238
immune system imbalances and, 284
neem oil, 291
nervous system, 35, 130, 133, 254–55, 256, 257, 263
neti pot rinses, 164, 285
nettles, 91, 95, 96, 121, 183, 184, 262, 284
neutral foods and herbs, 92, 93
imbalance patterns and, 60, 61, 63, 66, 67
in late summer, 205, 206, 209
topical use, 243
night sweats, 55, 60, 63, 68, 185–86, 239–40, 296, 328
nightshades, 282, 297
nonsteroidal anti-inflammatory drugs (NSAIDs), 266, 271–72, 295, 297, 299
nose, 47, 228
nut butters, 148, 150, 210
nutmeg, 90, 93, 95, 126–27, 211
nutrition, 19–20
cravings and, 74
five actions/properties, 60–69, 94–96
seasonal, 73–74, 117
temperatures, three categories of, 92–94
See also five flavors
nutritional supplements, 99–100
nuts and seeds, 82, 89, 93, 96, 304

seasonal, 118, 148, 180, 204, 230
Seed and Nut Pâté, 125
soaking and sprouting, 81
Sweet Nut Milk, 182, 211, 212

O

oats, 80, 89, 95, 96, 118, 126–27, 289
oatstraw, 91, 94, 256, 260
obsessive-compulsive disorder (OCD), 60, 66, 258
oils, 26, 76–77, 89, 93, 94, 204. *See also* individual types
oils, essential, 85, 107, 286, 291, 301
olive oil, 76, 77, 89, 93, 204
in broths and stocks, 120–21, 232
in pâtés, 125, 209
in salads and dressings, 124, 153
in smoothies, 154
onions, 90, 93, 118, 149, 204, 206, 229, 230
Basic Soup and Stew, 206–8
in broths and stocks, 120–21, 122–23, 232
green, 90, 118, 151–52, 204, 232
Lentil Pâté, 209
red, 234–35
orange peel, 181–82, 207, 275
oranges, 89, 92, 94, 154, 180
oregano, 93, 95, 125
oregano oil, 274, 275
osteoporosis, 131

P

pain, 297–98
acupuncture for, 23
acute, 298–99
bodywork for, 28, 35
calming sounds for, 134
chi and, 32
chronic, 65, 302–3
endometriosis and, 325
herbs for, 130
nature's opioids for, 304
stagnation and, 56
See also abdominal pain; joint pain
pancreas, 181–82, 198, 200
panic attacks, 56, 110, 257, 312
pantry cleaning, 73, 218, 247

cycles and rhythms of, 44–45
Five elements and, 47
syncing constitution with, 71
yin and yang in, 40, 105, 138, 167, 168
See also autumn; late summer; spring; summer; winter
seeds of Job's tears, 217, 291
sense-organs, 47. *See also* individual organ
serotonin, 249, 304
sesame oil, 26, 76, 77, 94, 151–52, 164, 243
sesame seeds, 81, 82, 89, 93, 96, 118, 148, 204
sexual fluids, 47, 175, 320, 321
shallots, 93, 118, 124, 153, 229, 232
shen (spirit), 113, 184, 263–64, 309
addiction and, 254
blood and, 177
disturbance, 173, 254, 261, 310
Shen Nong, 87, 239
shingles, 289
shrimp, 91, 94, 118, 122–23, 126–27, 148
siler, 291, 328
sinuses, 90, 146, 164, 189, 240, 275, 281
sinusitis, recurrent, 285–87
Sjogren's syndrome, 293–94
skin, 47, 55, 65, 68, 84, 146, 225, 228
asthma and, 292
autoimmune disease and, 294
with blood deficiency, 56
cleansing action of, 83
digestive imbalances and, 272
food intolerance and, 282
herbs for, 130–31, 159, 161, 187, 216, 239–40
seasonal cycles and, 44–45
See also acne; eczema
skin brushing, 83, 85, 107, 242–43
skullcap, 256, 265, 296, 308, 310
sleep, 55, 56
asthma and, 292
bedtimes and, 165
blood and, 177
chronic fatigue syndrome and, 308
emotional imbalances and, 258, 259, 261

fibromyalgia and, 303
imbalances in, 309–11
waking times, 191
women's health imbalances and, 316, 318, 324
See also dreams; insomnia
sleep apnea, 310
slippery elm, 94, 269, 270, 271, 272
small intestine bacterial overgrowth (SIBO), 174, 267
smoothies
Blood-Building Smoothie, 183
Detox Smoothie, 154
Soaking and Sprouting guide, 81
soil depletion, 99, 194, 283
Solomon's seal, 296
somatic experiencing, 255, 264
soups, broths, stocks, 306
Basic Soup and Stew, 206–8
Immunity Stock, 232
Medicinal Vegetable Broth, 120–21
Nourishing Bone Stock, 122–23
and stews, differences between, 208
sour taste, 47, 91–92, 148, 149
soy, 204, 285, 319, 327, 329
soy sauce, 91, 209
soybean oil, 77
soybeans, 93, 94, 180, 230
spearmint essential oil, 286
spinach, 94, 96, 124, 126–27, 183
spirituality, 17, 84, 101, 114, 199, 200, 222, 223, 225
spleen, 47, 66, 198
asthma and, 292
dampness and, 56
Earth and, 196, 200–201
herbs for, 128–30, 159, 162, 187, 214–15, 216, 217, 238, 239
menstruation and, 316
overworking and, 219
Pumpkin Spice Latte, 212
sweet and, 89
time of, 46
spleen chi deficiency, 66, 80, 201
adrenal fatigue and, 306
autoimmune disease and, 294
cancer and, 296
chronic fatigue syndrome and, 308
digestive imbalances and, 268, 270, 272, 275, 276, 277, 278

emotional imbalances and, 257, 258, 260, 262, 265
herbs for, 130, 158, 162, 188, 214, 215, 216, 217, 238, 239
immune system imbalances and, 284, 292
infertility and, 323
sleep imbalances and, 310
women's health imbalances and, 320, 324
spleen yang deficiency, 66, 128, 214, 215, 217, 238, 239, 272, 275, 278
spring, 45, 137–38
body in, 143–46
herbs and spices for, 158–62
nourishing practices in, 163–65
nutritional principles in, 148
transition to, 147–48, 158
See also Wood element
sprouting, 81, 149–50
St. John's wort, 256, 258, 260, 291, 303, 308, 319, 328
St. John's wort oil, 298
star anise, 93, 181–82
steroids, 227, 271, 273, 288, 293
Stevia, 212
stomach, 47, 67, 84, 198, 212
Earth and, 199
flu, 189
grains and, 80
headaches and, 299
hunger and, 196
sweet and, 89
time of, 46
ulcers, 67, 181
See also rebellious stomach chi
stomach chi deficiency, 293
stomach yin deficiency, 67, 68, 215, 216, 217, 269
stomachaches, 67, 69, 197, 214, 253
stress, 15, 41, 230, 281
acute and chronic, distinctions between, 250–52
adrenal fatigue and, 306
allergies and, 282
asthma and, 292
autoimmune disease and, 293
chronic, 113, 271
chronic fatigue syndrome and, 308
digestion and, 197, 219, 250, 253, 266, 273, 278

stress, *continued*
   five elements and, 252–53
   headaches and, 299
   heart and, 173
   herbs for, 130, 239–40
   infertility and, 322
   inflammation and, 289
   kidneys and, 112
   libido and, 321
   managing, 83, 252
   meditation for, 18
   Square Breathing for, 244
string beans, 89, 93, 180, 204, 206–8
sugar, 141, 230
   avoiding, 289, 304
   cravings, 197, 256, 272, 307
   natural, 194, 210
   refined, 89, 180, 204, 250, 267, 282, 297, 306, 315
   yeast overgrowth and, 273, 274
summer, 167–68, 179
   body in, 172–78
   herbs and spices for, 185–89
   nourishing practices in, 189–91
   nutritional principles in, 178–79
   See also Fire element
sunflower seeds, 81, 82, 89, 93, 118, 125, 149–50, 180, 204
sweating, 55, 83, 238, 312
sweet potatoes, 89, 93, 94, 95, 96, 118, 180, 204, 230
   Basic Soup and Stew, 206–8
   in broth, 120–21
   in congee, 126–27
sweet taste, 47, 89, 149, 194, 203, 204, 205
sweeteners, 77, 204, 212, 235
Swiss chard, 94, 148, 206–8

T
tachycardia, 185–86
tahini, 124
tai chi, 19, 250, 267, 282, 306
tamari, 91, 151–52, 209
tangerine peel, 162, 217, 265, 277, 298
Taoism, 15, 18, 20, 44, 87, 113, 140
teas
   Chaga Chai, 235–37
   for chemotherapy-related nausea, 296

Detox, 85, 155
Digestive, 277
Good Earth, 74, 256
green, 296
Happy Spirit, 184
rose hip, 240
Soothing Belly, 271
Warm Ginger Lemon, 156
tendons, 47, 144–45
throat, sore, 146, 159, 215, 216, 240, 269, 287, 308
thyme, 90, 93, 125, 207, 209, 233, 286
thyme essential oil, 285
thyroid diseases, 311–13
tiger warmer, 25, 26–28
tinnitus, 142, 185
tofu, 89, 94, 95, 151–52
tomatoes, 89, 92, 94, 180, 270, 282, 297
tongue, 47, 55, 178, 273, 274
   diagnosis using, 57–59, 60–69
   map of organs on, 59
tonifying action, 60, 62, 65, 68, 95, 149
topical formulas, 291, 298, 301, 302
trauma, 263–65
   acute, 61, 65
   addiction and, 254
   chronic fatigue syndrome and, 308
   emotional imbalance and, 260
   intergenerational, 112–13
   shen and, 173
   women's health and, 315
   See also post-traumatic stress disorder (PTSD)
tremors, 142, 146, 312
tribulus, 321
triple burner, 46, 47, 172, 175–76, 177
tui na, 34
tulsi (Holy Basil), 90, 184, 253, 258, 262, 265, 313
tumors, 88, 128, 161, 188, 295
turmeric, 90, 95, 118, 120–21, 149, 155, 180, 234–35. *See also* curcumin
turnips, 88, 90, 93, 118, 148, 180, 204, 206–8
tyrosine, 256, 307, 309, 313

U
ulcerative colitis, 293–94
urinary tract infections (UTIs), 110, 127, 161, 275, 295

V
valerian, 88, 96, 256, 258, 303, 311, 328
vanilla, 93, 95, 212
vanilla essential oil, 107
vegetables, 78, 304
   astringent, 95
   Basic Soup and Stew, 206–8
   bitter, 88
   blood-building, 96
   calming, 96
   Fermented Veggies, 233
   moistening, 94
   pungent, 90
   salty, 91
   seasonal, 118, 148, 180, 204, 230
   sour, 92
   sweet, 89
   three temperatures of, 93, 94
   tonifying, 95
vegetarianism, 82, 208
vertigo, 110, 146, 158
vervain, 256
vinegar, 87, 89
   apple cider, 122, 149, 155, 182, 207, 234–35, 290, 317
   in digestive bitters, 182
   rice, 209
   white wine, 232
vision boards, 164, 241
vodka, 181–82
vomiting, 67, 142, 189, 214, 215, 238, 267–68, 284

W
walking, 163, 196, 241, 270, 282
walnut oil, 77
walnuts, 81, 82, 89, 93, 118, 126, 204, 230
   in pâtés, 125, 209
   Sweet Nut Milk, 211
warming foods and herbs, 60, 62, 63, 66, 68, 93
   avoiding, 60, 61, 64, 65, 67, 68, 69
   seasonal,118, 149, 205, 231
   topical use, 243

ABOUT THE AUTHOR

— ◆ —

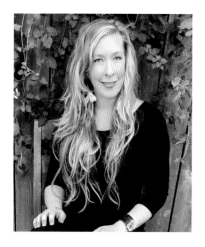

MINDI K. COUNTS, MA, LAc, is an integrative medical practitioner and five-element acupuncturist. Cofounder of the Inner Ocean Center for Healing, Mindi is a keynote speaker, retreat leader, and teacher. She is a contributing author to the *Trauma Toolkit* and *Singing Our Heart's Song*.

She is the founder of the international nonprofit Inner Ocean Empowerment Project, providing holistic health care and education through volunteer service missions to underserved populations around the world and in the United States. She was featured in Dr. Oz's *The Good Life* magazine for her work in Indian slum communities, Burmese refugee clinics, and earthquake-ravaged areas of Nepal.

Mindi is a graduate of Naropa University's contemplative psychology program and holds a master's degree in classical acupuncture from the Institute of Taoist Education and Acupuncture. She lives with her family and rescued dogs in the foothills of Colorado.